FIRST AID AND EMERGENCY CARE

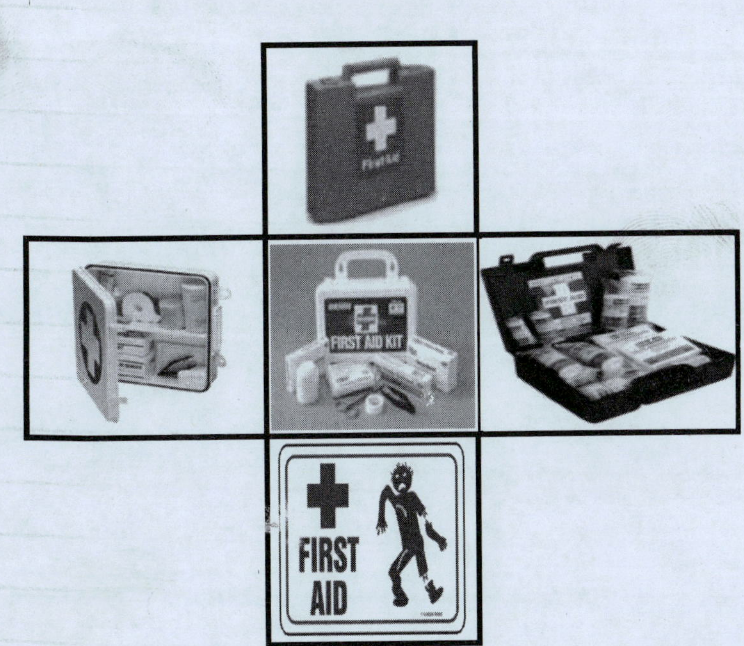

FIRST AID AND EMERGENCY CARE

N.C. Jain

M.A.(Psy.); M.Com.; L.L.B.; C.A.(I),; P.G.D.C.A.; P.G.D.M.

Ms. Saakshi

M.Sc.(Nsg.); P.G.D.C.A. (Aptech).

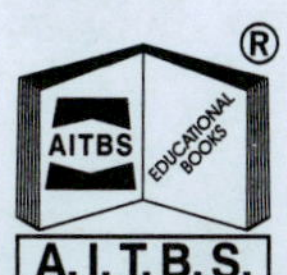

AITBS PUBLISHERS, INDIA

MEDICAL PUBLISHERS

J-5/6, Krishan Nagar, Delhi-110051 (INDIA)

Phone: 011-40167052, 49067602

E-mail: aitbsindia@gmail.com & aitbsindia@hotmail.com

First Edition : 2009
Revised Edition : 2015
Second Edition : 2027

ISBN: 978-81-7473-385-6

Published by:
Virender Kumar Arya for
AITBS Publishers, India
MEDICAL PUBLISHERS
J-5/6, Krishan Nagar, Delhi - 110051 (INDIA)
Phone: 011-40167052, 49067602
E-mail: aitbsindia@gmail.com & aitbsindia@hotmail.com

Printed by AITBS, Delhi

Dedicated To

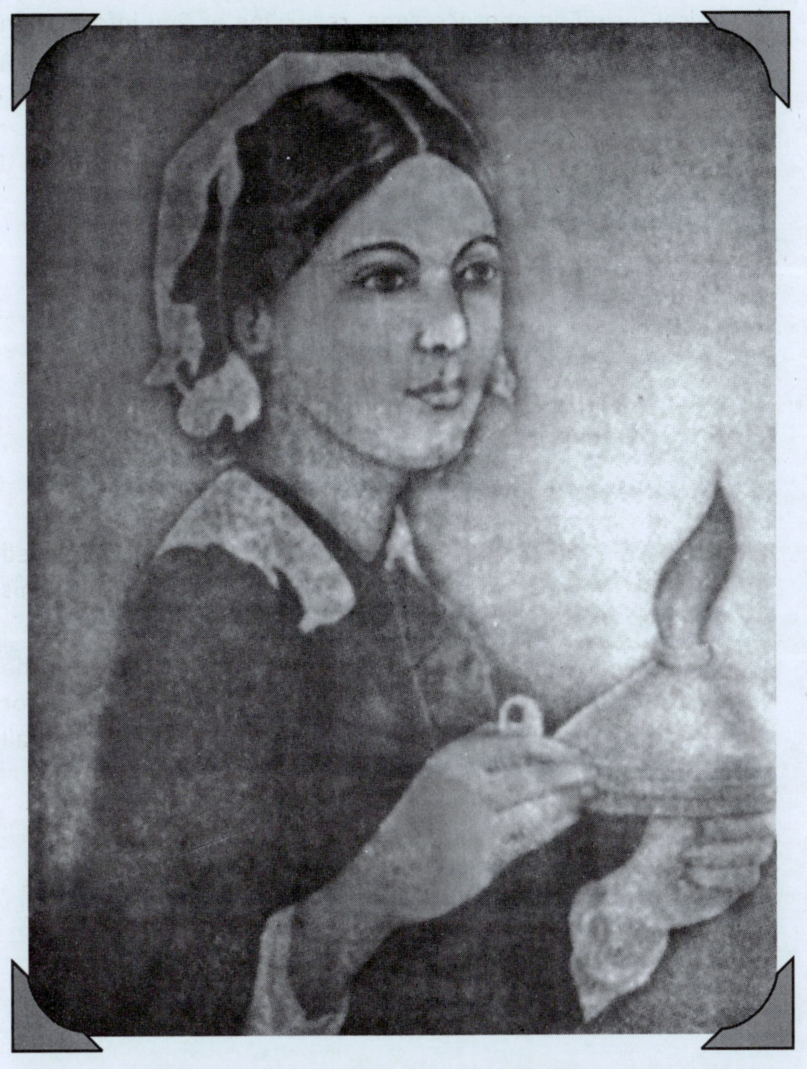

Miss Florence Nightingale

PIONEER OF MODERN NURSING

Born on:- 12th May 1820. Died on :- 13th August 1910

Preface

First aid is the emergency care given to the sick, injured, or wounded before being treated by medical personnel. The book 'First Aid and Emergency Care' aims to present a concise survey of the concepts and principles which are essentials of the first nursing course in first aid. The Army Dictionary defines first aid as "urgent and immediate lifesaving and other measures which can be performed for casualties by nonmedical personnel when medical personnel are not immediately available." Nonmedical soldiers have received basic first aid training and should remain skilled in the correct procedures for giving first aid. First aid is, like medicine, both an art and a science. Interest and some natural ability are necessary, but more fundamental is the need to learn the basic principles thoroughly, to revise, keep up to date, and look for new ideas.

The essential principles of emergency first aid have not changed over the years, but the emphasis has *cardiopulmonary resuscitation*, CPR, has been brought to the forefront. The full importance of those first four minutes has been well established: the need for urgent attention to airway, breathing, bleeding and circulation is now widely recognised. The basic principles of this life saving technique have been simplified and standardised. The book 'First Aid and Emergency Care' aims to present a concise survey of the concepts and principles which are essentials of the first nursing course in first aid. Indeed, it is rather a difficult task to present all the basic essentials of such a vast subject like first aid into a limited number of chapters and pages of a brief text. However, an attempt has been made to present what is essential from both the angle of the scope of the subject and the needs of the graduate and post-graduate courses of Indian universities. We must treat each A & E patient as an individual human being, acknowledging his/her physical, psychological and social needs, and striving to give integrated, individualised and rational care that attempts to meet all such needs.

We hope at least some of our nurses will develop a keen interest in this stimulating subject and pursue independent study, going in the end far beyond the scope and depth of the Indian Nursing Council syllabus on which this book is based.

We acknowledge the inspiration and blessings of our parents from the core of our heart and extend thanks to my husband and our family members for their moral support which helped us in the successful compilation of this book. Our gratitude is due to a large number of writers and authors of books on the subject of health economics, whose ideas and thoughts have imperceptibly influenced us in the preparation of this book.

Last, but not the least, we extend our sincere thanks to *Sh. Virender Kumar Arya*, of A.I.T.B.S. Publishers, India for his motivating guidance during the preparation of this book on several aspects.

Authors

Contents

Preface vii

SECTION – I

Introduction

Chapter: 1	Introduction to First Aid and Emergency	1–13
Chapter: 2	First Aid Kit and Emergency Equipment	14–18
Chapter: 3	Casualty Management	19–27
Chapter: 4	Resuscitation	28–46
Chapter: 5	Pregnancy and Childbirth	47–57

SECTION – II

Aanatomy

Chapter: 6	The Body as a Whole: (Regions and Cavity)	61–68
Chapter: 7	Cells, Tissue and Organs	69–76
Chapter: 8	The Skeletal System	77–91
Chapter: 9	Receptors: The Special Sense Organs	92–104
Chapter: 10	The Digestive System	105–115

Chapter: 11 The Circulatory System 116–125

Chapter: 12 The Nervous System 126–132

Chapter: 13 The Respiratory System 133–143

Chapter: 14 The Excretory System 144–151

Chapter: 15 The Reproductive System 152–166

SECTION – III

Clinical Practice

Chapter: 16 Burns and Scalds 169–181

Chapter: 17 Injuries, Wounds and Haemorrhage 182–201

Chapter: 18 Head Injury 202–208

Chapter: 19 Accidents: Road, Air and Fire 209–228

Chapter: 20 Impaired Consciousness and Drowing 229–236

Chapter: 21 Poisoining, Bites and Stings 237–247

Chapter: 22 Fractures: Bones and Joints 248–268

Chapter: 23 Bandage and Dressing 269–276

Chapter: 24 Effects of Heat 277–283

Chapter: 25 Effects of Cold 284–291

Chapter: 26 Handling and Transporting of Casualty 292–302

SECTION – IV

Emergency Management

Chapter: 27 Emergency Services 305–320

Chapter: 28 Ambulance 321–331

Chapter: 29 Major Disaster Management 332–346

Chapter: 30 Children in Accident and Emergency 347–358

Chapter: 31 Elderly People in Accident and Emergency 359–369

Chapter: 32 Eye Complaints and Emergencies 370–383

Chapter: 33 ENT and Dental Emergencies 384–395

Chapter: 34 Women's Health Problems in A & E 396–404

Chapter: 35 Medical Emergencies 405–484

Chapter: 36 Common Medical Problems 485–524

SECTION – V

Miscellaneous

Chapter: 37 Antiseptic: Their Usage 527–534

Chapter: 38 Nutrition 535–556

Chapter: 39 Sterilization 557–568

Chapter: 40 Violent Patient 569–578

Chapter: 41 Sexual Assault 579–583

Chapter: 42 Sign of Death 584–587

Index 588–590

SECTION-I

Introduction

Chapter: 1	Introduction to First Aid and Emergency	1–13
Chapter: 2	First Aid Kit and Emergency Equipment	14–18
Chapter: 3	Casualty Management	19–27
Chapter: 4	Resuscitation	28–46
Chapter: 5	Pregnancy and Childbirth	47–57

1 CHAPTER

INTRODUCTION TO FIRST AID AND EMERGENCY

INTRODUCTION

First Aid is the most important branch of medical science. First aid is, like medicine, both an art and a science. First aid is the immediate and temporary treatment given to the person who suffers an accident or any sudden illness before the medical help (aid) available, is called *First Aid.* First aid can also be defined as the immediate and temporary care given to an injured or sick person until the services of a qualified doctor are obtained. In order to save life and remove suffering proper and immediate care is absolutely necessary. The First aid is not an end by itself. It indicates that the person is in need of a "Secondary Aid".

General Esmarch (1823-1908) was the famous German Surgeon who first conceived the idea of "First aid". In 1877 St. John Ambulance Association of England was formed. In 1920, Red Cross Society of India was established. This is an age when technology has produced complicated machinery and swift means of transport. So, accidents are on the rise and produce devastating results with loss of life, injuries to body and mind. Under these circumstances, first aid has gained much importance. When the first aider reaches the spot of the accident, the causes of the accident may still be present and continues to exert harmful effects.

CONCEPT AND MEANING OF FIRST AID

First aid is the provision of limited care for an illness or injury, which is provided usually by a lay person to a sick or injured patient until definitive medical treatment can be accessed, or until the illness or injury is dealt with as not all illnesses or injuries will require a higher level of treatment. It generally consists of series of simple, sometimes life saving, medical techniques, that an individual, either with or without formal medical training, can be trained to perform with minimal equipment. The 3 main aims of first aid, commonly referred to as the "3 Ps" are:

(i) Preserve life

(ii) Prevent further injury

(iii) Promote recovery

In addition, some trainers may also advocate a 4th 'P' — Protect yourself, although this is not technically an 'aim' of providing first aid, and some people would consider that it is adequately covered by 'Prevent further injury' as this is to the casualty, yourself or others. Much of first aid is common sense, and people are almost certain to learn some elements as they go through their life such as knowing to apply an adhesive bandage to a small cut on a finger.

However, effective life-saving first aid needs hands-on training by experts, especially where it relates to potentially fatal illnesses and injuries, such as those that require Cardiopulmonary resuscitation (CPR), as the procedures may be invasive, and carry a risk of further injury to the patient - which the '3 aims' of first aid above, clearly try to avoid. As with any training, it is more useful if it occurs before an actual emergency, although in many countries, emergency ambulance dispatchers will give basic first aid instructions over the phone while the ambulance is on its way.

To be properly trained, a person must attend a course (hopefully leading to a qualification recognised in their country), but then, due to regular changes in procedures and protocols, based on updated clinical knowledge, must attend regular refresher courses or re-certification in order to ensure they are doing the best for their patient (and in some countries, to minimise the chance of being held liable for further injury or deterioration).

First aid training in first aid is often available through community organizations such as the Red Cross and St. John Ambulance, or through commercial providers, who will train people for a fee. This commercial training is most common for training of employees to perform first aid in their workplace. Many community organisations, such as the ones above, also provide a commercial service, which complements their community programmes.

KEY SKILLS TO FIRST AID

There are certain skills which can be regarded as core, regardless of where or how first aid is taught. First aiders are taught to focus on the 'ABC's of first aid before giving additional treatment:

(i) Airway
(ii) Breathing
(iii) Circulation

This means any first aider should first evaluate and attempt to treat problems with a casualty's airway. If the airway is open the first aider should then evaluate and attempt to treat problems with breathing followed by circulation (circulation of blood). Some instructors add a fourth step of "D" for Deadly Bleeds or Defibrillation. Variations on techniques to evaluate and maintain the ABCs depend on the skill level of the first aider. Once the ABCs are secured first aiders can begin more advanced treatments, if required. Some countries teach the same order of priority using the '3 Bs':

(i) Breathing

(ii) Bleeding

(iii) Bones

This means that any first aider should first seek to treat any problems with Breathing, before attempting to deal with a bleed or broken bone which is not to say that they should not be considered at the time — such as in the case of a spinal injury, where a variation on the technique can be used to open the airway.

LIFE PRESERVING

As the key skill to first aid is preserving life, the single most important training a first aider can receive is in the primary diagnosis and care of an unconscious or unresponsive patient. The most common mnemonic used to remember the procedure for this is ABC, which stands for Airway, Breathing and Circulation.

In order to save life, all persons require to have an open airway — a clear passage where air can move in through the mouth or nose through the pharynx and down in to the lungs, without obstruction. The people who are conscious will maintain their own airway automatically, but those who are unconscious (with a GCS of less than 8) may be unable to maintain a patent airway, as the part of the brain which autonomously controls in normal situations may not be functioning.

If an unconscious patient is lying on his or her back, the tongue may fall backward, obstructing the oropharynx (sometimes incorrectly called "swallowing" the tongue). This can be easily rectified by a first aider tipping the head backwards, which mechanically lifts the tongue clear.

If the patient was breathing, a first aider would normally then place them in the recovery position, with the patient leant over on their side, which also has the effect of clearing the tongue from the pharynx. It also avoids a common cause of death in unconscious patients, which is choking on regurgitated stomach contents.

The airway can also become blocked through a foreign object becoming lodged in the pharynx or larynx. It is generally called *choking*. The first aider will be taught to deal with this through a combination of 'back slaps' and 'abdominal thrusts'. Once the airway has been opened, the first aider would assess to see if the patient is breathing. If there is no breathing, or the patient is not breathing normally, such as agonal breathing, the first aider would undertake what is probably the most recognised first aid procedure — Cardiopulmonary resuscitation or CPR, which involves breathing for the patient, and manually massaging the heart to promote blood flow around the body.

PROMOTING RECOVERY

The first aider is also likely to be trained in dealing with injuries such as cuts, grazes or broken bones. They can deal with the situation in its entirety a small adhesive bandage on a paper cut, or need required to maintain the condition of something like a broken bone, until the next stage of definitive care usually an ambulance arrives.

IMPORTANCE OF FIRST AID

To give efficient first aid, one should have good knowledge of human anatomy and physiology of the human body and common sense and experience. The main importance of first aid are:

1. The immediate objective of first aid at a given situation is to save the life of the individual.
2. It is the first objective of first aid to reduce pain and prevent further injury or complication.
3. First aid should help to avoid further injury. It should correct situations which tend to increase the original injury.
4. The First aid should form a basis for subsequent treatment by the doctor or the hospital staff.

5. It can be done by supplying details of accident, injury and the first aid treatment given etc. The ultimate aim of First aid is to prevent disability and death.

It is necessary to obtain understanding of the working of the human body and its response to injury aid illness. This would be a good introduction to the study of medical science in a practical way.

LIMITATIONS OF FIRST AID

(i) The 'first aider' should be observant with the rules or objectives of first aid and act quickly and vigilantly.

(ii) He should inspire confidence in the patient and others closely related to the patient.

(iii) To save lives, there are three conditions that call for first aid

— Stoppage of breathing, severe bleeding and shock.

— If breathing movements are not proper, the lips, tongue and finger nails become blue. In such a situation, artificial respiration should be started immediately.

— If there is heavy bleeding, it may be from wounds through one or more large vessels. In this condition, pressure should be applied directly over the wound. For this, a clean handkerchief or a pad may be kept on the wound and pressed firmly with one or both hands, then apply a firm bandage.

— The third important factor to be attended immediately is *shock*. *Shock* accompanies severe injury or emotional disturbance. Cold and clammy skin, beads of perspiration on the forehead and palms. Pale face, nausea and vomiting are the common symptoms of shock.

Treatment— First take the casualty away from fire, live wires, moving machinery etc. Keep the patient in a safe and clear place. Do not allow people to crowd around the casualty. If the weather is extremely cold or hot or it is raining heavily, take the patient to a nearby room or a sheltered place. If there is no such facility, make use of an umbrella or a newspaper etc. The injured person should be made lie in a comfortable position on his back. His belt should be loosened, open the buttons of his shirt and trousers. Keep his legs in a natural position with toes facing up. The injured person should be kept comfortable but not hot. Water or other liquids should not be given to an unconscious person. The person should not be allowed to see his own injury. If there are wounds on the body, they should be cleaned gently and then dressed. In the case of burn victims, their clothes should not be pulled out. They should be cut with a clean scissors and removed. If there is bleeding, stop bleeding by pressure bandage. Use soft words and reassure the casualty. Send the patient to a hospital or a doctor by quickest means of transport. Inform the relatives of the patient, if possible. Always remember that you are only a first aider and not a doctor.

CONCEPT AND MEANING OF EMERGENCY

First aiders must always consider their own safety. Often the inexperienced or unthinking first aiders in the beat of the moment, put themselves at greater risk. Making sure of his own safety the first aider should approach the incident prepared to take charge if necessary. Bystanders, if any, can assist by going for help; if there are two they can be sent in opposite directions.

In the case of road traffic accidents the emergency services should be contacted first and told—

1. Location, road number, grid reference, landmarks;
2. Type of accident;
3. Number of vehicles involved;
4. Number of casualties;
5. Any casualties trapped; and
6. Special hazards — fire, chemical spillage, etc.

The aim of any treatment, whoever it is given by, is to prevent an existing condition deteriorating and provide, as far as is possible in the circumstances, the best conditions for recovery. The first essential in approaching an incident is to avoid panic. This applies to all involved, the first aider and through him the casualty and bystanders. This means that the first aider must have a calm and reassuring manner, even if he does not feel calm and reassured himself. By adopting this attitude a crisis situation is often defused and the first aid given that much more effective.

INCIDENT ASSESSMENT

A rapid assessment of the situation and a note of the number of casualties is first made. Each casualty should be looked at individually and an order of priority decided. There is a danger that the first casualty met with is the first to be treated; this attitude is not unnatural, but ignores the possibility that the second or third may be more severely injured. A mistaken order of priorities can be as dangerous as no first aid treatment being available at all. The casualty who is clamouring for attention may be in less danger than a silent motionless one.

PRIORITIES

First aiders should work on priorty basis. Airway problems and major bleeding always take precedence over fractures, minor wounds and hysteria. The first aider must check that each casualty

(a) has an adequate airway,
(b) is breathing,
(c) has no major bleeding, and
(d) is conscious.

If the answer to all of these is 'yes', he can he left in the care of a bystander. If the first aider is alone, each casualty will have to he left until all have been assessed.

Once this has been done it is necessary to decide who needs most help. This may not he the most seriously injured – a person who has been knocked out and only requires airway support will have his life saved by simple treatment given in time. The first aider may find it impossible to do anything effective for a casualty with severe multiple injuries.

UNCONSCIOUS CASUALTIES

They should be placed in the recovery position. If available, a bystander can be asked to hold the jaw forward to maintain an open airway and monitor pulse and respiration.

ROLE OF BYSTANDERS

Many people feel helpless in the face of an accident, but many also want to assist. Bystanders can be used to control traffic, get help and do specific tasks, e.g., apply pressure to a wound in a case of haemorrhage. By using bystanders in this way, their feelings of wanting to help can be employed to best advantage. The first aider can then be free to give his attention to the total situation.

WORKING ALONE

The alone first aider with one or more casualties should use the same guidelines as outlined above. After assessment the incident, he will have to decide whether to treat any or an before summoning help. In remote situations there may he the added problem of having to wait until rescued. It is vital that the first aider remain calm and think logically.

USE OF CLOTHES AND PROTECTIVE HEADGEAR

In many accidents, particularly road accidents, the injury will necessitate the removal of some of the casualty's clothes to make an effective assessment. Motorcyclists, for example, may have to have their helmets removed if there are airway problems, vomiting or severe bleeding from the head and neck. When removing the crash helmet it is advisable for the head and neck to he supported by an assistant.

Clothes that are not easily removable without disturbing the casualty unduly – for example, in cases of fracture – may be slit along the seams. Clothes which cover an injured part should never be tugged at repeatedly.

EXAMINATION OF THE CASUALTY

First check that the airway is adequate. Breathing which is noisy, sounding as though the casualty is snoring, means the airway is at least partially obstructed. Make sure he is breathing adequately (look at the chest – is it expanding? Feel for breath on the hand) and that he has a pulse. Adults breathe about 16 times a minute, babies about 30-40 times a minute. In the same way, the pulse rate varies with age, from 140 per minute at birth to around 60-80 in the adult. Remember the pulse rate will rise in shock states and when there is pain. Check for any characteristic smell on the breath e.g., acetone in diabetic coma.

Look at the casualty's colour. Cyaposis may indicate asphyxia. This may be due to the inhalation of vomit, teeth or dentures. Check that the mouth is empty. Full dentures may be left in the mouth only if the airway cannot be supported without them. As a good general rule, however, such a potentially dangerous foreign body should be removed.

Check for bleeding from the car and nose. Leakage of clear or straw-coloured fluid from them may indicate a fractured skull. Examine the pupils carefully. Do they get smaller on exposure to bright light (on opening the lid or on shining a torch in the eye)? When his eyelash is touched gently the casualty should blink. Check for any bleeding on the white of the eye – the eye will look bloodshot.

Feel the scalp below the hair and note any lacerations. Occasionally a fracture of the skull can he felt through a wound. Feel the contour of the cervical spine (the vertebrae of the neck). Is the contour smooth? If the casualty is conscious find out if there is any paid in the neck or any tenderness when finger pressure is applied over the bones. If there is, or if a neck injury is suspected, a cervical collar should be applied. In emergencies one can be made from a rolled-up newspaper bandaged round the neck.

Examine next the chest and the rest of the spine. Check that both sides of the chest move to the same extent with each breath. Look for any penetrating injuries or 'sucking wounds'. Make a note of any tender spots over the rib cage. If the airway is obstructed there will he an indrawing of the soft tissues between the ribs and under the rib margins. This is especially common in children. Examine the spine in the same way as the neck. If the casualty is supine this can he done by sliding a hand under the back. If at all possible, do not move a casualty with a spinal injury. If resuscitation is required, repositioning may be unavoidable. In this situation, the casualty should be moved 'in one piece' with the aid of several helpers.

Check the pelvic area by gently exerting pressure on both sides at the same time, so as to slightly compress the pelvic ring. Any sign of tenderness should lead one to suspect a fracture. Incontinence may he the result of fright, unconsciousness or a pelvic fracture. Examine the abdomen for wounds and bruising. Bowel may protrude from abdominal wounds. Examine the limbs in turn for any swelling, deformity or major bleeding. Note the shape and size of joints compared with the opposite side. Bleeding into a joint may result in profound swelling and severe pain. Remember that blood loss into limb fractures may be considerable and that there may be no external evidence of bleeding, the only signs being swelling over the fracture site, pain and shock.

Check for any warning medallions such as Medic-Alert around the wrist or neck. They can alert one to a particular condition or drug therapy, particularly steroids. There may be injection marks on the thighs or abdomen of diabetics. Drug addicts may have injection marks on the arms or, more rarely, legs.

Assess the level of consciousness in every casualty. Particularly note if he is becoming more or less responsive. Conscious level is best assessed by noting

(a) Eye opening
(b) Purposeful movement
(c) Spoken response

Following these stimuli:

(a) Spoken word

(b) Touch

(c) Pain (pinching the skin).

Test also for the eyelash reflex-touch the lash, it should cause blinking. Remember that in spinal injury the casualty may be unable to feel below the level of the injury yet may be fully conscious. In this case, touch and pinch him on the leg; if there is no response, move up the body until he can feel the stimulus.

Remember that fractures in the neck may also lead to difficulty with respiration.

It is vital to write down all these observations on paper, with the times at which they were made. Any history from the casualty or bystanders should also be recorded.

FURTHER INFORMATION

Always check through the pockets, handbag or luggage of an unconscious patient. In the presence of a witness. Look for information cards which indicate if the casualty is diabetic or on steroids. Look for hospital or GP's appointments cards, blood group cards, tablets, medicines, insulin or sugar.

GOLDEN RULES OF FIRST AID

1. Be calm and quick. Be methodical. Patiently, find out all major injuries and wounds and treat them suitably.
2. In case of failure of breathing, start artificial respiration immediately.
3. In order to control bleeding, press on the pressure points and press on the bleeding point with a pad and keep pressing at least for four minutes by watch. Do not remove the original pad instead keep adding fresh pads one on top of the other.
4. Do not allow a patient to go with a shock. If the shock is severe, patient is to be transferred to the hospital on top priority.
5. If the weather is fine, i.e., neither too hot or not too cold and without rain, treat the casualty in open. Otherwise move the casualty to nearby safer place like a verandah or some airy room. In extremes of weather general condition of the

casualty deteriorates very quickly e.g., a case of heat stroke lying on the road needs to be shifted to or needs cool place immediately.

6. Arrange for transport of the casualty to the nearest medical aid.
7. Use of first aid equipment. If standard first aid equipment is available, use it. Else first aider should improvise the equipment.
8. Do not allow people to crowd around the casualty. Allow fresh air.
9. Be careful in removing his clothes. Do not cause injury. Keep the body warm and avoid shock. Send the patient to a doctor or a hospital by the quickest means of transport. When serious accident takes place, inform the police.

STUDY–QUESTIONS

1. Explain the general principles of first-aid.
2. Discuss the importance and limitations of first-aid.

2

CHAPTER

FIRST AID KIT AND EMERGENCY EQUIPMENT

FIRST AID KIT

A first aid kit is a collection of supplies and equipment for use in giving first aid, particularly in a medical emergency. Most first aid kits contain bandages for controlling bleeding, personal protective equipment such as gloves and a breathing barrier for performing rescue breathing and CPR (cardiopulmonary resuscitation), and sometimes instructions on how to perform first aid.

Several store bought first aid kits, especially the cheap ones, are very poor in terms of quality, quantity, and selection of items, and are only suited for treating very minor injuries. A homemade kit, if properly prepared, is generally better and sometimes cheaper than most commercial kits.

Casualty should be well equipped for making the jo easy. At home, school, buses, factories and cars there should be a first aid kit or bag kept ready for emergencies. Infact the contents of a first aid kit will vary according to the duties to be performed and the special needs of the occasion. The following list provide a basis for selecting equipment for:

One list of items for a first aid kit are as follows:

— Adhesive bandages are one of the most commonly used items in a first aid kit.

DRESSING MATERIALS (STERILE, APPLIED DIRECTLY TO WOUND)

— Pads

— Sterile eye pads

— Sterile gauze pads

— Sterile nonadherent pads

— Burn dressing (sterile pad soaked in a cooling gel)

BANDAGES (STERILITY IS NOT NECESSARY, USED TO SECURE A DRESSING)

— Gauze Roller bandages — absorbent, breathable, and often elastic

— Elastic bandages — used for sprains, and pressure bandages

— Adhesive, elastic roller bandages — Very effective pressure bandages or durable, waterproof bandaging

— Triangular bandages — used as slings, tourniquets, to tie splints, and many other uses

Sometimes dressings and bandages are combined, in which case they must be sterile.

— Adhesive bandages (band-aids, sticking plasters)

— Straight adhesive bandages

— Butterfly (knuckle) bandages

— Disposable gloves should be provided in a first aid kit.

TOOLS AND INSTRUMENTS

— Adhesive tape, hypoallergenic

— Trauma shears, for cutting clothing and general use

— Tweezers

— Irrigation syringe, for cleaning wounds

— Rubber suction bulb, for clearing the airway of an unconscious patient

— If treating snakebites is a concern. This is the only snakebite kit generally recognised as not causing further damage and possibly reducing the effects of a snakebite.

EQUIPMENT

A torch (flashlight) is a useful addition to a first aid kit, especially one placed in a vehicle

— Personal Protective Equipment (PPE)
— Gloves, disposable non- latex
— CPR mask or other breathing barrier such as a face shield
— Eye cup or small plastic cup
— Torch (also known as a flashlight)
— Instant-acting chemical cold packs
— Sterile eye wash (commonly saline)
— Sterile saline may also be used for cleaning wounds where clean tap water is not available.
— Swabs, sterile non-woven
— Space blanket (lightweight plastic foil blanket, sometimes called "emergency blanket")
— Alcohol rub (hand sanitizer) or antiseptic hand wipes
— Thermometer
— Penlight

MEDICATION

Single use packets of medications, ointments, and antiseptics will prolong shelf life, decrease contamination risk, reduce risk of leakage (usually), and save space (for small quantities).

— Antiseptics/antimicrobial.
— Povidone iodine wipes — very effective and painless, but messy. It can also be used to purify water.
— Benzalkonium Chloride — painless, effective, often includes anesthetic.
— Alcohol pads — should not be used on open cuts or wounds, since they cause tissue damage and delay healing. They can

be used to prep unbroken skin for injections etc. or to disinfect equipment such as thermometers. While not a medical use, alcohol pads are also useful as a solvent to remove ink, adhesives, etc.

— Antibiotic ointment — single, double, or triple antibiotic ointment in petroleum jelly base antiseptic/anesthetic ointment or spray.

— Anti-itch ointment (especially for outdoor kits).

— Hydrocortisone cream.

— Antihistamine cream, such as benadryl.

— Calamine lotion.

— Painkillers/fever reducers.

— Acetaminophen.

— Ibuprofen - anti-inflammatory, often more effective that acetaminophen.

— Aspirin — one 300 mg Aspirin tablet may be given to a patient suffering a heart attack, to be chewed slowly.

— Antihistamines —can treat allergies and allergic reactions, including life-threatening anaphylactic shock.

— Diphenhydramine (brand name Benadryl).

— Aloe vera gel — used for a wide variety of skin problems, including burns, sunburns, itching, and dry skin.

— Burn gel — a water based gel that acts as a cooling agent and often includes a mild anesthetic such as lidocaine and, sometimes, an antiseptic such as tea tree oil.

— Epinephrine auto-injector (brand name Epipen) — Often included in kits for wilderness use and in places like summer camps, to treat anaphylactic shock.

— Poison treatments.

— Activated charcoal.

— Syrup of ipecac.

— QuikClot is a hemostatic agent sometimes included in first aid kits, especially military kits, to control severe bleeding.

Improvised uses — Many first aid items can have improvised uses in a survival situation. For example, alcohol pads and petroleum jelly based ointments can be used as a fire-starting aid in an emergency, and the latter can even be used as an improvised lubricant for certain mechanical devices, and adhesive tapes and bandages can be used for repairs. These alternate uses can be an important consideration when picking items for a kit that may be used in wilderness or survival situations.

IMPROVISATION

First aid can be performed without a first aid kit. Any cloth (preferably as clean as possible) can be used as a bandage. Duct tape could also be used to secure a dressing. Common household items such as a magazine or even sticks can be used for splints. Direct pressure to stop bleeding can be applied with a hand if nothing else presents itself. Obviously it is better to have proper equipment, but improvised equipment has saved many lives.

TRAUMA BAG/FIRST RESPONDER BAG

Emergency responders use a more advanced medical kit called a trauma bag or a first responder bag. The contents are more high quality and the quantity of supplies is more than a basic first aid kit.

STUDY–QUESTION

Explain the first-aid kit and emergency equipments.

***

3

CHAPTER

Casualty Managment

INTRODUCTION

Casualty management can be organised according to environment, arrival, permission, examination, scope of treatment, multiple casualties, medical aid and relationship with police. Casualty services or Accident and Emergency Services is the place where serious patients have their first interaction with the hospital. This is the place which never sleeps and runs round the clock and, no doubt it tells about the functioning of any hospital, so one must be careful the way a patient is treated in casualty will let him decide whether to continue the treatment in that hospital or to take their patient for treatment to another hospital. If any hospital wants to increase its admission, it should give the best treatment at the first interaction.

Casualty department that is required to render a comprehensive range of services right from the elementary first aid and general outpatient services to sophisticated management of surgical and medical emergencies and full scale trauma care. Nowaday's people and general practitioner have increasingly come to accept that hospital emergency department is the safest place to refer trauma and other life threatening cases that cannot be tackled in ordinary way.

A well-designed emergency department is an important source of revenue for the hospital. Based on the needs of the patient and their relatives the casualty department must be located on the ground floor with an easy access for patients and ambulance. There should be separate entrance for casualty so that approach to the department is very easy. If casualty is located at the higher level then a ramp should cross it so that the ambulance could be taken right to the casualty entrance.

INFRASTRUCTURE AND DESIGN OF CASUALTY

1. Casualty department shall be such that it can handle a wide range of cases in the most economical and efficient manner in terms of space, equipment and supplies.
2. There should be separate entrances for casualty so that approach to the department is very easy. If casualty is located at the higher level than a room should cross it so that the ambulance could be taken to the casualty entrance.
2. Medical stores should be located near the casualty and must remain open 24 hours and must keep all the necessary drugs and equipments for this a pharmacist should be in touch with the doctors and keep the items with their consultation.
3. Adequate space to keep wheelchair and stretchers, so that patient is shifted to casualty or out to the ward at the earliest, but this space should be away from the normal passage.
4. Spacious waiting hall with attached toilets should be provided close to the casualty where the attendants could wait till their patient is being taken care of.
5. Reception-cum-enquiry-cum-billing counter should be close to the casualty, preferably at the entrance of the casualty there should be a separate counter for the casualty so that valuable time is not wasted standing in a queue, as investigations will be delayed due to lack of registration number, if there is a common counter then preference must be given to the casualty patients.

6. Ancillary services like laboratory, blood bank and radiology department must be located in a close proximity to casualty.
7. Entrance shall be well lighted up and must bear a sign board—"CASUALTY", "24 HOURS EMERGENCY", or "ACCIDENT AND EMERGENCY SERVICES". So that no time is wasted in locating the department.
8. A telephone booth should be located at an easily reachable distance from casualty.
9. Provision for safe drinking water is essential.
10. A.T.M. bank facility if provided is very beneficial.
11. Adequate parking space must be provided close to the casualty, so that relatives have easy access to their vehicle as they might have to go to different places to get some help.
12. A security room or a police control room must be close to casualty to control the crowd in case of mass casualty or otherwise if required.
13. Provision for a canteen is a must.
14. Government authorities should ensure the issuing of easily recognisable mobile numbers with specially made distinct mobile instruments and make it mandatory to be kept operational at all Emergencies for use in relation to needs of patients or their attendants.

CASUALTY SETUP

An accident and emergency department needs a staff with a high degree skill and well experienced as this is no place to experiment. This department provides 24 hours service, so a well-trained staff must be posted in casualty. This department is either a separate one with a senior most casualty medical officer being in charge and reporting to the medical superintendent of the hospital or is attached to the surgical unit where H.O.D. of that department looks after management and the functioning of casualty in consultation with C.M.O. *(Casualty Medical Officer).*

C.M.O. is the pillar of casualty department and so no junior doctor should be deployed as a C.M.O. The C.M.O. is the first person to interact with any patient who is brought in to casualty and hence holds a lot of responsibility.

In serious case one must try to maintain 'AIRWAY, BREATHING AND CIRCULATION' first and then take further history. Remember quick action of yours could save many lives. Give primary treatment to the patient to get the urgent investigations done, and send a call to the specialist concerned with the case, do not hesitate to take specialist advice whenever needed and one must manage the case till the specialist reaches casualty.

The C.M.O. must have with him telephone numbers of specialists, senior officials of the hospital, local fire station, police post, nearby higher centres, railway station, etc., so that he may contact these without delay. The C.M.O. has a great role to play in cases of medico legal importance.

In case of any mis-happening or misadventure you must inform the higher authority at the earliest, as something might not be under jurisdiction and control of yours and they may come out with a solution that is more effective. C.M.O. must not leave the casualty without making any alternative arrangement and must be available in casualty throughout his duty or should only leave after mentioning his whereabouts, as his absence might prove fatal to some patient. He must always try to improve the functioning of the casualty and must try to solve any problem, he must not have attitude of "I want to just do my duty, the rest is the headache of hospital and management."

AREAS OF CASUALTY SETUP

(i) Casualty Reception/Enquiry

Casualty reception/enquiry functions round the clock, all the enquiry regarding hospital is given here and admission ticket is made. Billing of patient is done here.

(ii) Nursing Station

One each in casualty OPD and observation room. This is working place for the staff nurse, where they keep all the emergency drugs in an almirah or a shelf, this area is used to load the syringe before dispensing and for doing the paper work of a patient.

(iii) Observation Room/Casualty Ward

This is a place where patients are kept for recovery from the acute illness and later on shifted to the wards or discharged from there, but no patients should be kept here unnecessarily as beds might be needed for some other patient. This ward is divided in medical and surgical cubicles for convenience to the respective departments.

(iv) Examination Room/Casualty OPD

This is the examination or OPD room, where casualty medical officer is present along with other medical and paramedical staff. Nowadays casualties are being made centrally air-conditioned. Provision for hand washing must be provided inside casualty and toilets for staff shall be provided nearby. Patients are first brought to this area, so the entrance to this area should be spacious and preferably two entrances should be there. There must be provision of central oxygen and suction if not then keep oxygen cylinders and suction machines.

Every casualty OPD must have: BP apparatus, ECG machines, De-fibrillator, Cardiac monitor, Pulse-oximeter, X-ray view box, Refrigerator, Portable ventilator (optional), Nebulishing machine.

(v) Dressing Room/Plaster Room

This is an area where plaster is applied to the patients and dressing is done, so that from here either the patient is discharged or sent to a ward.

(vi) Casualty OT/MOT

Hospital should have emergency OT which should run round the clock. It should be well equipped and provision to operate upon at least two cases at a time. In MOT procedures like suturing, incision and drainage, thoracocentesis, tracheostomics are performed.

(vii) Duty Room for CMO

Duty room should be very close to the casualty, so that he can reach casualty without delay. This room should have an attached toilet.

(viii) Junior Doctor

These are junior residents posted in casualty and are generally deployed in casualty of a big setup and where there are a large number of patients visiting casualty. They have a very important role to play when a large number of serious patients are lying in casualty. In a few hospitals the junior-residents of various clinical branches are posted in casualty to help in managing these cases.

(ix) Staff Nurse

Casualty must have an adequate number of staff nurses and all should be well trained, as they are the ones who can make your job easy or else can mess up everything. They must be very polite and soft spoken. It's the responsibility of the staff nurse to keep an adequate stock of emergency drugs in casualty and get it indented before stock lasts. They must maintain and keep updated the records and documents.

(x) Ward Boys

They are suppose to assist the staff nurse in managing patients and to shift the patient in or out of the casualty and follow any other orders given to them.

(xi) OT Technician

They look after casualty OT and keep it ready to take any patient for surgery whenever required.

(xii) Receptionist

Must be posted round the clock. They should know the local language and should be very soft spoken.

MEDICAL EMERGENCIES

(i) Acute Myocardial Infraction

The most common complaint is acute chest pain, which is usually severe and prolonged. Pain is typically constricting in nature, reterosternal and radiate to left arm and back of the scapula, many patients may just come with complaint of pain in the epigastric region. Such patients are treated as a case of gastritis and later on when the diagnosis is made its already too late, and comes with this type of complaint get an ECG done, there is no harm in getting it done and excluding any ischimic pain than to commit a blunder. This pain is many times associated with severe sweating mainly over the fore head, nausea, or vomiting.

Do ECG, as this is the first investigation that help you in diagnosis. In ECG sometimes the changes might not occur for 24-48 hours, so always have a high degree of suspicion and admit the case.

(ii) Hypertensive Crisis

This is sudden increase in the arterial pressure even to a very high level (280–170 mm of Hg). The most common symptoms are severe headache, nausea or vomiting, palpitation, giddiness etc.

(iii) Bronchial Asthma

The most common symptoms are severe dysponea, tachyponea with a struggle to breath it, wheeze is audible from distance. In few cases it may come with bluish discoloration of the lips, finger tips or whole skin.

(iv) Hyper Pyrexia

Usually the temperature goes above 104° F. The symptoms are high degree fever, associated with sweating, headache, giddiness, confusion, trachycardia, tachyponea.

Treatment—Keep patient in the cool air temperature preferably in the A.C. room. Tepid sponge wash. Correct any dehydration by giving I.V. fluids.

(v) Acute Pancreatitis

Pain abdomen mainly over the epigastric region throbbing in nature radiating to the back, nausea or vomiting, sometimes severe dehydration. For this treatment get abdominal and chest X-ray done try to look for cut-off sign, and/or sentinel loop. Ultrasound and C.T. scan may confirm the diagnosis. History of chronic alcoholism in most of the patients.

(vi) Acute Gastro Enteritis

The symptoms are vomiting, diarrhoea, abdominal cramps, weakness, dehydration, loss of skin texture and depressed anterior frontenella in case of infants.

Treatment—In case of mild dehydration recommend ORS, but if dehydration is moderate to severe, give I.V. fluids — DNS is mainly used. We can give multivitamin.

(vii) Meningitis

The symptoms are high degree fever of small or long duration associated with sweating, nausea or vomiting, neck rigidity. For this, treat fever with cold tepid sponging, give injection paracetamol.

(viii) Epilepsy

This a brief disorder of cerebral function due to sudden electrical discharge of cerebral neurons and is usually associated with disturbance of consciousness. In this case, patient will either have an attack of its in front of you or will be brought to you after the patient had the attack. History of frothing.

Treatment—If the patient comes to you with actual fits in such case turn the head of the patient to other side to prevent any aspiration. Loosen all the cloths around the chest. Do not try to open the mouth with tongue depressor or with your finger, patient might bite your finger or you may injure his tongue/ gums instead padded be inserted. Give oxygen by mask.

(ix) Renal Colic

The symptoms are sudden severe pain in the loin that radiates to the lumber region or/and to the groin and in the testicles. Nausea or vomiting, retention of urine.

(x) Excessive Crying Child

This is very common complaint in the infant age group as they are not able to express anything and if they have any problem they just cry.

Treatment—Firstly ask the following from mother: feed of the baby, passing urine, passing stool, any history of UTI, any insect bite, dentition, emotional sufferings. In few cases, you will find that baby is not able to suck the mother milk, this could be due to the blocked nostrils. If the baby has not passed urine check for stenosed meatus, you might need to pass an infant feeding tube and evacuate the bladder. If the baby has not passed stools give neotomic enema.

STUDY–QUESTIONS

1. What do you understand by casualty management?
2. Explain casualty design and infrastructure in brief.
3. Write short notes on the following:
   (a) Acute Myocardial Intraction;
   (b) Bronchial Asthma;
   (c) Excessive Crying Child; and
   (d) Epilepsy.

***

4

CHAPTER

Resuscitation

INTRODUCTION

Resuscitation is the combination of the techniques used for sustaining lives of those patients whose spontaneous breathing and heart is stopped. This is also termed as *Cardiac Pulmonary Resuscitation (CPR)*. This is an emergency procedure every doctor must be aware of it. The basics of CPR is the same to maintain airway breathing and circulation of the patients who have a cardio pulmonary arrest.

The arrival in Accident and Emergency (A & E) of a critically injured patient is potentially one of the most difficult situations that can confront an A & E nurse, especially as several patients often arrive together from the same incident. The requirement, therefore, is for a plan of action, known to all members of the A & E team, which will identify and prioritise the major life-threatening problems and the interventions required around these problems. Such a plan involves the well-known ABC checklist of resuscitation — Airway, Breathing and Circulation — and continues with Consciousness (head injury), Spinal injury and Abdominal injury. A rapid primary survey must be carried out of these critical areas. At all times during resuscitation, the universal precautions for the prevention of blood-borne disease must be observed.

CHECKING AIRWAY

First important thing is to check any foreign body in the airway and it must be immediately removed. If the patient's airway is obstructed, all other considerations are of secondary importance and immediate intervention to clear the airway is required. Common causes of obstruction are vomitus, blood, inhaled material such as food or dentures, and soft tissue trauma affecting the neck or respiratory tract. This trauma can be caused by the inhalation of flames or of hot or noxious gases leading to burns of the trachea, by insect stings in the upper respiratory tract, or by a blow to the neck. The unconscious patient will be far less able to protect his or her airway than the patient who is conscious.

ASSESSING THE PATIENT

Airway obstruction is the first step in assessing the A & E patient. Obvious respiratory distress, cyanosis, stridor, the history of the incident and the patient's level of consciousness are all relevant facts in assessing airway patency. The sound of the patient's voice is also important. Is it hoarse? Laryngoscopy should not be performed as it may provoke spasm of the epiglottis or vocal cords. Shining a pen torch into the open mouth is the most appropriate way to examine the upper respiratory tract. Frequency and depth of respirations are important parameters for the nurse to record.

INTERVENTION

The first intervention is to clear the airway for the patient. This can be done manually with the aid of forceps or a gloved hand or with the aid of a wide bore, rigid sucker. Dentures often cause obstruction. In the case of an unconscious patient, the airway can be readily cleared by the chin lift or jaw thrust method. This action will pull the tongue away from the posterior pharynx. In the event of an unsuccessful injury the team should assume a cervical injury until proven otherwise and the head and neck should be stabilized in a correct alignment. *Watson* cites evidence to indicate there is a 5 to 10% chance of cervical injury in cases of blunt trauma to the head region. This emphasizes the importance of immobilizing the neck.

In serious cases of trauma to the neck region leading to an airway obstruction not amenable to clearance by manual or suction methods e.g., soft tissue swelling, the medical is what is required.

Once the airway is clear, the next intervention is to maintain its patency. The unconscious patient can be turned into the lateral position. Great care, however, is needed if there is any suspicion of a spinal injury and, in such cases, patients are best left flat with other means used to maintain their airway. One

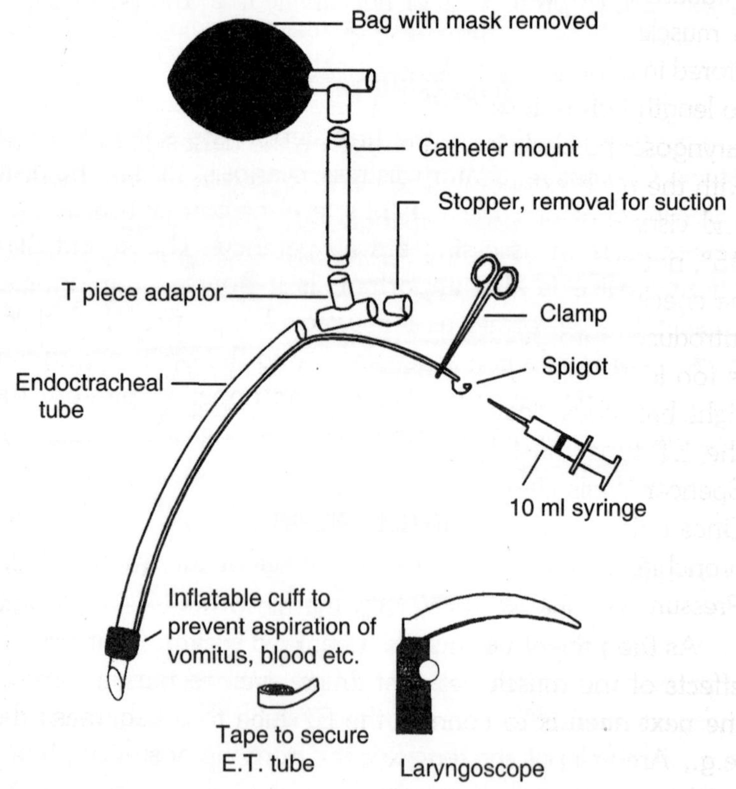

Fig. 4.1: *Equipment for intubation and IPPV.*

simple means of doing this is the oropharyngeal airway which will keep the tongue clear of the airway and which will also allow pharyngeal suction to be readily carried out with a long flexible suction catheter. The airway is introduced 'upside-down' into the mouth and then rotated into the correct position as it is slid over the back of the tongue.

Intubation is the most satisfactory way of maintaining the airwayn. In most hospitals, this is a medical task, although ambulance crews are now trained to intubate, and with the development of A & E clinical nurse specialists, it could easily become part of the nurse's role.

At present the A & E nurse must know how to assist with intubation (see Fig. 4.1 for equipment). The first requirement is a muscle relaxant drug, usually suxamethonium, which will be stored in a fridge. The endotracheal tube will often require cutting to length before insertion, so scissors should be kept ready. The laryngoscope blade is then passed on the right side of the midline with the neck extended. The blade is used to elevate the tongue and visualise the glottic opening by pulling forward the jaw at 45°, not by levering on the front teeth. The laryngoscope should be checked every morning to ensure it is working. The tube is introduced into the glottic opening by the right hand. If the tube is too long, there is a danger that it will be introduced into the right bronchus, leaving the left lung unventilated. The cuff of the ET tube must be inflated using a 10 ml syringe, and a Spencer Wells clamp is used to ensure the air stays in the cuff. Once inflated, the cuff protects the airway from aspiration, deep bronchial suction is possible and efficient Intermittent Positive Pressure Ventilation (IPPV) may be performed.

As the patient will now be unable to breathe, because of the effects of the muscle relaxant drugs given to permit intubation, the next need is to connect the ET tube to a bag/mask device (e.g., Ambu bag) and an oxygen source via an adaptor and a catheter mount. It is essential that the A & E nurse has the correct equipment to hand immediately, can connect it together promptly and if need be, can take over ventilating the patient.

The nurse should not forget the need for tape to tie and secure the ET tube in place.

EVALUATION

Evaluation of the patency of the airway after intervention is crucial. The nurse should check the following:

— Does the patient's colour improve?
— What happens to the respiratory rate?
— Does the chest expand with ventilation in the case of an intubated patient? And is there air entry to both lungs?

BREATHING

When the airway is cleared and maintained clear, the next questions are—can the patient breathe normally? And if not, how can the patient be helped to meet this most basic self-care demand? If the patient is making no respiratory effort, the procedure for respiratory arrest must be initiated at once with IPPV. However, the patient may be attempting to breathe but may be suffering from chest trauma which is interfering with normal respiration. If this trauma is serious, it may quickly prove fatal.

A common problem associated with serious chest trauma is *pneumothorax* in which air gains entry to the potential space of the pleura surrounding a lung. This will lead to the lung's collapse. A *pneumothorax* can arise spontaneously, without any trauma, due to the rupture of a weakness in the wall of the lung (Fig. 4.2a).

The most serious form of pneumothorax is a tension pneumothorax in which the hole into the pleura acts like a one-way flap valve, permitting air entry to the pleural space but prohibiting any escape of air (Fig. 4.2b). The result is a progressive build-up of pressure in the pleural space which will not only collapse the lung on the affected side, but will exert pressure on the uninjured side, leading to mediastinal shift, possible nipping of major blood vessels and collapse of the other lung.

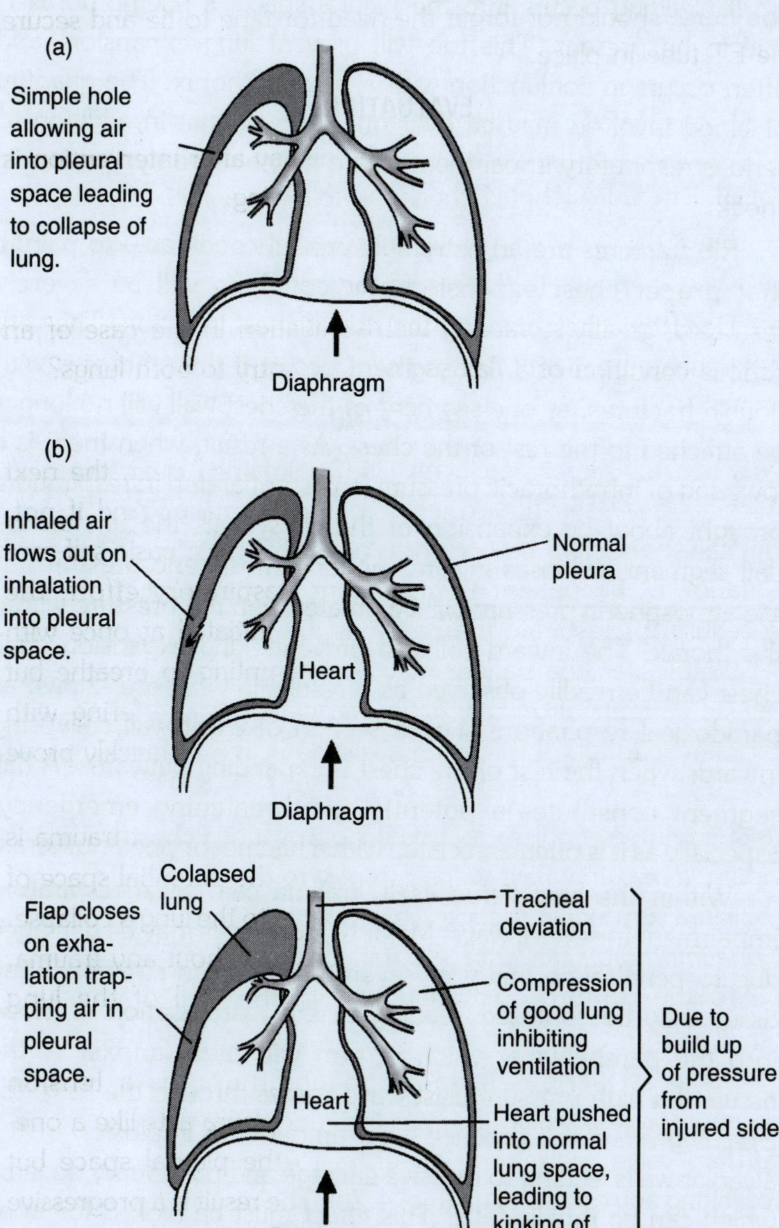

Fig. 4.2: *(a) Spontaneous pneumothorax. (b) Tension pneumothorax.*

If bleeding occurs into the pleural space, a haemothorax is said to be present. This too will prevent lung expansion, and often occurs in conjunction with a pneumothorax. The quantity of blood involved may be over one litre, so that in addition to serious respiratory impairment, there may also be hypovolaemic shock.

Rib fractures are an extremely painful condition—so painful that proper chest expansion and coughing will be severely restricted, greatly increasing the risk of chest infection. The very serious condition of a flail segment occurs if there are ribs with double fractures, as one segment of the chest wall will no longer be attached to the rest of the chest. As a result, when there is a lowering of intrathoracic pressure (an essential step in respiration) brought about by expansion of the chest wall, the unattached flail segment collapses inwards under atmospheric pressure, as the atmospheric pressure will be greater than the pressure within the thorax. The inward collapse prevents lung expansion. Flail chest can be readily observed as it results in what are known as paradoxical respirations, i.e., a section of chest wall collapsing inwards when the rest of the chest is expanding outwards. A flail segment constitutes a potential life-threatening emergency, especially as it is often associated with a haemo–or pneumothorax.

Within the lung tissue itself, trauma can cause respiratory impairment in several ways. Major blood vessels may be damaged due to penetrating injury or severe deceleration stresses. Lung tissue may be contused, leading to the extravasation of blood into the parenchyma which in turn will cause anoxia of the tissue. If a high pressure blast wave passes through the lung, the *Spaiding effect* will produce what amounts to implosion of the alveolar walls leading to massive damage and pulmonary oedema which can be rapidly fatal. This effect must be looked for in all victims of explosions. Finally, there is the possibility of the inhalation of material deep into the lung tissue. This material can range from water in drowning victims to noxious gases in burns cases.

ASSESSMENT

The chest must be fully visualised for examination. If necessary, clothing should be cut off. The respiratory rate must be recorded, together with the depth and pattern of the respirations. The following should be watched for:

- Evidence of cyanosis.
- Notably shallow or deep respirations.
- The use of accessory muscles of respiration.
- *Cheyne-Stokes* breathing.
- Gulping, 'air hunger' type breathing (an indication of hypovolaemic shock).
- Stridor (an indication of airway obstruction).
- Pain (an indication of fractured ribs).

The chest wall should be examined for evidence of trauma, bruising and wounds. Crepitus, indicating rib fractures, may be inadvertently elicited while palpating for bony tenderness (the cardinal sign of a fracture). Surgical emphysema may be perceived as a crackling feeling. This is caused by air escaping into the tissues, typically into the upper part of the chest wall. Paradoxical respirations will usually be apparent if there is a flail segment.

Pulse oximetry is a widely used non-invasive monitoring procedure which measures arterial oxyhaemoglobin saturation (SaO_2) and therefore gives important information about the supply of oxygen to body tissues. It does not, however, provide the information about ventilatory status which might come from arterial blood gases, *e.g.*, CO_2 tension or acid-base balance, and its accuracy is compromised by a range of factors such as patient motion, abnormal haemoglobin, dark skin pigmentation or nail polish. Adequate tissue oxygenation, according to *Durren*, requires an SaO_2 of over 90 per cent and adequate haemoglobin levels.

The medical staff's assessment will include the standard percussion and stethoscopic exam, chest X-rays (the area of lung collapse in pneumothorax is seen on an X-ray as a blank area without lung markings separating the lung margin from the chest wall) and arterial blood gases.

INTERVENTION

If the patient is not breathing, IPPV must be commenced at once. Cardiac compression, however, should be withheld until an assessment has been made of cardiac output and the EGG. Using an oropharyngeal airway and a bag/mask connected to an oxygen supply, the A & E nurse should be able to ventilate the patient adequately. *Watson*, suggests more effective ventilation occurs if a second person secures the mask on the face, as in this way a more airtight seal is achieved.

If the patient is exhibiting respiratory distress, 100 per cent oxygen should be applied by mask at 61/min. If possible, the sitting-upright position should be adopted to assist respiration. Chest injuries are very painful; the nurse may relieve such pain by the administration of Entonox, which is 50 per cent oxygen and 50 per cent nitrous oxide.

If the patient is conscious, it is likely that he or she will require a great deal of psychological support as difficulty in breathing is a very frightening experience. It is suggested that such a patient should not be left alone at any time, for, in addition to the risk of deterioration going unnoticed, it may provoke great fear in the patient.

The need for pulse oximetry and continual monitoring of respiratory rate and effort cannot be overemphasized as this will give first warning of a deterioration in respiratory function. Cyanosis is a very late sign, and in a significant proportion of the population, i.e., the non-Caucasian population, it is an unlikely sign at all. In non-Caucasians, cyanosis can be seen in the mucous membranes. Drowsiness and confusion are associated with respiratory failure and are due to cerebral hypoxia. In multiple trauma victims, however, it may not be possible to differentiate between when these signs are caused by head injury and when they are due to respiratory failure.

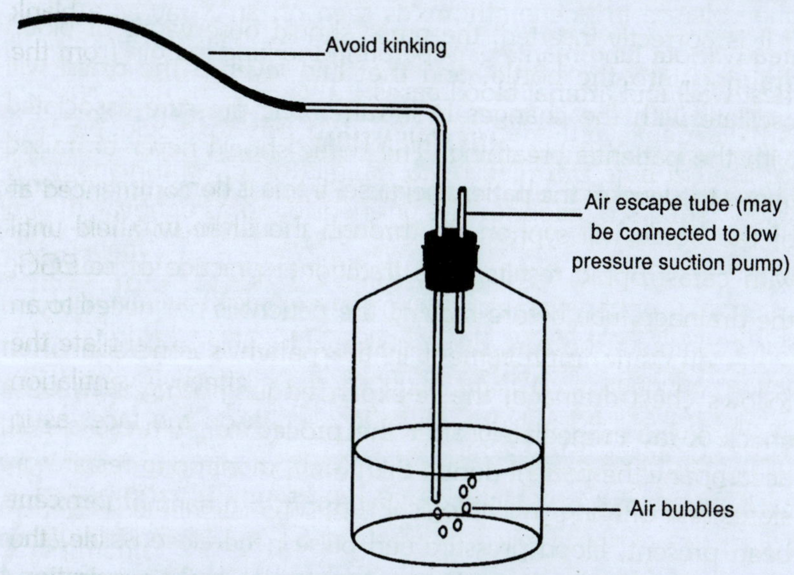

Fig. 4.3: *Simplified diagram of chest drainage.*

The remaining area of nursing care for respiratory problems concerns supporting medical intervention. In the case of a pneumo–thorax or haemothorax, the requirement is for a rapidly introduced chest drain, together with an underwater seal, to drain off the air or blood that is compressing the lung (Fig. 4.3). Most of the equipment for this procedure should be ready in advance in the form of a CSSD pack in the resuscitation room. Great stress should be laid on asepsis during the procedure. Iodine in spirit is usually used as a skin preparation. Local anaesthetic will be administered around the area, followed by a small incision with a scalpel to facilitate the introduction of the chest drain. The nurse should have the bottle ready with a litre of sterile water and should ensure that the tubing is connected the correct way, i.e., the drain coming from the patient must be connected to the tube that ends underwater.

Negative pressure is usually applied to the system by means of a specialised suction pump to facilitate drainage of blood. The chest drain will be sutured in place and the area around it should be dressed with a keyhole dressing secured with elastoplast.

If it is correctly inserted, the nurse should observe air or blood draining into the bottle, and the fluid level in the drain will oscillate with the changes in intrathoracic pressure associated with the patient's breathing. The bottle should never be raised above the level of the patient because, if this is done, the contents of the bottle will syphon off through the drain into the chest with catastrophic results. The traditional practice of clamping the drainage tube before moving the patient is not necessary.

A dramatic improvement in the patient's condition often follows chest drainage, the re-expanded lung being seen on a check X-ray immediately after the procedure. A nurse should accompany the patient during this X-ray, monitoring respiratory status and offering psychological support. If a haemothorax has been present, blood pressure and pulse need close observation because of the danger of hypovolaemic shock. The quantity of blood draining into the bottle needs to be recorded accurately.

In dealing with a large flail segment, it is likely that IPPV will be required, although the medical staff will not automatically resort to this measure; the patient's clinical condition is the key indication. The patient will require intubation for IPPV.

EVALUATION

The effectiveness of interventions to improve breathing must be carefully evaluated. Simple mistakes can occur, such as having the oxygen mask connected to an oxygen point that is not turned on or to an empty cylinder. The chest drain can become kinked or blocked by clots and can, therefore, stop functioning. Patients may be placed in the correct position to help their breathing, but that is no guarantee that they will stay there. They have a tendency to slip down the trolley.

Airway and breathing problems are very dramatic and desperate situations. It is very easy, therefore, for some simple error to occur with potentially fatal results. Continual evaluation must be the rule to be absolutely sure that things are going to plan and that the patient is benefiting from our interventions to assist the self-care demand of normal breathing.

TABLE 4.1

Classification of Shock by Cause

1. Hypovolaemic

(a) Haemorrhagic — Blood loss due to soft tissue bleeding, fractures, wounds, etc.

(b) Burns — Loss of plasma in burn exudate.

(c) Dehydration — Major body fluid loss, e.g., due to prolonged vomiting, diarrhoea,or metabolic disorders such as diabetic ketoacidosis.

2. Cardiogenic

Failure of cardiac pump leading to inadequate cardiac output although the blood volume is normal, e.g., after myocardial infaretion.

3. Vasogenic

(a) Septic—Endotoxins from gram-negative bacteria can cause massive vasodilatation in certain infective conditions.

(b) Anaphylactic—Severe allergic reaction; histamine release increases capillary permeability and leads to dilatation of capillaries and arterioles.

(c) Neurogenic—Loss of sympathetic control leading to dilatation of venuies, capillaries and arterioles.

CIRCULATION

The next priority in the resuscitation is circulation. Here the principal concern is the possibility of cardiac arrest or of insufficient circulation leading to shock. Therefore, while attention is being paid to the patient's airway and breathing, a nurse should also be assessing the patient's circulation.

The pathology of shock is very complex and there remains much still to be learnt of its nature. However, the main common denominator in all types of shock is reduced cellular perfusion, i.e., insufficient oxygen reaches the tissues of the body. If this condition is not corrected, it will eventually set in train a series of complex physiological changes which will result in irreversible shock and death. There are three main types of shock—*hypovolaemic*, *cardiogenic* and *vasogenic*.

In *hypovolaemic shock*, the problem is that there is a loss of fluid from the circulation.

In *cardiogenic shock*, there is a failure of the pump, although the blood volume is not affected.

While in *vasogenic shock*, the blood volume is again not affected but rather the arterioles and capillaries dilate, leading to diminished venous return and hence diminished cardiac output, which in turn leads to decreased tissue perfusion, i.e., shock.

The body has compensating mechanisms against shock which come into operation after injury, and which can give rise to misleadingly normal blood pressures in the A & E patient. The main result of these mechanisms is vaso-constriction.

Decreased renal perfusion leads to the release of renin which in turn leads, via the plasma protein angiotensinogen to angiotensin, a powerful vasoconstrictor at the micro-circulatory level. In addition, there is adrenaline and noradrenaline release, both of which are vasoconstrictors. This may allow patients to compensate for circulatory loss for some time with a normal blood pressure, especially if they are young and have, therefore, more elastic walls to their blood vessels.

Significant changes will occur in the urine output of the shocked patient. The reduction in circulating volume will reduce glomerular filtration and hence urine formation. Furthermore, the hormone aldosterone and the anti-diuretic hormone will be released as part of the compensatory effect, both of which will diminish urine output. In hypovolaemic shock, urine output may be less than 30 ml/h. This is a critical level since output below this value is indicative of renal failure. Hypovolaemic shock is, therefore, the major cause of acute renal failure.

ASSESSMENT

In assessing the patient's circulation, we first of all need to know if the heart is beating and if it is, whether it is producing an effective circulation. The A & E nurse needs, therefore, to take the patient's pulse, noting both *rate* and *rhythm*. The absence of a radial pulse indicates that systolic blood pressure is below 80. If the patient is unresponsive and making no apparent respiratory effort, the carotid pulse should be palpated and, if absent, a state of cardiac arrest assumed. The alarm should be raised first and then CPR initiated.

If the patient has a cardiac output, the next step is to assess the risk of shock. Continual monitoring of blood pressure is required, and the nurse should bear in mind the possibility of compensated shock as outlined above. Blood pressure should preferably be monitored by the same nurse so that any differences will reflect real differences in blood pressure rather than different hearing abilities or any other subjective factors that can make blood pressure readings unreliable.

Respiratory rate and pulse are other key parameters in the development of shock. Both will rise, the respiratory rate in response to the body's need to try to increase tissue oxygenation and the pulse in response to the failing blood pressure. The condition of the skin should be noted as the increased production of adrenaline and the resulting vasoconstriction will lead to a cool, pale and moist skin. The time for capillary refill to occur after blanching a digit by momentarily squeezing the extremity should be less than 2 seconds. A longer time is an indication of likely shock.

If the patient is conscious or if witnesses are present, a history of the accident is required. The history will often indicate the risk of injuries that may produce hypovolaemia, e.g., trauma to the right upper quadrant of the abdomen will alert the nurse to the risk of liver damage. The patient's mental state should also be assessed as psychological support is very important.

INTERVENTION

If there is no cardiac output, CPR must be commenced immediately. After clearing the airway the patient's lungs should be slowly inflated twice with oxygen using a bag/mask device before chest compressions are commenced to produce an effective circulation. If a bag/mask is not available, 'mouth-to-mouth' expired air respiration should be commenced with two slow breaths. It should be remembered that there has been no demonstrated case of HIV transmission by this route and *Zideman* considers there is no realistic risk of AIDS infection as a result of mouth-to-mouth resuscitation, as long as blood is not present in the saliva. This view is supported by *Baskett*.

The nurse should place both hands together on the sternum at a point some two fingers' width up from its lower end (xiphisternum). The fingers should be interlocked and the arms held straight, the aim being to use about half the nurse's body weight to compress the sternum by 4-5 cm. A rate of about 60 compressions per minute carried out correctly will give a cardiac output of between 33 per cent and 50per cent of normal, sufficient to prevent cerebral damage and permit the medical staff to attempt various techniques aimed at restarting the heart.

It is probable that the output produced in this way owes as much to a general rise in intrathoracic pressure and compression of the great vessels of the chest as it does to actual compression of the heart. For this reason, if equipment is available as it is in hospital, chest compression and ventilation may proceed independently as greater pressures will be generated in this way. A rate of 12-14 ventilations along with 60-80 chest compressions per minute should be aimed at although it is difficult to count precisely in the intense activity that surrounds a CPR attempt. Alternatively, a 5:1 ratio of compressions to ventilations is required in two persons life support, or 15:2 in single person CPR.

The patient should be connected to an ECG monitor as soon as possible in order that cardiac activity may be monitored. The ECG and the presence or absence of cardiac output, as measured by a carotid or femoral pulse, will determine the medical treatment that follows. Effective CPR must be maintained at all times to ensure an oxygenated blood supply continuously reaches the patient's brain.

In a cardiac arrest the three most likely cardiac arrhythmias to be found are—asystole, ventricular fibrillation or electromechanical dissociation.

In *asystole,* there is no cardiac electrical activity (straight line on the ECG) while in *electromechanical dissociation,* the ECG looks normal except that unfortunately the heart is not responding and producing any contractions; cardiac output is therefore nil. *Ventricular fibrillation* is a condition where there is uncoordinated electrical discharge throughout the ventricles and is the most common cause of cardiac arrest.

The result is that the myocardial muscle only quivers instead of carrying out its normal coordinated contraction and cardiac output effectively ceases. Giving an electrical shock, defibrillation aims to produce a simultaneous depolarization of all the myocardial cells, thus allowing them to repolarize at the same time and hopefully restore normal coordinated electrical and muscular activity. Resuscitation guidelines are aimed at ensuring defibrillation occurs at the earliest possible opportunity as prospects for success decrease at 5 per cent per minute of CPR.

In young children a different approach is required — the heel of one hand only for a small child, and two thumbs for a baby. The rate needs to be 80 to 100 compressions per minute, and the respiration rate correspondingly quicker but also more shallow.

The nurse will usually be responsible for drawing up and recording various drugs in a CPR attempt. It will greatly expedite the proceedings if nursing staff knows what is likely to be asked for and have the drugs to hand.

The nurse needs to know how to charge the defibrillator and to apply conducting pads to the chest in the correct positions (sternum and apex of the heart). If necessary, the nurse should be prepared to defibrillate if the nursing and medical staff have agreed to that being part of the nurse's role. The golden rule is to make sure that nobody is touching the trolley or else they too will receive a shock (200 to 360 joules).

If CPR is successful in re-establishing cardiac output, continual ECG monitoring is required, and further drug therapy may be needed to stabilize the patient's rhythm.

Asystole does not respond to defibrillation, however *Chamberlain* points out the need to be sure asystole is correctly diagnosed and is not misread from the monitor as it may actually be very fine. If in doubt, defibrillation is recommended.

The most common cause of shock in the A & E department is *hypovolaemia*. Immediate nursing interventions should be to elevate the foot of the trolley to try to increase the volume of blood in the vital heart-lung-brain circulation, to administer high concentration oxygen to assist tissue oxygenation, to control any obvious bleeding with pressure dressings and to offer psychological support to the patient.

As hypovolaemic shock is the type of shock most commonly seen in A & E, and as it requires large scale circulating volume replacement therapy, the nurse must be prepared to offer support to the medical staff in carrying out such potentially life-saving measures. Cannulation of the internal jugular or subclavian vein with a wide bore cannula will be carried out as well as establishing a peripheral line. Accurate fluid balance charts are required as there may be three drips running at once, together with CVP monitoring.

Clear fluids alone, such as normal saline, are not satisfactory as they are easily excreted by the kidneys and can leak from damaged capillaries. Therefore, in resuscitating the hypovolaemic patient, colloidal solutions such as Haemaccel or Gelofusin are used as a temporary measure until whole blood is grouped and cross-matched. These IV solutions have such large molecules that they are not readily filtered out by the kidneys, and due to the osmotic pressure they exert, fluid is moved from the intracellular compartment into the circulation. Crystalloid solutions such as Ringer lactate may also be used to restore interstitial fluid loss (*Baskett*). An IVI warming coil should be available as such is the volume of fluid likely to be given that it may cause hypothermia if not pre-warmed to body temperature. To facilitate the giving of large volumes of fluid in short times, some form of pump is required. A simple device like a sphygmanometer cuff can be inflated around the IVI bag to force the fluid in quickly.

A supply of '*O' Rhesus negative blood* should be available for emergency transfusion if one is needed while the patient's blood is being grouped and cross-matched. Catheterisation of the patient may be required in order to monitor urine output accurately on an hourly basis.

One form of effective treatment of shock used is *MAST—(Medical Anti-Shock Trousers).* MAST is a cross between a pair of trousers and a sphygmomanometer cuff inflated with a foot pump. It is an inflatable pair of trousers that has the effect of splinting lower limb fractures, controlling lower limb bleeding and, most importantly, autotransfusing the patient with a litre or so of ready-warmed, compatible blood, by squeezing it out of the less essential lower limbs into the vital heart-lung-brain circulation. It is only a temporary device and needs very careful deflation, but MAST can bring about a dramatic improvement in a patient's condition in A & E. *Randall* described the use of MAST in A & E on seven patients suffering from leaking aortic aneurysm or multiple trauma who had no measurable BP. Their condition greatly improved in the short term and a BP became recordable. However, only two survived surgery. MAST in A & E can therefore be life-saving in some cases.

EVALUATION

Continual monitoring of vital signs is essential to evaluate the progress of the shocked patient. Urine output must be carefully watched as acute renal failure is a grave sign (urine output less than 30 ml/h *Hudak* and *Gallo*. If the patient is becoming more alert and the skin is feeling warmer, IV replacement therapy is likely to be improving the situation. Repeated checks should be made that the pressure dressing really is controlling bleeding. Is there another wound that has been missed at the first assessment, or is there evidence of internal haemorrhage? The nurse caring for the patient must be alert to these possibilities if care is to be effectively evaluated.

STUDY–QUESTIONS

1. Write short notes on the following:
   (a) Hypovolaemic
   (b) Vasogenic
   (c) Cardiogenic
   (d) Breathing and
   (e) Circulation.

5 CHAPTER PREGNANCY AND CHILDBIRTH

PREGNANCY

Pregnancy is the period from conception to the birth of the baby. After fertilization, the combined egg and sperm cells begins to split repeatedly into two and is called an *embryo*. Some development of the embryo is necessary before it can implant into the lining of the womb. So if fertilization has occurred too near the point where the Fallopian tubes enters the womb, there may be insufficient time for the ovum to develop to the stage at which it can implant. In this case, the pregnancy ends at that point. Although pregnancy is a continuous, slow process of embryonic and then fetal growth, doctors and nurses find it convenient to divide the whole gestation period arbitrarily into three periods, each of three months, called *trimesters*. In addition to using hormone tests, doctors can confirm pregnancy by noting certain physical changes (sign) and by taking a history of a few symptoms.

CHILDBIRTH

Childbirth (also called labour, birth, partus or parturition) is the culmination of a human pregnancy or gestation period with the delivery of one or more newborn infants from a woman's uterus. The process of human childbirth is categorized in three stages of labour. The first stage accomplishes the shortening and then the dilation of the cervix. It is deemed to have started when the cervix is 3 cm long, and ends with full dilation. The second stage starts when the cervix is fully dilated and ends with the expulsion of the fetus. In the third stage, the placenta detaches from the uterine wall and is expelled through the birth canal. The latent phase of labour causes confusion with many. Latent phase may last many days and the contractions are an intensification of the Braxton-Hicks contractions that start around 26 weeks gestation. Cervical effacement may be accomplished fully. Latent phase ends with the onset of active first stage; when the cervix is three cm. dilated.

STAGES OF NORMAL HUMAN BIRTH

LATENT PHASE

The latent phase of labour causes confusion with many. Latent phase may last many days and the contractions are an intensification of the Braxton-Hicks contractions that start around 26 weeks gestation. Cervical effacement occurs the the closing weeks of pregnancy and is usually complete or near complete, by the end of latent phase. Cervical effacement is the incorporation of the cervix to form the lower segment of the cervix. The muscular portion of the uterus is the upper segment, and is made of non-striated muscle. The lower segment of the uterus has no muscles and is comprised of the cervix itself, which becomes massively stretched and thinned out. This cervical effacement will usually be accomplished fully prior to the onset of labour. The degree of cervical effacement may be felt during a vaginal examination. A 'long' cervix implies that not much has been taken into the lower segment, and vice versa for a 'short' cervix. Latent phase ends with the onset of active first stage; when the cervix is three cm. dilated.

FIRST STAGE: CONTRACTIONS

The first stage of labour is an active stage and should not be confused with the latent phase of labour. The first stage of labour starts classically when the effaced cervix is 3 cm dilated. There is variation in this point as some patients may present a little before this point with active contraction, or later, without regular contractions. The onset of actual labour is defined when the cervix begins to progressively dilate. Rupture of the membranes, or a blood stained 'show' may or may not occur at around this stage.

Uterine muscles form opposing spirals from the top of the upper segment of the uterus to its junction with the lower segment. During effacement, the cervix becomes incorporated into the lower segment. During a contraction, these muscles contract causing shortening of the upper segment and drawing upwards of the lower segment, in a gradual expulsive motion. This draws the cervix up over the baby's head. Full dilatation is reached when the cervix is the size of the baby's head; at around 10cm dilation for a term baby.

The duration of labour varies widely, but active phase averages some 8 hours for women giving birth to their first child "primiparae" and 4 hours for women who have already given birth "multiparae".

SECOND STAGE: DELIVERY

This stage begins when the cervix is fully dilated, and ends when the baby is finally delivered. At the beginning of the normal second stage, the head is fully engaged in the pelvis; the widest diameter of the head has successfully passed through the pelvic brim. Ideally it has successfully also passed below the interspinous diameter. This is the narrowest part of the pelvis. If these have been accomplished, all that will remain is for the fetal head to pass below the pubic arch and out though the introitus. This is assisted by the additional maternal efforts of "bearing down." The fetal head is seen to 'crown' as the labia part. At this point the woman may feel a burning or stinging sensation.

Delivery of the fetal head signals the successful completion of the fourth mechanism of labour (delivery by extension), and is followed by the fifth and sixth mechanisms (restitution and external rotation).

Abnormalities of second stage

Delays in second stage may be caused by:

- — malpresentaion of the fetal head;
- — failure of descent of the fetal head through the pelvic brim or the interspinous diameter;
- — poor uterine contraction strength;
- — a big baby and a small pelvis.

These factors will lead to prolongation of the second stage of labour. Secondary changes may be observed: swelling of the tissues, maternal exhaustion, fetal heart rate abnormalities. Left untreated, severe complications include death of mother or baby, and genitovaginal fistula. These are commonly seen in Third World countries where births are often unattended or attended by poorly trained community members.

THIRD STAGE: PLACENTA

In this stage, the uterus expels the placenta (afterbirth). Maternal blood loss is limited by the compression of the spiral arteries of the uterus as they pass though the lattice-like uterine muscles of the upper segment. Normal blood loss is less than 600 ml.

Management of third stage

Third stage is managed either expectantly or actively. Active management utilizes oxytocic agents to augment uterine muscular contraction. This contraction acts both to shear off the placental attachment and to compress the spiral arteries. Controlled cord traction assists with rapid delivery of the placenta. Expectant management allows the placenta to be expelled without assistance.

AFTER THE BIRTH

Medical professionals typically recommend breastfeeding of the first milk, colostrum, to reduce postpartum bleeding/ hemorrhage in the mother, and to pass immunities and other benefits to the baby. Parents usually bestow the infant its given name soon after birth. Often people visit and bring a gift for the baby.Many cultures feature initiation rites for newborns, such as naming ceremonies, baptism, and others.

Mothers are often allowed a period where they are relieved of their normal duties to recover from childbirth. The length of this period varies. In China it is 30 days and is referred to as "doing the month" or "sitting month". In other countries taking time off from work to care for a newborn is called "maternity leave" and varies from a few days to several months.

INDUCTION OF LABOUR

If there is a significant medical risk to continuing the pregnancy, induction may be necessary. There is a increased risk of uterine rupture in women that have had a previous cesarean section, who undergo induction.

VARIATIONS

When the amniotic sac has not ruptured during labour or pushing, the infant can be born with the membranes intact. This is referred to as "being born in the caul." The caul is harmless and its membranes are easily broken and wiped away. In medieval times, and in some cultures still today, a caul was seen as a sign of good fortune for the baby, even giving the child psychic gifts such as clairvoyance, and in some cultures was seen as protection against drowning. The caul was often impressed onto paper and stored away as an heirloom for the child. With the advent of modern interventive obstetrics, premature artificial rupture of the membranes has become common, so babies are rarely born in the caul.

PAIN

Pain levels reported by labouring women vary widely. This variation is not dissimilar for perceived pain in other situations. Pain levels seem to be influenced by fear and anxiety levels, experience with prior childbirth, cultural ideas of childbirth and pain, mobility during labour and the support given during labour.

NON-MEDICAL PAIN CONTROL

Some women believe that analgesic medication is unnatural, or believe that it may harm the child. They still can alleviate labour pain using psychological preparation, education, massage, hypnosis, or water therapy in a tub or shower. Some women like to have someone to support them during labour and birth, such as the woman's mother, a sister, the father of the baby, a close friend, a partner or a doula. Some women deliver in a squatting or crawling position in order to more effectively push during the second stage and so that gravity can aid the descent of the baby through the birth canal.

The human body also has its own method of pain control for labour and childbirth in the form of beta-endorphins. As a naturally occurring opiate, beta-endorphin has properties similar to pethidine, morphine, and heroin, and has been shown to work on the same receptors of the brain. Like oxytocin, beta-endorphin is secreted from the pituitary gland, and high levels are present during sex, pregnancy, birth, and breastfeeding. This hormone can induce feelings of pleasure and euphoria during childbirth.

Meditation and mind medicine techniques for the use of pain control during labour and delivery. These techniques are used in conjunction with progressive muscle relaxation and many other forms of relaxation for the mind and body to aid in pain control for women during childbirth. These techniques are a form of natural pain control. One such technique is the use of hypnosis in childbirth. This technique is a form of meditation that empowers and liberates the woman by uplifting her body and its natural process to welcoming her new child into the world.

MEDICAL PAIN CONTROL

In some countries of Europe, doctors commonly prescribe inhaled nitrous oxide gas for pain control; in the UK, midwives may use this gas without a doctor's prescription. Pethidine (with or without promethazine) may be used early in labour, as well as other opioids, but if given too close to birth there is a risk of respiratory depression in the infant.

Popular medical pain control in hospitals include the regional anesthetics epidural blocks, and spinal anaesthesia. Doctors and many parents favor the epidural block because medication does not enter the woman's circulatory system, thus it does not cross the placenta and enter the bloodstream of the fetus. Some studies find that although epidural use can lengthen the labour and increase the need for operative intervention, it has no adverse effect on perinatal outcome, and is a safe and effective method of pain control.

Different measures for pain control have varying degrees of success and side effects to the woman and her baby. The risks of medical pain control should be balanced against the fact that childbirth can be extremely painful, and anesthetics are an effective and generally safe way to control pain.

COMPLICATIONS AND RISKS OF BIRTH

Infant deaths (neonatal deaths from birth to 28 days, or perinatal deaths if including fetal deaths at 28 weeks gestation and later) are around 1% in modernized countries. The maternal mortatlity (MMR) rate varies from 9/100,000 live births in the US and Europe, to 900/100,000 live births in Sub-Saharan Africa. The "natural" mortality rate of childbirth—where nothing is done to avert maternal death—has been estimated as being between 1,000 and 1,500 deaths per 100,000 births.

The most important factors affecting mortality in childbirth are adequate nutrition and access to quality medical care ("access" is affected both by the cost of available care, and distance from health services). "Medical care" in this context does not refer specifically to treatment in hospitals, but simply routine prenatal care and the presence, at the birth, of an attendant with birthing skills. Birthing complication may be maternal or fetal, and long term or short term.

MATERNAL RISKS

HEMORRHAGE

Hemorrhage is still the biggest killer of birthing mothers in the world today especially in the developing world. Heavy blood loss leads to hypovolemic shock, insufficient perfusion of vital organs and death if not rapidly treated. Blood transfusion may be life saving. Rare sequelae include Hypopituitarism Sheehan's syndrome.

INFECTION

Infection remains a major cause if mortality and morbidity in the developing world today. The work of Ignaz Semmelweis was seminal in the pathophysiology and treatment of puerperal fever and saved many lives.

VAGINAL BIRTH INJURY

Vaginal birth injury with visible tears or episiotomies are common. Internal tissue tearing as well as nerve damage to the pelvic structures lead in a proportion of women to problems with prolapse, incontinence of stool or urine and sexual dysfunction. Fifteen percent of women become incontinent, to some degree, of stool or urine after normal delivery, this number rising considerably after these women reach menopause. Vaginal birth injury is a necessary, but not sufficient, cause of all non hysterectomy related prolapse in later life. Risk factors for significant vaginal birth injury include: a baby weighing more than nine pounds, the use of forceps or vacuum for delivery. These markers are more likely to be signals for other abnormalities as forceps or vacuum are not used in normal deliveries. It needS to repair large tears after delivery.

PELVIC GIRDLE PAIN

Hormones and enzymes work together to produce ligamentous relaxation and widening of the symphysis pubis during the last trimester of pregnancy. Most girdle pain occurs before birthing, and is know as diastasis of the pubic symphysis. Predisposing factors for girdle pain include maternal obesity.

FETAL COMPLICATIONS

INTRAPARTUM ASPHYXIA

The term Fetal distress is emotive and misleading. True intrapartum asphyxia is the impairment of oxygen to the brain and vital tissues during the progress of labour. This may exist in a pregnancy already impaired by maternal or fetal disease, or may rarely arise de novo in labour. True intrapartum asphyxia is not as common as previously believed, and is usually accompanied by multiple other symptoms during the immediate period after delivery. Monitoring might show up problems during birthing, but the interpretation and use of monitoring devices is complex and prone to misinterpretation.

MECHANICAL FETAL INJURY

Risk factors for fetal birth injury include fetal macrosomia (big baby), maternal obesity, the need for instrumental delivery, and an inexperienced attendant. Specific situtations that can contribute to birth injury include breech presentation and shoulder dystocia. Most fetal birth injuries resolve without long term harm, but brachial plexus injury may lead to Erb's palsy.

NEONATAL INFECTION

Neonates are prone to infection in the first month of life. Some organisms such as S. agalactiae (Group B Steptococcus) or (GBS) are more prone to cause these occasionally fatal infections. Risk factors for GBS infection include:prematurity, a sibling who has had a GBS infection, and prolonged labour or rupture of membranes

INSTRUMENTAL DELIVERY (FORCEPS AND VENTOUSE)

— The woman will have her legs supported in stirrups.

— If an anaesthetic is not already in place it will be given.

— Episiotomy might be needed.

— A Trial Forceps might be performed, which is abandoned in favor of a caesarean section if delivery is not optimal.

TWINS.AND MULTIPLE BIRTHS

Twins can be delivered vaginally. In some cases twin delivery is done in a larger delivery room or in theatre, just in case complications occur e.g.;

— Both twins born vaginally - one comes normally but the other is breech and/or helped by a forceps/ventouse delivery

— One twin born vaginally and the other by caesarean section.

— If the twins are joined at any part of the body — called conjoined twins, delivery is mostly by caesarean section.

PROFESSIONS ASSOCIATED WITH CHILDBIRTH

Midwives may be licensed and registered, or may be lay practitioners. Jurisdictions with legislated midwives will typically have a registering and disciplinary body, such as a College of Midwifery. Midwives are trained a licensed to provide care to low risk pregnant mothers. Registered midwives are trained to assist at births, either through direct-entry or nurse-midwifery programs. Lay midwives, who are usually not licensed or registered, typically gain experience with other experienced lay midwives.

Obstetricians are experts in dealing with normal and abnormal births and pathological labour conditions. Obstetricians are trained surgeons, so they can undertake surgical procedures relating to childbirth. Such procedures include cesarean sections, episiotomies, or assisted delivery.

Most Obstetricians also provide gynecological care, and may have a primary, well woman, care element to their practices. Maternal-fetal medicine specialists are experts in managing and treating high-risk pregnancy and delivery. They are usually obstetricians

Obstetric nurses assist midwives, doctors, women, and babies prior to, during, and after the birth process, in the hospital system. Some midwives are also obstetric nurses. Obstetric nurses hold various certifications and typically undergo additional obstetric training in addition to standard nursing training

Doulas are assistants who support mothers during pregnancy, labour, birth, and postpartum. They are not medical attendants; rather, they provide emotional support and non-medical pain relief for women during labour.

STUDY–QUESTIONS

Write short notes on the following:

(a) Pregnancy

(b) Childbirth

(c) Complications and risks of birth.

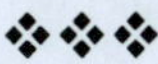

SECTION-II

Anatomy

Chapter: 6	The Body as a Whole (Regions and Cavity)	61–68
Chapter: 7	Cells, Tissue and Organs	69–76
Chapter: 8	The Skeletal System	77–91
Chapter: 9	Receptors: The Special Sense Organs	92–104
Chapter: 10	The Digestive System	105–115
Chapter: 11	The Circulatory System	116–125
Chapter: 12	The Nervous System	126–132
Chapter: 13	The Respiratory System	133–143
Chapter: 14	The Excretory System	144–151
Chapter: 15	The Reproductive System	152–165

CHAPTER 6

The Body as a Whole (Regions and Cavity)

INTRODUCTION

The human body is the entire physical structure of a human being. The human body consists of a head, neck, torso, two arms and two legs. The average height of an adult human is about 1.6 m (5 to 6 feet) tall. This size is largely determined by genes. Body type and body composition are influenced by postnatal factors such as diet and exercise. The human body is often called a "body". The body of a dead person is called a "corpse" or "cadaver".

The human body consists of systems, organs, tissues and cells. Human *anatomy* studies structures and systems of the human body and *physiology* studies the workings of the human body. Ecology focuses on the distribution and abundance of the bodies and how the distribution and abundance are affected by interactions between bodies and its environment.

Human anatomy is primarily the scientific study of the morphology of the adult human body. It is subdivided into gross anatomy and microscopic anatomy. Gross anatomy (also called topographical anatomy, regional anatomy, or anthropotomy) is the study of anatomical structures that can be seen by unaided vision. Microscopic anatomy is the study of minute anatomical structures assisted with microscopes, which includes histology (the study of the organisation of tissues), and cytology (the study of cells).

In some of its facets human anatomy is closely related to embryology, comparative anatomy and comparative embryology, through common roots in evolution; for example, much of the human body maintains the ancient segmental pattern that is present in all vertebrates with basic units being repeated, which is particularly obvious in the vertebral column and in the ribcage, and can be traced from very early embryos.

HUMAN BODY

The human body consists of:

CELLS

Cells have long been recognized as the simplest units of living matter that can maintain life and reproduce themselves. The human body, which is made up of numerous cells, begins as a single, newly fertilized cell.

TISSUES

Tissues are somewhat more complex units than cells. By definition, a tissue is an organization of a great many similar cells with varying amounts and kinds of nonliving, intercellular substance between them.

ORGANS

Organs are more complex units than tissues. An organ is an organization of several different kinds of tissues so arranged that together they can perform a special function. For example, the stomach is an organization of muscle, connective, epithelial, and nervous tissues. Muscle and connective tissues form its wall, epithelial and connective tissues form its lining, and nervous tissue extends throughout both its wall and its lining.

SYSTEMS

Systems are the most complex of the component units of the human body. A system is an organization of varying numbers and kinds of organs so arranged that together they can perform complex functions for the body. The major systems of the human body are:

- Circulatory system— the blood circulation with heart, arteries and veins.
- Digestive system—processing food with mouth, oesophagus, stomach and intestines.
- Endocrine system—communicating within the body using · hormones
- Urinary system—eliminating wastes from the body.
- Immune system—defending against disease-causing agents.
- Integumentary system—skin, hair and nails.
- Lymphatic system
- Muscular system—moving the body with muscles.
- Nervous system—collecting, transferring and processing information with brain and nerves.
- Reproductive system—the sex organs.
- Respiratory system—the organs used for breathing, the lungs
- Skeletal system—structural support and protection through bones

ANATOMY AND PHYSIOLOGY

Anatomy is the branch of biology that is the consideration of the structure of living things. It is a general term that can include human anatomy, animal anatomy (zootomy) and plant anatomy (phytotomy). In some of its facets anatomy is closely related to embryology, comparative anatomy and comparative embryology, through common roots in evolution. Anatomy is subdivided into:

Gross anatomy—It is also called topographical anatomy, regional anatomy, or anthropotomy. It is the study of anatomical structures that can be seen by unaided vision.

Microscopic anatomy—It is the study of minute anatomical structures assisted with microscopes, which includes histology (the study of the organisation of tissues), and cytology (the study of cells).

Systemic anatomy—It covers specific systems of the body, such as the system of nerves, spinal cord, and brain or the system of heart, blood and blood vessels.

Regional anatomy—It concerns with a specific region of the body such as the head, neck, chest or abdomen. Another kind of anatomy is the developmental anatomy that deals with the study of development from fertilized egg to adult form. Pathological anatomy is the study of structural changes caused by disease.

The history of anatomy has been characterized, over time, by a continually developing understanding of the functions of organs and structures in the body. Methods have also advanced dramatically, advancing from examination of animals through dissection of cadavers (dead human bodies) to technologically complex techniques developed in the 20th century.

Superficial anatomy—It is also called surface anatomy. It is important in anatomy being the study of anatomical landmarks that can be readily seen from the contours or the surface of the body. With knowledge of superficial anatomy, physicians or veterinary surgeons gauge the position and anatomy of the associated deeper structures.

Human anatomy—It includes gross human anatomy and histology. It is primarily the scientific study of the morphology of the adult human body.

Generally, students of certain biological sciences, paramedics, physiotherapists, nurses and medical students learn gross anatomy and microscopic anatomy from anatomical models, skeletons, textbooks, diagrams, photographs, lectures and tutorials. The study of microscopic anatomy (or histology) can be aided by practical experience examining histological preparations (or slides) under a microscope; and in addition, medical students generally also learn gross anatomy with practical experience of dissection and inspection of cadavers (dead human bodies).

Human anatomy, physiology and biochemistry are complementary basic medical sciences. Human anatomy can be taught regionally or systemically; that is, respectively, studying anatomy by bodily regions such as the head and chest, or studying by specific systems, such as the nervous or respiratory systems. A thorough working knowledge of anatomy is required by all medical doctors, especially surgeons, and doctors working in some diagnostic specialities, such as histopathology and radiology.

Academic human anatomists are usually employed by universities, medical schools or teaching hospitals. They are often involved in teaching anatomy, and research into certain systems, organs, tissues or cells.

Other Branches

Comparative anatomy relates to the comparison of anatomical structures (both gross and microscopic) in different animals.

Anthropological anatomy or physical anthropology relates to the comparison of the anatomy of different races of humans.

Artistic anatomy relates to anatomic studies for artistic reasons.

Physiology is the study of the mechanical, physical, and biochemical functions of living organisms.

Physiology has traditionally been divided between plant physiology and animal physiology but the principles of physiology are universal, no matter what particular organism is being studied. For example, what is learned about the physiology of yeast cells may also apply to human cells.

The field of animal physiology extends the tools and methods of human physiology to non-human animal species. Plant physiology also borrows techniques from both fields. Its scope of subjects is at least as diverse as the tree of life itself. Due to this diversity of subjects, research in animal physiology tends to concentrate on understanding how physiological traits changed throughout the evolutionary history of animals. Other major branches of scientific study that have grown out of physiology research include biochemistry, biophysics, paleobiology, biomechanics, and pharmacology.

DIRECTIONAL TERMS OF THE HUMAN BODY

Directional terms describe the positions of structures relative to other structures or locations in the body.

- Superior or cranial: toward the head end of the body; upper (example, the hand is part of the superior extremity).
- Inferior or caudal: away from the head; lower (example, the foot is part of the inferior extremity).
- Anterior or ventral: front (example, the kneecap is located on the anterior side of the leg).
- Posterior or dorsal: back (example, the shoulder blades are located on the posterior side of the body).
- Medial: toward the midline of the body (example, the middle toe is located at the medial side of the foot).
- Lateral: away from the midline of the body (example, the little toe is located at the lateral side of the foot).
- Proximal: toward or nearest the trunk or the point of origin of a part (example, the proximal end of the femur joins with the pelvic bone).
- Distal: away from or farthest from the trunk or the point or origin of a part (example, the hand is located at the distal end of the forearm).

PLANES OF THE BODY

Medical professionals often refer to sections of the body in terms of anatomical planes (flat surfaces). These planes are imaginary lines - vertical or horizontal - drawn through an upright body. The terms are used to describe a specific body part.

(i) Coronal Plane (Frontal Plane): A verticle plane running from side to side; divides the body or any of its parts into anterior and posterior portions.

(ii) Sagittal Plane (Lateral Plane): A verticle plane running from front to back; divides the body or any of its parts into right and left sides.

(iii) Axial Plane (Transverse Plane): A horizontal plane; divides the body or any of its parts into upper and lower parts.

(iv) Median plane: Sagittal plane through the midline of the body; divides the body or any of its parts into right and left halves.

THE BODY CAVITY

The cavities, or spaces, of the body contain the internal organs, or viscera. The two main cavities are called the ventral and dorsal cavities. The ventral is the larger cavity and is subdivided into two parts (thoracic and abdominopelvic cavities) by the diaphragm, a dome-shaped respiratory muscle.

Thoracic Cavity

The upper ventral, thoracic, or chest cavity contains the heart, lungs, trachea, esophagus, large blood vessels, and nerves. The thoracic cavity is bound laterally by the ribs (covered by costal pleura) and the diaphragm caudally (covered by diaphragmatic pleura).

Abdominal and Pelvic Cavity

The lower part of the ventral (abdominopelvic) cavity can be further divided into two portions: abdominal portion and pelvic portion. The abdominal cavity contains most of the gastrointestinal tract as well as the kidneys and adrenal glands. The abdominal cavity is bound cranially by the diaphragm, laterally by the body

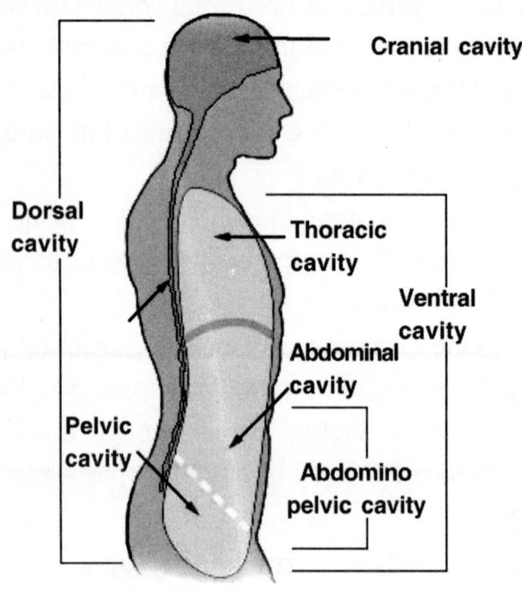

Fig. 6.1: *Body cavity.*

wall, and caudally by the pelvic cavity. The pelvic cavity contains most of the urogenital system as well as the rectum. The pelvic cavity is bounded cranially by the abdominal cavity, dorsally by the sacrum, and laterally by the pelvis.

Dorsal cavity

The smaller of the two main cavities is called the dorsal cavity. As its name implies, it contains organs lying more posterior in the body. The dorsal cavity, again, can be divided into two portions. The upper portion, or the cranial cavity, houses the brain, and the lower portion, or vertebral canal houses the spinal cord.

STUDY–QUESTION

Explain the different types of body cavity in human body.

7 CHAPTER

CELLS, TISSUE AND ORGANS

CELLS

Cells are the microscopic fundamental units of all living things. Some organisms are made up of just one cell means *unicelluler* (e.g. bacteria and protozoans), but animals, including human beings, are *multicellular*. An adult human body is composed of about 100,000,000,000,000 cells. Each cell has basic requirements to sustain it, and the body's organ systems are largely built around providing the many trillions of cells with those basic needs (such as oxygen, food, and waste removal). There are about 200 different kinds of specialized cells in the human body.

Cell (plasma) Membrane

The boundary of the cell is sometimes called the plasma membrane. It separates internal metabolic events from the external environment and controls the movement of materials into and out of the cell. This membrane is very selective about what it allows to pass through; this characteristic is referred to as selective permeability.

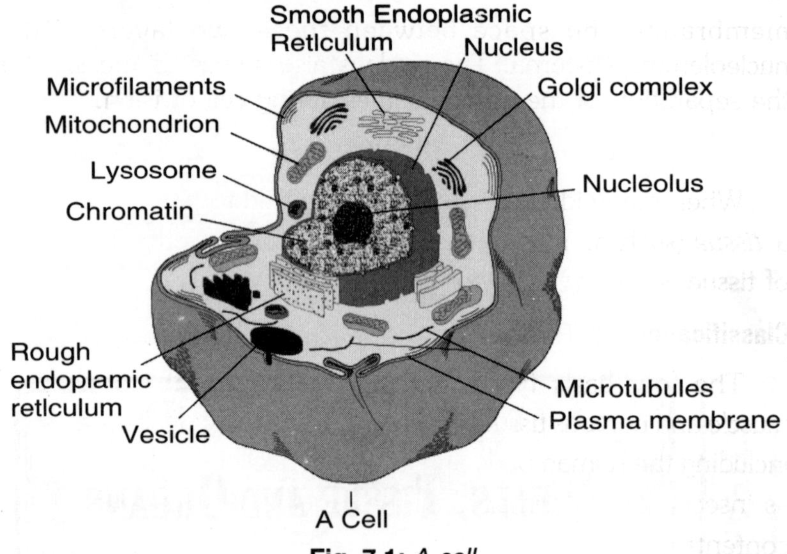

Fig. 7.1: *A cell.*

Cytoplasm

The gel-like material within the cell membrane is referred to as the cytoplasm. It is a fluid matrix, the cytosol, which consists of 80 per cent to 90 per cent water, salts, organic molecules and many enzymes that catalyze reactions, along with dissolved substances such as proteins and nutrients. The cytoplasm plays an important role in a cell, serving as a "molecular soup" in which organelles are suspended and held together by a fatty membrane.

Organelles (little organs)

Organelles are bodies embedded in the cytoplasm that serve to physically separate the various metabolic activities that occur within cells. The organelles are each like separate little factories, each organelle is responsible for producing a certain product that is used elsewhere in the cell or body.

Nucleus

The nucleus is the largest of the cells organelles. Cells can have more than one nucleus or lack a nucleus all together. Skeletal muscle cells contain more than one nucleus whereas red blood cells do not contain a nucleus at all. The nucleus is bounded by the nuclear envelope, a phospholipid bilayer similar to the plasma membrane. The space between these two layers is the nucleolemma Cisterna. The nucleus also serves as the site for the separation of the chromosomes during cell division.

TISSUES

When many identical cells are organized together it is called a *tissue* (such as muscle tissue, nervous tissue, etc). The study of tissue is known as *histology*.

Classification of Tissues

The four basic types of tissue are epithelial, connective, muscle and nervous tissue. They exist in the body of all organisms, including the human body and lower multicellular organisms such as insects. These compose all the organs, structures and other contents.

- *Epithelium tissue* — Tissues composed of layers of cells that cover organ surfaces such as surface of the skin and inner lining of digestive tract: the tissues that serve for protection, secretion, and absorption.
- *Connective tissue* — As the name suggests, connective tissue holds everything together. Connective tissue is characterized by the separation of the cells by an inorganic material, which is called extracellular matrix. Bone and blood are connective tissues.
- *Muscle tissue* — Muscle cells contain contractile filaments that move past each other and change the size of the cell. Muscle tissue also is separated into three distinct categories: visceral or smooth muscle, which is found in the inner linings of organs; skeletal muscle, which is found attached to bone in order for mobility to take place; and cardiac muscle which is found in the heart.
- *Nervous tissue* — Cells forming the brain, spinal cord and peripheral nervous system. The nervous system forms an integrated communication network throughout the body.

It is divided into a central part called the central nervous system (CNS), which includes the brain and spinal cord and a peripheral nervous system (PNS).

MUSCLE TISSUES

Muscle is contractile tissue of the body and is derived from the mesodermal layer of embryonic germ cells. It is classified as skeletal, cardiac, or smooth muscle, and its function is to produce force and cause motion, either locomotion or movement within internal organs. Much of muscle contraction occurs without conscious thought and is necessary for survival, like the contraction of the heart, or peristalsis (which pushes food through the digestive system). Voluntary muscle contraction is used to move the body, and can be finely controlled, like movements of the eye, or gross movements like the quadriceps muscle of the thigh. There are two broad types of voluntary muscle fibers, slow twitch and fast twitch. Slow twitch fibers contract for long periods of time but with little force while fast twitch fibers contract quickly and powerfully but fatigue very rapidly.

There are three types of muscle:

- *Skeletal muscle* or "*voluntary muscle*"— It is anchored by tendons to bone and is used to affect skeletal movement such as locomotion and in maintaining posture. Though this postural control is generally maintained as a subconscious reflex, the muscles responsible react to conscious control like non-postural muscles. An average adult male is made up of 40-50 per cent of skeletal muscle and an average adult female is made up of 30-40 per cent.
- *Smooth muscle* or "*involuntary muscle*"— It is found within the walls of organs and structures such as the esophagus, stomach, intestines, bronchi, uterus, urethra, bladder, and blood vessels, and unlike skeletal muscle, smooth muscle is not under conscious control.
- *Cardiac muscle* — It is also an "involuntary muscle" but is a specialized kind of muscle found only within the heart.

Cardiac and skeletal muscles are "striated" in that they contain sarcomeres and are packed into highly-regular arrangements of bundles; smooth muscle has neither. While skeletal muscles are arranged in regular, parallel bundles, cardiac muscle connects at branching, irregular angles (called intercalated discs). Striated muscle contracts and relaxes in short, intense bursts, whereas smooth muscle sustains longer or even near-permanent contractions.

VISCERAL SMOOTH MUSCLE

It occurs mainly in the walls of hollow visceral (internal) organs such as the intestines and uterus. This type has low-resistance bridges between individual fibres and the fibres thus function in a syncytial fashion as impulses spread from fibre to fibre. Like cardiac muscle, there are peacemaker cells, responsible for spontaneous activity of this type of muscle. The spontaneous discharge of impulses is largely responsible for the wavelike motions called *peristalsis*.

ORGANS

The word organ is derived from Latin word *organum*, means instrument, tool; usually there is a main tissue and sporadic tissues. In biology, an organ is a group of tissues that perform a specific function or group of functions. The main tissue is the one that is unique for the specific organ. For example, main tissue in the heart is the myocardium, while sporadic are the nervous, blood, connective etc.

ORGANS OF THE HUMAN BODY BY REGION

HEAD AND NECK

- brain
- face
- ears
- orbit
- eye

- mouth
- tongue
- teeth
- lips
- nose
- scalp
- larynx
- pharynx
- salivary glands
- meninges
- thyroid
- parathyroid gland

BACK

- vertebra
- spinal cord

ABDOMEN

- peritoneum
- stomach
- duodenum
- intestine
- colon
- liver
- spleen
- pancreas
- kidney
- adrenal gland
- appendix
- skin
- gall bladder

PELVIS AND PERINEUM

- pelvis

- sacrum
- coccyx
- ovaries
- Fallopian tube
- uterus
- vulva
- clitoris
- perineum
- urinary bladder
- testicles
- rectum
- penis

UPPER LIMBS/LOWER LIMBS

- muscle
- skeleton
- nerves
- hand
- wrist
- elbow
- shoulder
- hip
- knee
- ankle

ORGAN SYSTEMS

Organ system is a group of related organs. Organs within a system may be related in any number of ways, but relationships of function are most commonly used. For example, the urinary system comprises organs that work together to produce, store, and carry urine.

The functions of organ systems often share significant overlap. For instance, the nervous and endocrine system both operate via a shared organ, the hypothalamus. For this reason, the two systems are combined and studied as the neuroendocrine system. The same is true for the musculoskeletal system, which involves the relationship between the muscular the skeletal system and the digestive system.

LIST OF MAJOR HUMAN ORGAN SYSTEMS

There are typically considered to be eleven major organ systems of the human body.

- Digestive system — Absorption of nutrients and excretion of waste.
- Skeletal system — Support and movement, lymphocyte production
- Muscular system — Support and movement, production of heat
- Nervous system — Integration and coordination through electrochemical signals
- Endocrine system — Integration and coordination through hormones
- Cardiovascular system — Internal transport
- Respiratory system — Elimination of CO_2 and absorption of O_2
- Reproductive system — Production of offspring.
- Lymphatic system — Regulate fluids and immunity
- Urinary system — Excretion of nitrogenous waste, and maintain homeostasis of electrolytes.

STUDY–QUESTIONS

Explain the following terms:

(a) Cells

(b) Tissues

(c) Organs.

8 CHAPTER

THE SKELETAL SYSTEM

SKELETAL SYSTEM

The skeletal system is laso known as skeleton system. This is the biological system providing physical support in living organisms. Skeletal systems are commonly divided into three types—external (an *exoskeleton*), internal (an *endoskeleton*), and fluid based (a hydrostatic skeleton), although hydrostatic skeletal systems may be classified separately from the other two, because they lack hardened support structures. An internal skeletal system compries of rigid or semi-rigid structures, within the body, moved by the muscular system. If the structures are mineralized or ossified, as they are in humans and other mammals, they are referred to as bones.

Cartilage is another common component of skeletal systems, supporting and supplementing the skeleton. The human ear and nose are shaped by cartilage. Some organisms have a skeleton consisting entirely of cartilage and without any calcified bones at all, for example sharks. The bones or other rigid structures are connected by ligaments and connected to the muscular system via tendons.The skeletal system can be divided into *axial* and *appendicular* divisions.

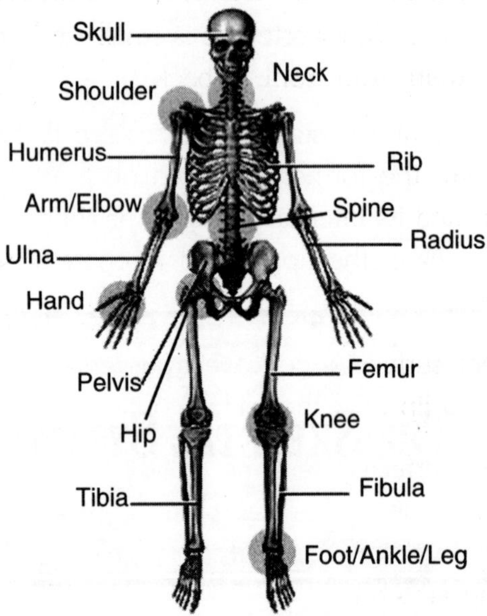

Fig. 8.1: *The skeletal system.*

1. THE SKULL

The skull is a bony structure found in many animals which serves as the general framework for the head. The skull supports the structures of the face and protects the head against injury. The skull can be subdivided into two parts: the cranium and the mandible. A skull that is missing a mandible is only a cranium; this is the source of a very commonly made error in terminology. Those animals having skulls are called craniates.

Protection of the brain is only one part of the function of a bony skull. For example, a fixed distance between the eyes is essential for stereoscopic vision, and a fixed position for the ears helps the brain to use auditory cues to judge direction and distance of sounds. In some animals, the skull also has a defensive function e.g., horned ungulates; the frontal bone is where horns are mounted.

CERVICAL VERTEBRAE

In vertebrates, cervical vertebrae (singular: vertebra) are those vertebrae immediately behind (caudal to) the skull. These are the general characteristics of the third through sixth cervical vertebrae.

The first, second, and seventh vertebrae are extraordinary.

(i) The body of these four vertebrae is small, and broader from side to side than from front to back.

- The anterior and posterior surfaces are flattened and of equal depth; the former is placed on a lower level than the latter, and its inferior border is prolonged downward, so as to overlap the upper and forepart of the vertebra below.
- The upper surface is concave transversely, and presents a projecting lip on either side;
- The lower surface is concave from front to back, convex from side to side, and presents laterally shallow concavities which receive the corresponding projecting lips of the underlying vertebra.

(ii) The pedicles are directed laterally and backward, and are attached to the body midway between its upper and lower borders, so that the superior vertebral notch is as deep as the inferior, but it is, at the same time, narrower.

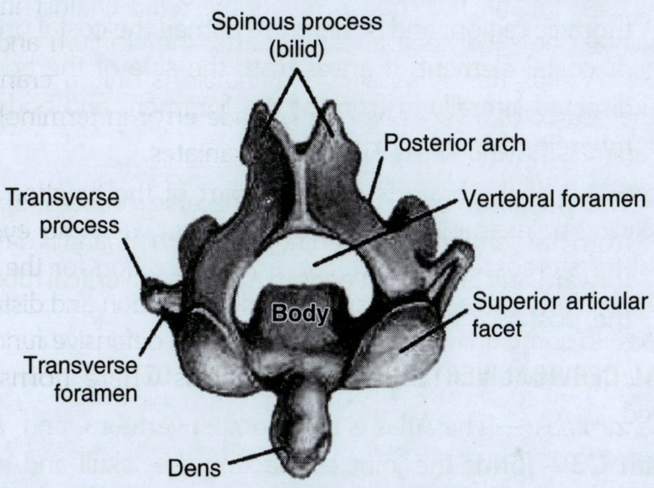

Fig. 8.2: *Cervical vertebrae .*

(iii) The laminae are narrow, and thinner above than below; the vertebral foramen is large, and of a triangular form.

(iv) The spinous process is short and bifid, the two divisions being often of unequal size.

(v) The superior and inferior articular processes of neighboring vertebrae often fuse on either or both sides to form an articular pillar, a column of bone which projects laterally from the junction of the pedicle and lamina.

(vi) The articular facets are flat and of an oval form:
- the *superior* face backward, upward, and slightly medially.
- the *inferior* face forward, downward, and slightly laterally.

(vii) The transverse processes are each pierced by the foramen transversarium, which, in the upper six vertebrae, gives passage to the vertebral artery and vein, as well as a plexus of sympathetic nerves. Each process consists of an anterior and a posterior part. These two parts are joined, outside the foramen, by a bar of bone which exhibits a deep sulcus on its upper surface for the passage of the corresponding spinal nerve.

- The anterior portion is the homologue of the rib in the thoracic region, and is therefore named the costal process or costal element. It arises from the side of the body, is directed laterally in front of the foramen, and ends in a tubercle, the anterior tubercle.

- The posterior part, the true transverse process, springs from the vertebral arch behind the foramen, and is directed forward and laterally; it ends in a flattened vertical tubercle, the posterior tubercle.

SPECIAL CERVICAL VERTEBRAE (C1, C2, AND C7)

- *C1 or atlas* —The Atlas is the topmost vertebra, and along with C2 – forms the joint connecting the skull and spine. Its chief peculiarity is that it has no body, and this is due to the fact that the body of the atlas has fused with that of the next vertebra.

- *C2 or axis* — It forms the pivot upon which C1 rotates. The most distinctive characteristic of this bone is the strong odontoid process (dens) which rises perpendicularly from the upper surface of the body. The body is deeper in front than behind, and prolonged downward anteriorly so as to overlap the upper and front part of the third vertebra.
- *C7 or vertebra prominens* — The most distinctive characteristic of this vertebra is the existence of a long and prominent spinous process, hence the name *vertebra prominens*. In some subjects, the seventh cervical vertebra is associated with an abnormal pair of ribs, known as cervical ribs. These ribs are usually small, but may occasionally compress blood vessels (such as the subclavian artery) or nerves in the brachial plexus, causing unpleasant symptoms.

The Thorax

The skeleton of the chest, or thorax, consists of the thoracic vertebrae, the ribs, and the sternum. The ribs, or costae, and the sternum form the rib cage and establish the contours of the thoracic cavity. The rib cage protects the heart, lungs, and other internal organs and serves as a base for muscles involved with respiration.

Thoracic Vertebrae

There are 12 thoracic vertebrae. A typical thoracic vertebra has a distinctive heart-shaped body that is more massive than that of a cervical vertebra. Each thoracic vertebra articulates with ribs, via articulations located along the dorsolateral surfaces of the centrum.

The Ribs and Sternum

The ribs are elongate, flattened bones that originate on or between the thoracic vertebrae and end within the wall of the thoracic cavity. There are 12 pairs of ribs. The first 7 pairs are called true, or vertebrosternal, ribs. They reach the anterior body wall and connect to the sternum via separate cartilagenous extensions, the costal cartilages Ribs 8-12 are called the false ribs because they do not attach directly to the sternum. The costal cartilages of rib 8-10, the vertebrochondral ribs, fuse together. This cartilage merges with the costal cartilage of rib 7 before it reaches the sternum. The last two pairs of ribs are called floating ribs because they have no connection with the sternum.

APPENDICULAR SKELETON

1. THE PECTORAL GIRDLE (UPPER LIMB)

The pectoral girdle is the set of bones which connect the upper limb to the axial skeleton on each side. It consists of the clavicle and scapula in humans and, in those species with three bones in the pectoral girdle, the coracoid. Some mammalian species e.g. dog and horse have evolved to have only the scapula.

In humans, the only joints between shoulder girdle and axial skeleton are the sternoclavicular joints on each side. No joint exists between each scapula and the thoracic cage, instead the muscular connection between the two permits relatively great mobility of the shoulder girdle in relation to the pelvic girdle. In those species having only the scapula, no joint exists between the forelimb and the thorax, the only attachment being muscular.

(i) The Clavicle

In human anatomy, the clavicle or collar bone is classified as a long bone that makes up part of the shoulder girdle (pectoral girdle). It receives its name from the Latin clavicula ("little key") because the bone rotates along its axis like a key when the shoulder is abducted. (This movement is palpable with the opposite hand). In some people, particularly females who may have less fat in this region, the location of the bone is clearly visible as it creates a bulge in the skin.

The clavicle is a doubly-curved long bone (the only horizontal long bone in the human body) that connects the arm (upper limb) to the body (trunk), located directly above the first rib.

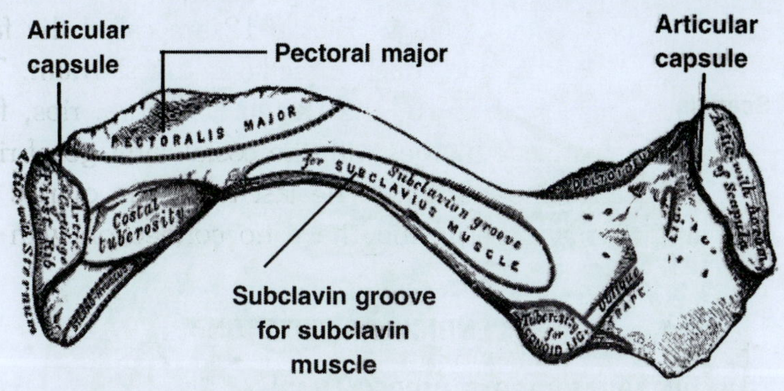

Fig. 8.3: *Clavicle.*

Medially, it articulates with the manubrium of the sternum (breastbone) at the sternoclavicular joint. At its lateral end it articulates with the acromion of the scapula (shoulder blade) at the acromioclavicular joint. It has a rounded medial end and a flattened lateral end.

From the roughly pyramidal sternal end, each clavicle curves laterally and posteriorly for roughly half its length. It then forms a smooth posterior curve to articulate with a process of the scapula (acromion). The flat, acromial end of the clavicle is broader than the sternal end. The acromial end has a rough inferior surface that bears prominent lines and tubercles. These surface features are attachment sites for muscles and ligaments of the shoulder.

(ii) The Scapula

In anatomy, the scapula, or shoulder blade, is the bone that connects the humerus (arm bone) with the clavicle (collar bone). The scapula forms the posterior part of the shoulder girdle. In humans, it is a flat bone, roughly triangular in shape. It has two surfaces, three borders, and three angles.

The anterior (front) side of the scapula shows the fossa subscapularis (subscapular fossa) to which the subscapularis muscle attaches. In animals, this side is referred to as medial or costal

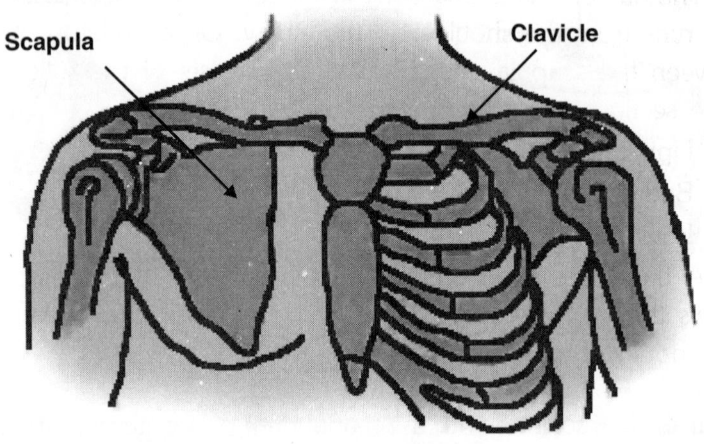

Fig. 8.4: *Pectoral girdle.*

(since it faces the ribs and the middle part of the animal) and also shows the facies serrata, for the insertion of the ventral serratus muscle.

The posterior side (lateral in animals) of the scapula is divided by a bony projection, the spina scapulae (opposite to the fossa subscapularis) into the supraspinous fossa and the infraspinous fossa. This projection is called the spine of the scapula. It begins flat at the base of the shoulder bone, ascends in distal direction to its peak at about the middle of the scapula, this peak is called tuber scapulae. After this peak the spina scapulae steeply decays in height. For humans and carnivores and bovinae the spina runs into a forward pointing hook called *acromion*, which continues past the main part of the bone.

Another hook-like projection comes off the lateral angle of the scapula, and is called the coracoid process. The end of this hook is the site of attachment of many muscles, such as the coracobrachialis muscle. Near the base of the coracoid process, so also on the lateral angle, there is a depression called the glenoid cavity. This forms the socket that the head of the humerus articulates with.

2. THE HUMERUS

The humerus is a long bone in the arm or fore-legs (animals) that runs from the shoulder to the elbow. On a skeleton, it fits between the scapula and the ulna. It consists of the following three sections:

- Upper extremity of humerus
- Body of humerus
- Lower extremity of humerus

A bursa lies between the scapula and the chest wall, and allows the scapula to move over the chest wall. Movements of the shoulder are actually often combined movements of the glenohumeral joint as well as movement of the scapula on the chest wall.

The distal end of the humerus (at the elbow) creates a hinge joint with the ulna, allowing only flexion and extension. This happens on the trochlea of the humerus. Two pits at this end of the humerus (the coronoid fossa and the olecranon fossa) allow the ulna room to move, but prevent it from over-flexing/ extending.

There is also a pivot joint between the capitulum (sometimes called the capitellum) of the humerus, and the head of the radius. This allows the hand to pronate and supinate (turn to face downwards or upwards).

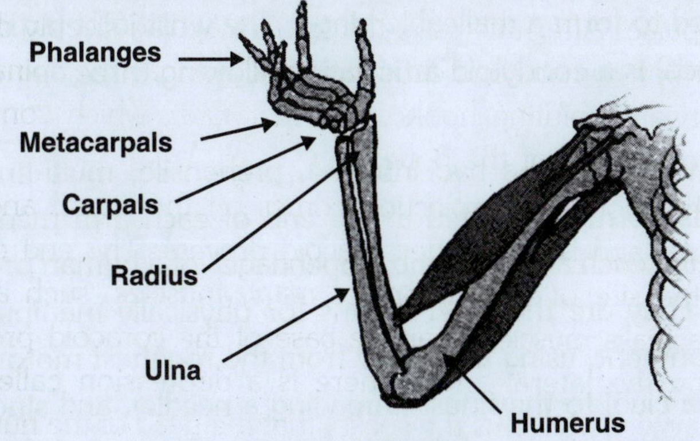

Fig. 8.5: *Humerus.*

(a) The Ulna

The ulna (elbow bone) is a long bone, prismatic in form, placed at the medial side of the forearm, parallel with the radius.The ulna articulates with:

- the humerus, at the right side elbow as a hinge joint.
- the radius, near the elbow as a pivot joint, this allows the radius to cross over the ulna in pronation.
- the distal radius, where it fits into the ulna notch.
- the radius along its length via the interosseous membrane that forms a syndesmoses joint.

(b) The Radius

The radius is the bone of the forearm that extends from the outside of the limb to the phlangx (lateral) of the elbow to the thumb side of the wrist. The radius is situated on the lateral side of the ulna, which exceeds it in length and size. It is a long bone, prismatic in form and slightly curved longitudinally. The radius articulates with the capitulum of the humerus.

(c) The Wrist and Hand

In human anatomy, the wrist is the flexible and narrower connection between the forearm and the palm. The wrist is essentially a double row of small short bones, called carpals, intertwined to form a malleable hinge. The wrist-joint (articulatio radiocarpea) is a condyloid articulation allowing three degrees of freedom.

The hands are the two intricate, prehensile, multi-fingered body parts normally located at the end of each arm medically: "terminating each anterior limb/appendage" of a human or other primate. They are the chief organs for physically manipulating the environment, using anywhere from the roughest motor skills (wielding a club) to the finest (threading a needle), and since the fingertips contain some of the densest areas of nerve endings on the human body, they are also the richest source of tactile feedback so that sense of touch is intimately associated with human hands. Like other paired organs (eyes, ears, legs), each hand is dominantly controlled by the opposing brain hemisphere, and thus handedness, or preferred hand choice for single-handed activities such as writing with a pen, reflects a significant individual trait.

3. THE LOWER LIMB

(i) The Pelvis

The pelvis (pl. pelvises or pelves) is the bony structure located at the base of the spine (properly known as the caudal end). It is part of the appendicular skeleton. Each os coxae (hipbone) consists of three bones: the illium, ischium, and the pubis.

The illium is the largest and upper most part, the ischium is the posterior-inferior (back-lower) part, and the pubis is the anterior (front) part of the hipbone. The two hipbones are joined anteriorly at the symphysis pubis and posteriorly to the sacrum. The pelvis incorporates the socket portion of the hip joint for each leg (in bipeds) or hind leg (in quadrupeds). It forms the lower limb (or hind-limb) girdle of the skeleton.

(ii) The Femur

The femur is the thigh bone. In humans, it is the longest most voluminous, and strongest bone. It forms part of the hip and part of the knee.

The word femur is Latin for thigh. Theoretically in strict usage, femur bone is more proper than femur, as in classical Latin femur means "thigh", and os femoris means the bone within it. In medical Latin its genitive is always femoris, but in classical Latin its genitive is often feminis, and should not be confused with case forms of femina, which means "woman".

(iii) The Tibia

The tibia is a long bone with an expanded upper end which articulates with the femur. Its upper surface has two smooth areas. The central portion is raised with attachment areas for the strong cruciate ligaments and the meniscal cartilages. The shaft of the bone is triangular, and its medial side, flat and smooth lies immediately under the skin, easily felt as the shin bone. The lower surface with the prominent medial malicolus articulates with the upper surface of the talus.

(iv) The Fibula

The fibula is a thin, twisted bone with many surfaces for the attachment of muscles. The prominent head articulates with the tibia. A large nerve passes close to the neck at the upper end and is easily damaged by pressure. The expanded lower portion, the lateral malleolus, is joined to the tibia by a strong interosscous ligament. The lateral ligament attaches the fibula to the bones of the foot and is often sprained.

(v) The Foot

The foot has seven tarsal bones: the talus, os caleis, navicular, cuboid and three cunciform bones. These are small bones which glide over each other for short distances. The five metatarsals have the phalanges attached to them. The great toe has two phalanges whst the others have three. They form a flexible platform with longitudinal and transverse arches which adjust to weight and movement.

BONE MARROW

Bone marrow (or *medulla ossea*) is the soft tissue found in the hollow interior of bones. In adults, marrow in large bones produces new blood cells. There are two types of bone marrow *red marrow* (also known as myeloid tissue) and *yellow marrow.* Red blood cells, platelets and most white blood cells arise in red marrow; some white blood cells develop in yellow marrow. The color of yellow marrow is due to the much higher number of fat cells. Both types of bone marrow contain numerous blood vessels and capillaries.

At birth, all bone marrow is red. With age, more and more of it is converted to the yellow type. Adults have on average about 2.6 kg (5.7 lb) of bone marrow, with about half of it being red. Red marrow is found mainly in the flat bones such as hip bone, breast bone, skull, ribs, vertebrae and shoulder blades, and in the cancellous ("spongy") material at the proximal ends of the long bones femur and humerus. Yellow marrow is found in the hollow interior of the middle portion of long bones. In cases of severe blood loss, the body can convert yellow marrow back to red marrow in order to increase blood cell production.

JOINTS

There are three basic types of joints in the human skeletal structure. They are classified as fibrous joints, cartilaginous joints, and synovial joints. Joints are defined anatomically as the conjuncture between two bones, the meeting place in a less strict definition. Fibrous joints are bound together by fibrous tissue which connects from each opposing side of the joint. Cartilage binds the joints defined as cartilaginous joints. And of course synovial joints are determined by their structure as free moving joints lubricated with synovial fluid.

The skeletal system has numerous responsibilities, one of which is to allow the body ambulation throughout its environment without assistance. The bones provide the structure of the skeleton while the joints are responsible for its ability, or lack thereof, to move about freely. Joints are also referred to as articulations. Joints are a member of the skeletal system, but they are complex and require a vast amount of knowledge to understand them in health and an even greater understanding to fix them when they are in poor health.

Direction of movement as well as the range of motion that a joint permits the skeleton is determined entirely on its structural basis. Flexibility between various joints vary greatly, and in certain forms of movement, some joints may need to become stiff while other joints are in full swing. This cohesive action between the joints allows for stability as well as balance. All joint action is required for all movement, such as walking and writing require the joints to provide equal cohesiveness as sports, simply at a different rate of speed.

The study of joints is scientifically known as *anthrology.* Kinesiology varies from anthrology, as it is the applied studies of motion while anthrology is the study of joints, their structure, their functions, and the determinations in creating variation in the event of a dysfunction. Kinesiology deals more with the relationship between the muscles and the joints and the mechanics associated with human motion.

Human motion is created through cohesive actions of muscle, blood flow, joint motion, air flow, oxygenation, and other elemental bodily systems which must work as a unit in order to provide the structure of motion desired.

Each joints structure provides basic adapted pros and cons within each basic type of joint. While some joints provide ample motion they are more prone to dysfunction. Discerning the joint types and their relationship to the body is the first basic step to understanding the process which is skeletal motion.

Fibrous joints are held fast by connective tissue which can be described as fibrous. They are devoid of joint cavities. Cartilaginous joints are also devoid of joints cavities and use cartilage as their basic form of securing the joints together. Synovial joints can often be capped with cartilage or assisted by ligaments or tendons, but are free moving joints that are distinguished by their joint cavities which are filled with synovial fluids.

STUDY–QUESTIONS

Write short notes on the following:

(a) Cervical Vertebrae

(b) Skulll

(c) Pectoral Girdal

(d) Pelvis

(e) Bone Marrow

(f) Joints

(g) Fibrous Joints

(h) Cartilaginous Joints

(i) Synovial Joints.

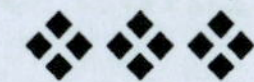

9

CHAPTER

RECEPTORS: THE SPECIAL SENSE ORGANS

RECEPTORS

Receptors are the specialised cells meant to perceive fluctuating conditions outside and to some extent inside the body. Receptors are supplied with nerve fibres of sensory or afferent nerve. Most of what is known about sense organs has been gathered from studies of man. The receptors which are most familiar are the: photoreceptors, phonoreceptor, olfactoreceptors, gustatoreceptors and tangoreceptors.

KINDS OF RECEPTORS

(A) EXTERNAL RECEPTORS

These are receptors which are usually found outside the body but may also be found inside the body. Exteroreceptros receive informations from external environment. This category includes:

1. Photoreceptors — Light
2. Phonoreceptors — Hearing
3. Olfactoreceptors — Smell
4. Gustatoreceptor — Taste

5. Tangoreceptors	—	Touch, pressure
6. Thermo-receptors	—	Temperature
(i) Caloreceptors	—	Heat
(ii) Frigidoreceptors	—	Cold
7. Rheoreceptors	—	Current of water/air
8. Galvanoreceptors	—	Electric current
9. Telereceptors	—	Distance receptors (vision/hearing)
10. Proprioreceptors	—	Muscle position.

(B) INTERNAL RECEPTORS

These are found within the body and are responsive to the changes of internal environment or body. This category includes:

1. Stato-receptors	—	Equilibrium
2. Algesi-receptors	—	Pain
3. Intero-receptors	—	Hunger, Thirst etc.

The receptors found in skin, joints, skeletal muscles and internal organs are the general *sensory receptors*. These are more or less diffused over a large area. Those receptors which are localized are the *special sensory receptors* (eyes, ears etc.).

PHOTO-RECEPTOR OR EYE

Eyes are organs of vision that detect light. Different kinds of light-sensitive organs are found in a variety of organisms. The simplest eyes do nothing but detect whether the surroundings are light or dark, while more complex eyes can distinguish shapes and colors. The visual fields of some such complex eyes largely overlap, to allow better depth perception (binocular vision), as in humans; and others are placed so as to minimize the overlap, such as in rabbits and chameleons.

The structure of the mammalian eye can be divided into three main layers or tunics whose names reflect their basic functions: the fibrous tunic, the vascular tunic, and the nervous tunic.

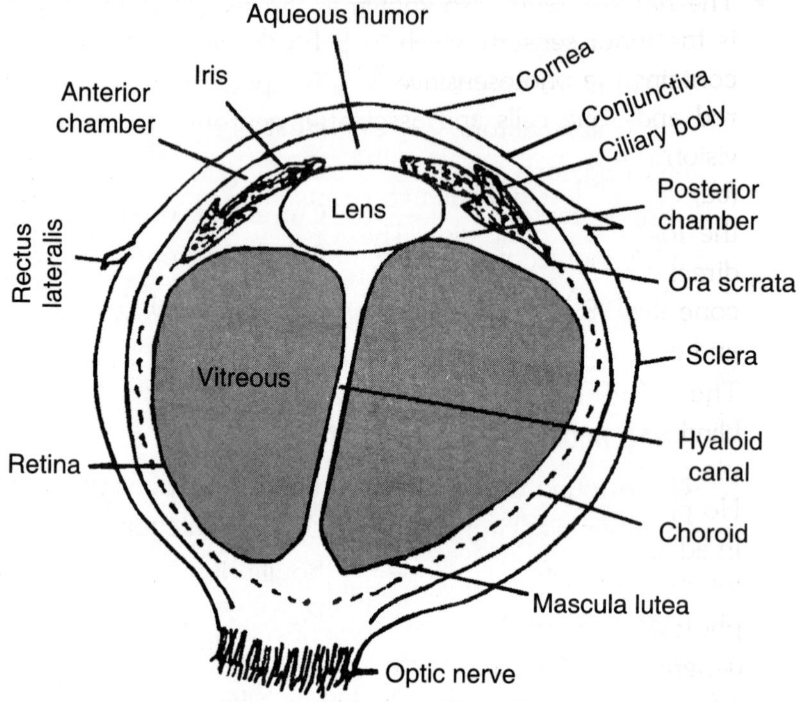

Fig. 9.1: *Human eye ball.*

- The *fibrous tunic*, also known as the *tunica fibrosa oculi*, is the outer layer of the eyeball consisting of the *cornea* and *sclera*. The sclera gives the eye most of its white color. It consists of dense connective tissue filled with the protein collagen to both protect the inner components of the eye and maintain its shape.
- The *vascular tunic*, also known as the *tunica vasculosa oculi*, is the middle vascularized layer which includes the *iris*, *ciliary body*, and *choroid*. The choroid contains blood vessels that supply the retinal cells with necessary oxygen and remove the waste products of respiration. The choroid gives the inner eye a dark color, which prevents disruptive reflections within the eye.

- The *nervous tunic*, also known as the *tunica nervosa oculi*, is the inner sensory which includes the *retina*. The retina contains the photosensitive rod and cone cells and associated neurons. To maximise vision and light absorption, the retina is a relatively smooth (but curved) layer. It has two points at which it is different; the fovea and optic disc. The fovea is a dip in the retina directly opposite the lens, which is densely packed with cone cells. It is largely responsible for color vision in humans, and enables high acuity, such as is necessary in reading. The optic disc, sometimes referred to as the anatomical blind spot, is a point on the retina where the optic nerve pierces the retina to connect to the nerve cells on its inside. No photosensitive cells exist at this point, it is thus "blind". In addition to the *rods and cones*, a small proportion (about 2% in humans) of the ganglion cells in the retina are photosensitive through the pigment melanopsin. They are generally most excitable by blue light, about 470 nm. Their information is sent to the SCN (suprachiasmatic nuclei), not to the visual center, through the retinohypothalamic tract, not via the optic nerve. It is these light signals which regulate circadian rhythms in mammals and several other animals. Many, but not all, totally blind individuals have their circadian rhythms adjusted daily in this way.

Anterior and Posterior Segments

The mammalian eye can also be divided into two main segments: the *anterior segment* and the *posterior segment.*

Anterior segment—The anterior segment is the front third of the eye that includes the structures in front of the vitreous humour: the cornea, iris, ciliary body, and lens. Within the anterior segment are two fluid-filled spaces: the anterior chamber and the posterior chamber. The anterior chamber is the space between the posterior surface of the cornea (i.e. the corneal endothelium) and the iris, whereas the posterior chamber is between the iris and the front face of the vitreous.

The *cornea* and *lens* help to converge light rays to focus onto the retina. The lens, behind the iris, is a convex, springy disk which focuses light, through the second humour, onto the retina. It is attached to the ciliary body via a ring of suspensory ligaments known as the *Zonule of Zinn.* To clearly see an object far away, the ciliary muscle is relaxed, which stretches the fibers connecting it with the lens, flattening the lens. When the ciliary muscle contracts, the tension of the fibers decrease (imagine that the distance between the tip of a triangle to its base, is less than the tip of the triangle to the other two tips.) which lets the lens bounce back a more convex and round shape. Humans gradually lose this flexibility with age, resulting in the inability to focus on nearby objects, which is known as presbyopia. There are other refraction errors arising from the shape of the cornea and lens, and from the length of the eyeball. These include myopia, hyperopia, and astigmatism. The iris, between the lens and the first humour, is a pigmented ring of fibrovascular tissue and muscle fibres. Light must first pass though the centre of the iris, the pupil. The size of the pupil is actively adjusted by the circular and radial muscles to maintain a relatively constant level of light entering the eye. Too much light being let in could damage the retina; too little light makes sight difficult.

All of the individual components through which light travels within the eye before reaching the retina are transparent, minimising dimming of the light. Light enters the eye from an external medium such as air or water, passes through the cornea, and into the first of two humours, the aqueous humour. Most of the light refraction occurs at the cornea which has a fixed curvature. The first humour is a clear mass which connects the cornea with the lens of the eye, helps maintain the convex shape of the cornea (necessary to the convergence of light at the lens) and provides the corneal endothelium with nutrients.

Posterior segment—The posterior segment is the back two-thirds of the eye that includes the anterior hyaloid membrane and all structures behind it: the vitreous humor, retina, choroid, and optic nerve. On the other side of the lens is the second humour, the vitreous humour, which is bounded on all sides: by the lens, ciliary body, suspensory ligaments and by the retina. It lets light through without refraction, helps maintain the shape of the eye and suspends the delicate lens. In some animals, the retina contains a reflective layer (the tapetum lucidum) which increases the amount of light each photosensitive cell perceives, allowing the animal to see better under low light conditions.

PHYSIOLOGY OF VISION

The formation of an image on the retina requires four basic processes, all concerned with focusing light rays:

(i) refraction of the light rays;
(ii) accommodation of the lenses;
(iii) constriction of the pupil; and
(iv) convergence of the eyes.

Accommodation and pupil size are functions of the smooth muscle cells of the ciliary muscle and the dilator and splincter muscles of the iris. They are termed intrinsic eye muscles since they are inside the eyeball. Convergence is a function of the voluntary muscles attached to the outside of the eyeball called the extinsic eye muscles.

The normal eye, known as an emmetropic eye, can sufficiently refract light rays from an object 6 m (20 ft.) away to focus a clear object on the retina. Many individuals, however, do not have this ability because of abnormalities related to improper refraction. Among these abnormalities are myopia (near sightedness), hypermyopia (farsightedness), and astigmatism (irregularities in the surface of lens or cornea). Binocular vision is best developed in man. In human being, the vision is binocular as well as stereoscopic that gives three dimensional effect.

PHONORECEPTOR OR EAR

The ear is the sense organ that detects sounds. The vertebrate ear shows a common biology from fish to humans, with variations

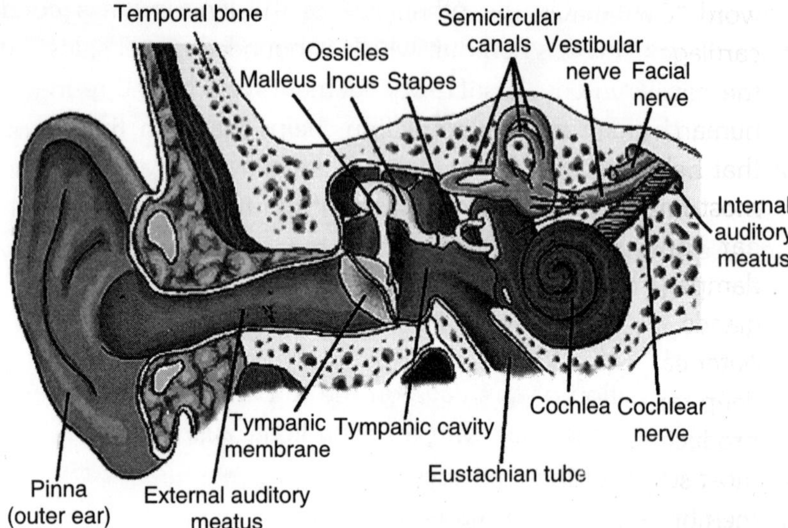

Fig. 9.2: *The ear.*

in structure according to order and species. It not only acts as a receiver for sound, but plays a major role in the sense of balance and body position. The ear is part of the auditory system. In most animals, the visible ear is a flap of tissue that is also called the pinna. The pinna may be all that *shows* of the ear, but it serves only the first of many steps in hearing and plays no role in the sense of balance. In people, the pinna is often called the *auricle*. Vertebrates have a pair of ears, placed symmetrically on opposite sides of the head. This arrangement aids in the ability to localize sound sources.

STRUCTURE OF THE EAR

There are three parts of the ear: Outer ear, middle ear, and inner ear.

1. OUTER EAR

The outer ear is the most external portion of the ear. The outer ear includes the *pinna* (also called auricle), the *ear canal*, and the very most superficial layer of the *ear drum* (also called the tympanic membrane). In humans, and almost all vertebrates, the only visible portion of the ear is the outer ear. Although the word "ear" may properly refer to the pinna (the flesh covered cartilage appendage on either side of the head), this portion of the ear is *not* vital for hearing. The complicated design of the human outer ear does help capture sound (and imposes filtering that helps distinguish the direction of the sound source), but the most important functional aspect of the human outer ear is the ear canal itself. Unless the canal is open, hearing will be dampened. Ear wax (medical name - cerumen) is produced by glands in the skin of the outer portion of the ear canal. This outer ear canal skin is applied to cartilage; the thinner skin of the deep canal lies on the bone of the skull. Only the thicker cerumen-producing ear canal skin has hairs. The outer ear ends at the most superficial layer of the tympanic membrane. The tympanic membrane is commonly called the ear drum.

The pinna helps direct sound through the ear canal to the tympanic membrane (eardrum). The framework of the auricle consists of a single piece of yellow fibrocartilage with a complicated relief on the anterior, concave side and a fairly smooth configuration on the posterior, convex side. The Darwinian tubercle, which is present in some people, lies in the descending part of the helix and corresponds to the true ear tip of the long-eared mammals. The lobule merely contains subcutaneous tissue. In some animals with mobile pinnae (like the horse), each pinna can be aimed independently to better receive the sound. For these animals, the pinnae help localize the direction of the sound source. Human beings localize sound within the central nervous system, by comparing arrival-time differences and loudness from each ear, in brain circuits that are connected to both ears.

2. MIDDLE EAR

The middle ear, an air-filled cavity behind the ear drum (tympanic membrane), includes the three ear bones or ossicles: the malleus (or hammer), incus (or anvil), and stapes (or stirrup). The opening of the Eustachian tube is also within the middle ear. The malleus has a long process (the manubrium, or handle) that is attached to the mobile portion of the eardrum. The incus is the bridge between the malleus and stapes. The stapes is the smallest named bone in the human body. The three bones are arranged so that movement of the tympanic membrane causes movement of the malleus, which causes movement of the incus, which causes movement of the stapes. When the stapes footplate pushes on the oval window, it causes movement of fluid within the cochlea (a portion of the inner ear).

In humans and other land animals, the middle ear (like the ear canal) is normally filled with air. Unlike the open ear canal, however, the air of the middle ear is not in direct contact with the atmosphere outside the body. The Eustachian tube connects from the chamber of the middle ear to the back of the pharynx. The middle ear is very much like a specialized paranasal sinus, called the tympanic cavity; it, like the paranasal sinuses, is a hollow mucosa-lined cavity in the skull that is ventilated through the nose. The mastoid portion of the human temporal bone, which can be felt as a bump in the skull behind the pinna, also contains air, which is ventilated through the middle ear.

Components of the Middle Ear

Normally, the Eustachian tube is collapsed, but it gapes open both with swallowing and with positive pressure. When taking off in an airplane, the surrounding air pressure goes from higher (on the ground) to lower (in the sky). The air in the middle ear expands as the plane gains altitude, and pushes its way into the back of the nose and mouth. On the way down, the volume of air in the middle ear shrinks, and a slight vacuum is produced. *Active* opening of the Eustachian tube is required to equalize the pressure between the middle ear and the surrounding atmosphere as the plane descends. The diver also experiences this change in pressure, but with greater rates of pressure change; active opening of the Eustachian tube is required more frequently as the diver goes *deeper* into higher pressure.

The arrangement of the tympanic membrane and ossicles works to efficiently couple the sound from the opening of the ear canal to the cochlea. There are several simple mechanisms that combine to increase the sound pressure. The first is the "hydraulic principle". The surface area of the tympanic membrane is many times that of the stapes footplate. Sound energy strikes the tympanic membrane and is concentrated to the smaller footplate. A second mechanism is the "lever principle". The dimensions of the articulating ear ossicles lead to an increase in the force applied to the stapes footplate compared with that applied to the malleus. A third mechanism channels the sound pressure to one end of the cochlea, and protects the other end from being struck by sound waves. In humans, this is called "round window protection", and will be more fully discussed in the next section.

Abnormalities such as impacted ear wax (occlusion of the external ear canal), fixed or missing ossicles, or holes in the tympanic membrane generally produce conductive hearing loss. Conductive hearing loss may also result from middle ear inflammation causing fluid build-up in the normally air-filled space. Tympanoplasty is the general name of the operation to repair the middle ear's tympanic membrane and ossicles. Grafts from muscle fascia are ordinarily used to rebuild an intact ear drum. Sometimes artificial ear bones are placed to substitute for damaged ones, or a disrupted ossicular chain is rebuilt in order to conduct sound effectively.

3. INNER EAR: COCHLEA, VESTIBULE, AND SEMI-CIRCULAR CANALS

The inner ear includes both the organ of hearing (the cochlea) and a sense organ that is attuned to the effects of both gravity and motion (labyrinth or vestibular apparatus). The balance portion of the inner ear consists of three semi-circular canals and the vestibule. The inner ear is encased in the hardest bone of the body. Within this ivory hard bone, there are fluid-filled hollows. Within the cochlea are three fluid filled spaces: the tympanic canal, the vestibular canal, and the middle canal. The eighth cranial nerve comes from the brain stem to enter the inner ear. When sound strikes the ear drum, the movement is transferred to the footplate of the stapes, which presses into one of the fluid-filled ducts of the cochlea. The fluid inside this duct is moved, flowing against the receptor cells of the Organ of Corti, which fire. These stimulate the spiral ganglion, which sends information through the auditory portion of the eighth cranial nerve to the brain.

Hair cells are also the receptor cells involved in balance, although the hair cells of the auditory and vestibular systems of the ear are not identical. Vestibular hair cells are stimulated by movement of fluid in the semicircular canals and the utricle and saccule. Firing of vestibular hair cells stimulates the Vestibular portion of the eighth cranial nerve. Man can hear 16,000 to 20,000 vibrations per second whereas dog upto 40,000 vibrations per second. Bat receives ultrasonic sound waves that is why it has the thickest auditory nerve made up of 30,000 neurons.

Injury to or disease of the auditory system causes either conduction, nerve or central deafness. Conduction deafness is caused by the ruptured tympanic membrane or improper function of the ear ossicles. Nerve deafness follows degeneration of hair cells in the organ of Corti or damage to the cochlear nerve. Central deafness is caused by damage to central auditory pathways or to the primary auditory cortax.

OLFACTION

Olfaction (also known as olfactics) refers to the *sense of smell.* Smell may refer to:

- Olfaction, the sense of smell, that is, the ability of humans and other animals to perceive odors.
- Odor, what is smelled, that is, the chemical compounds themselves that are detected in very low concentration by the sense of olfaction.

The chemicals themselves which activate the olfactory system, generally at very low concentrations, are called odors.

OLFACTION AND TASTE

Olfaction, taste and trigeminal receptors together contribute to flavor. The human tongue can distinguish only among five distinct qualities of taste, while the nose can distinguish among hundreds of substances, even in minute quantities. Olfaction amplifies the sense of taste, as can be proven by a simple "kitchen" experiment. If peeled pieces of apple are placed in one bowl, and peeled pieces of potato in another, and then the nostrils are held completely closed while a piece from one bowl is sampled, the taste of apple and potato are indistinguishable.

DISORDERS OF OLFACTION

The following are disorders of olfaction:

- Anosmia - lack of ability to smell
- Hyposmia - decreased ability to smell
- Phantosmia - "hallucinated smell", often unpleasant in nature
- Dysosmia - things smell differently than they should
- Hyperosmia - an abnormally acute sense of smell

GUSTATO-RECEPTORS OR TONGUE

Gustato-receptors form the organs of taste and the ability to taste the material is called gustation. These receptors are located in taste-buds. A taste bud is composed of cells sensitive to one specific taste modality. Despite the many substances we seem to taste, there are basically only four taste sensations: sour, salt, sweet and bitter. Each of four tastes is due to a different response to different chemicals. Although the tip of the tongue reacts to all four taste sensations, it is highly sensitive to sweet and salty substances. The posterior portion of the tongue is highly sensitive to bitter substances. The lateral edges of the tongue are more sensitive to sour substance. Except specific areas concerned with four basic tastes, rest of the tongue is insensitive to various chemicals. For gustatory cells to be stimulated, the substances we taste must be in solution in the saliva, so they can enter the taste pores.

TANGORECEPTORS (TOUCH)

Touch, also called tactition or mechanoreception, is the sense of pressure perception, generally in the skin. There are a variety of pressure receptors that respond to variations in pressure (firm, brushing, sustained, etc). The inability to feel anything or almost anything is called anesthesia. Paresthesia is a sensation of tingling, pricking, or numbness of a person's skin with no apparent long term physical effect.

Touch may be considered one of five human senses; however, when a person touches something or somebody this gives rise to various feelings: the perception of pressure (hence shape, softness, texture, vibration, etc.), relative temperature and sometimes pain. Thus the term "touch" is actually the combined term for several senses. In medicine, the colloquial term "touch" is usually replaced with somatic senses, to better reflect the variety of mechanisms involved.

THERMO RECEPTORS

Thermoception is the sense of heat and the absence of heat (cold), also by the skin and including internal skin passages. There is some disagreement about how many senses this actually represents - the thermoceptors in the skin are quite different from the homeostatic thermoceptors in the brain (hypothalamus) which provide feedback on internal body temperature.

STUDY–QUESTIONS

1. Explain the different types of sense organs.
2. Describe the accessory structures of the eye.
3. Explain the various types receptors.
4. Write short notes on:
   (a) Glaucoma
   (b) Myopia
   (c) Astigmatism and
   (d) Diabetic.

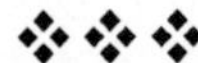

10

CHAPTER

THE DIGESTIVE SYSTEM

DIGESTIVE SYSTEM

The digestive tract is the system of organs within multicellular animals that takes in food, digests it to extract energy and nutrients, and expels the remaining waste. The major functions of the Gastro-Intestinal (GI) tract are ingestion, digestion, absorption, and excretion.

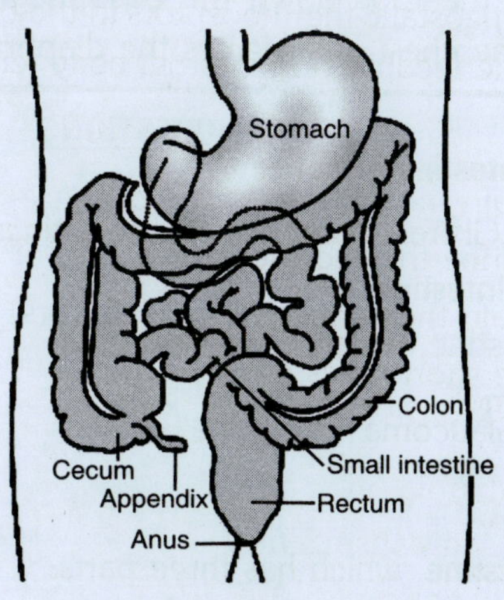

Fig. 10.1: *Digestive System.*

The GI tract ditfers substantially from animal to animal. Some animals have multi-chambered stomachs, while some animals' stomachs contain a single chamber. In a normal human adult male, the GI tract is approximately 6.5 meters (20 feet) long and consists of the upper and lower GI tracts. The tract may also be divided into foregut, midgut, and hindgut, reflecting the embryological origin of each segment of the tract.

GENERAL ORGANISATION OF THE ALIMENTARY CANAL

On the basis of physiological division of labour, the alimentary canal can be divided into:

1. INGRESSIVE ZONE

Upper Gastrointestinal Tract

The upper GI tract consists of the mouth, pharynx, esophagus, and stomach.

- The mouth contains the buccal mucosa, which contains the openings of the salivary glands; the tongue; and the teeth.
- Behind the mouth lies the pharynx, which leads to a hollow muscular tube, the oesophagus.
- Peristalsis takes place, which is the contraction of muscles to propel the food down the oesophagus which extends through the chest and pierces the diaphragm to reach the stomach.

Lower Gastrointestinal Tract

The lower GI tract comprises the intestines and anus.

- Bowel or intestine
- Small intestine, which has three parts:
- Duodenum
- Jejunum
- Ileum
- Large intestine, which has three parts:

Cecum (the vermiform appendix is attached to the cecum).
Colon (ascending colon, transverse colon, descending colon and sigmoid flexure) and Rectum

- Anus

Accessory Organs

Accessory organs to the alimentary canal include the liver, gallbladder, and pancreas. The liver secretes bile into the small intestine via the biliary system, employing the gallbladder as a reservoir. Apart from storing and concentrating bile, the gallbladder has no other specific function. The pancreas secretes an isosmotic fluid containing bicarbonate and several enzymes, including trypsin, chymotrypsin, lipase, and pancreatic amylase, as well as nucleolytic enzymes (deoxyribonuclease and ribonuclease), into the small intestine. Both of these secretory organs aid in digestion.

2. PROGRESSIVE ZONE

It includes the pharynx, oesophagus and stomach. It forwards the food taken in and passes in through the preliminary stages of modification.

Pharynx

The pharynx (plural: pharynges) is the part of the neck and throat situated immediately posterior to the mouth and nasal cavity, and cranial, or superior, to the esophagus, larynx, and trachea. In human being the pharynx is divided into three regions by the palate:

(a) oral pharynx ventral to the soft palate;
(b) nasal pharynx dorsal to the soft palate receiving the opening of the eustachian tube;
(c) laryngeal pharynx surrounding the glottis.

It is part of the digestive system and respiratory system of many organisms. Because both food and air pass through the pharynx, a flap of connective tissue called the epiglottis closes

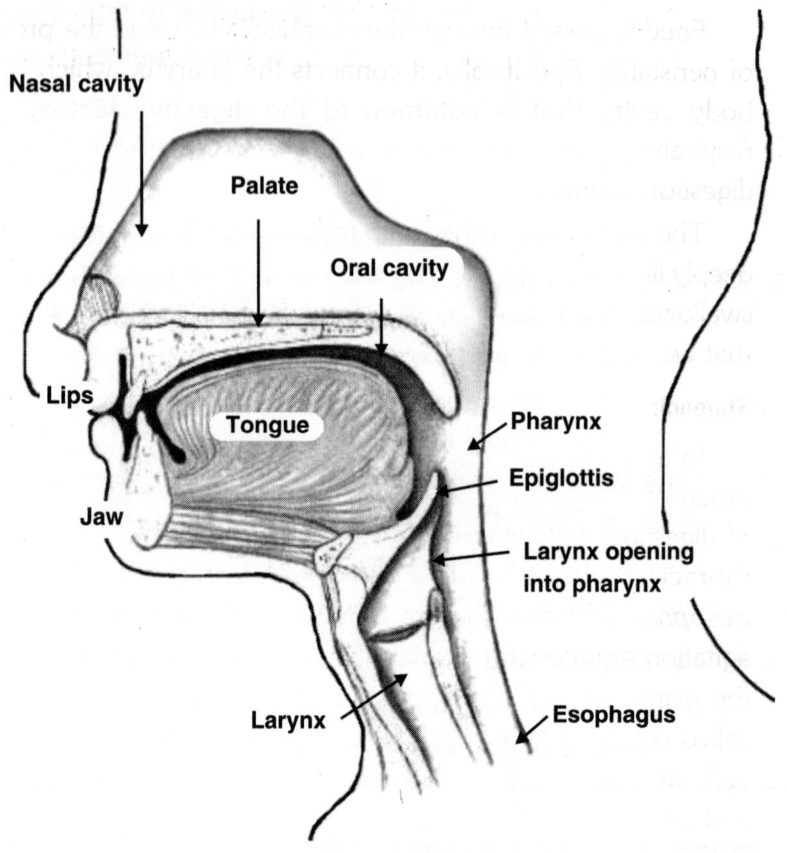

Fig. 10.2: *Progressive zone.*

over the trachea when food is swallowed to prevent choking or aspiration. In humans the pharynx is important in vocalization.

Oesophagus

The esophagus (also spelled oesophagus/œsophagus, or gullet is an organ in vertebrates which consists of a muscular tube through which food passes from the pharynx to the stomach. In humans, the esophagus is continuous with the laryngeal part of the pharynx at the level of the C6 vertebra. The esophagus has a length of approximately 25 cm (1 ft) and a diameter of about 2 cm (0.75 in.) Except during swallowing, normal muscular tone keeps the lumen closed, and the mucosa and submucosa are thrown into large folds.

Food is passed through the esophagus by using the process of peristalsis. Specifically, it connects the pharynx, which is the body cavity that is common to the digestive factory and respiratory system with the stomach, where the second stage of digestion is initiated.

The esophagus is lined with mucous membrane, and is more deeply lined with muscle that acts with peristaltic action to move swallowed food down to the stomach. The swallowing sound that we hear is the esophagus at work.

Stomach

In anatomy, the stomach is a bean-shaped hollow muscular organ of the gastrointestinal tract involved in the second phase of digestion, following mastication. The oesophagus leaves the thoracic cavity through an opening in the diaphragm, the *oesophageal hiatus*, before emptying into the *stomach*. The agitation of ingested materials with the *gastric juices* secreted by the glands of the stomach produces a viscous, soupy mixture called *chyme*. The stomach has three primary functions : (1) the bulk storage of ingested matter, (2) the mechanical distortion and breakdown of resistant material and (3) the disruption of chemical bonds through the action of acids and enzymes.

3. DEGRESSIVE ZONE

Small Intestine

The small intestine is the part of the gastrointestinal tract (gut) between the stomach and the large intestine and includes the *duodenum, jejunum*, and *ileum*. It is where the vast majority of digestion takes place. Ducts from the liver, gall bladder, and the pancreas (a long, narrow thin gland lying back of and below the stomach) Open into the duodenum, generally through a common orifice about 7.5 cm from the pylorus. The gall bladder provides a reservoir for the storage of bile, which is continually secreted by the liver.

4. EGRESSIVE ZONE

Separating the ileum and the colon is the ileocecal spincter, which is normally closed. It serves two functions : (1) to delay passage of chyme from the small intestine and (2) to prevent regurgitation of material from the colon into the small intestine.

Large Intestine

The large intestine, an organ which is now more commonly referred to by its Greek name, the colon, is the last part of the digestive system: the final stage of the alimentary canal in vertebrate animals. Its function is to absorb the remaining water from indigestible food matter, stores these unusable food matter (wastes) and then eliminates the wastes from the body.

The large intestine starts in the right iliac region of the pelvis, just at or below the right waist. Joined to the bottom end of the small intestine, it consists of the cecum and colon. The large intestine is about 1.5 meters long, which is about one-fifth of the whole length of the intestinal canal.

THE LIVER

The liver is an organ present in vertebrates and some other animals. It plays a major role in metabolism and has a number of functions in the body, including glycogen storage, decomposition of red blood cells, plasma protein synthesis, and detoxification. This organ also is the largest gland in the human body. It lies below the diaphragm in the thoracic region of the abdomen.[2] It produces bile, an alkaline compound which aids in digestion, via the emulsification of lipids. It also performs and regulates a wide variety of high-volume biochemical reactions requiring specialized tissues.

BILE

Bile (or gall) is a bitter, yellow or green alkaline fluid secreted by hepatocytes from the liver of most vertebrates. In many species, it is stored in the gallbladder between meals and upon eating is discharged into the *duodenum* where it excretes waste and aids the process of digestion of lipids.

Bile is produced by hepatocytes in the liver, draining through the many bile ducts that penetrate the liver. During this process, the epithelial cells add a watery solution that is rich in bicarbonates that dilutes and increases alkalinity of the solution. Bile then flows into the common hepatic duct, which joins with the cystic duct from the gallbladder to form the common bile duct. The common bile duct in turn joins with the pancreatic duct to empty into the duodenum. If the sphincter of Oddi is closed, bile is prevented from draining into the intestine and instead flows into the gall bladder, where it is stored and concentrated to up to five times its original potency between meals. This concentration occurs through the absorption of water and small electrolytes, while retaining all the original organic molecules. Cholesterol is also released with the bile, dissolved in the acids and fats found in the concentrated solution. When food is released by the stomach into the duodenum in the form of chyme, the gallbladder releases the concentrated bile to complete digestion.

The human liver can produce close to one litre of bile per day (depending on body size). 95 per cent of the salts secreted in bile are reabsorbed in the terminal ileum and re-used. Blood from the ileum flows directly to the hepatic portal vein and returns to the liver where the hepatocytes resorb the salts and return them to the bile ducts to be re-used, sometimes two to three times with each meal.

Physiological Functions

Bile acts to some extent as a detergent, helping to emulsify fats (increasing surface area to help enzyme action), and thus aids in their absorption in the small intestine. The most important compounds are the salts of taurocholic acid and deoxycholic acid. Bile salts combine with phospholipids to break down fat globules in the process of emulsification by associating its hydrophobic side with lipids and the hydrophilic side with water. Emulsified droplets then are organized into many micelles which increases absorption. Since bile increases the absorption of fats, it is an important part of the absorption of the fat-soluble vitamins D, E, K and A. Besides its digestive function, bile serves as the route of excretion for the hemoglobin breakdown product (bilirubin) created by breakdown of erythrocytes, which are conjugated by glucuronidation in the liver ; it also neutralises any excess stomach acid before it enters the ileum, the final section of the small intestine. Bile salts are also bacteriocidal to the invading microbes that enter with food.

Bile from slaughtered animals can be mixed with soap. This mixture, applied to textiles a few hours before washing, is a traditional and rather effective method for removing various kinds of tough stains called bile soap.

THE PANCREAS

The pancreas is a gland organ in the digestive and endocrine systems of vertebrates. It is both exocrine (secreting pancreatic juice containing digestive enzymes) and endocrine (producing several important hormones, including insulin, glucagon, and somatostatin).

Endocrine

There are four main types of cells in the islets of Langerhans. They are relatively difficult to distinguish using standard staining techniques, but they can be classified by their secretion: α (secrete glucagon), β (secrete insulin), δ (secrete somatostatin and gastrin), and PP cells (secrete pancreatic polypeptide).

The islets are a compact collection of endocrine cells arranged in clusters and cords and are crisscrossed by a dense network of capillaries. The capillaries of the islets are lined by layers of endocrine cells in direct contact with vessels, and most endocrine cells are in direct contact with blood vessels, by either cytoplasmic processes or by direct apposition.

Exocrine

There are two main types of exocrine pancreatic cells, responsible for two main classes of secretions:

Name of cells	*Exocrine secretion*	*Primary signal*
Centroacinar cells	bicarbonate ions	Secretin
	digestive enzymes	
Acinar cells	pancreatic amylase, pancreatic lipase, trypsinogen, chymotrypsinogen, etc.	CCK

ROLE OF BACTERIA IN INTESTINE

The intestine of the new born child is bacteriologically sterile and the material excreted from it, is a semifluid greenish mass known as meconium. Sterility persists for a few days only thereafter the intestine is invaded and colonized by ingested bacteria.

ABSORPTION

The term absorption is derived from a Latin word — *absorber* — means to suck in i.e. taking in of nutritive materials through living cells or tissue within the body of an organism. The food which has already been digested, is passed through the layer of cells into the blood and lymphatic vessels and then distributed. The basic process followed in absorption is diffusion but it has been indicated that diffusion and osmotic laws are not followed very strictly as the hexose sugar diffuses more rapidly than the pentose sugar in the body. Therefore, the differential absorption is taking place.

FAECES AND DEFECATION

Feces, faeces, or fæces (see spelling differences) is a waste product from an animal's digestive tract expelled through the anus (or cloaca) during defecation.

Defecation—Mass peristalic movement pushes faecal matter into the rectum. The resulting distension of the rectal wall stimulates pressure-sensitive receptors initiating are reflex which is gastrocolic reflex for defecation, which is emptying of the rectum.

In humans, defecation may occur (depending on the individual and the circumstances) from once every two or three days to several times a day. Hardening of the feces may cause prolonged interruption in the routine and is called constipation.

Human fecal matter varies significantly in appearance, depending on diet and health. Normally it is semisolid, with a mucus coating. Its brown coloration comes from a combination of bile and bilirubin, which comes from dead red blood cells.

In newborn babies, fecal matter is initially yellow/green after the meconium. This coloration comes from the presence of bile alone. In time, as the body starts expelling bilirubin from dead red blood cells, it acquires its familiar brown appearance, unless the baby is breast feeding, in which case it remains soft, pale yellowish, and not-unpleasantly scented until the baby begins to eat significant amounts of other food.

Throughout the life of an ordinary human, one may experience many types of feces. A "green" stool is from rapid transit of feces through the intestines (or the consumption of certain blue or green food dyes in quantity), and "clay-like" appearance to the feces is the result of a lack of bilirubin.

Bile overload is very rare, and not a health threat. Problems as simple as serious diarrhea can cause blood in one's stool. Black stools caused by blood usually indicate a problem in the intestines (the black is digested blood), whereas red streaks of blood in stool are usually caused by bleeding in the rectum or anus.

Food may sometimes make an appearance in the feces. Common undigested foods found in human feces are seeds, nuts, corn and beans, mainly because of their high Dietary fiber content. Artificial food coloring in some processed foods such as highly colorful packaged breakfast cereals can also cause unusual feces coloring if eaten in sufficient quantities.

11 CHAPTER
THE CIRCULATORY SYSTEM

HUMAN CIRCULATORY SYSTEM

The circulatory system (or cardiovascular system) is an organ system that moves nutrients, gases, and wastes to and from cells, and helps stabilize body temperature and pH to maintain homeostasis. While humans, as well as other vertebrates have a closed circulatory system, some invertebrate groups have open circulatory system. The most primitive animal phyla lack circulatory systems.

The main components of the human circulatory system are the heart, the blood, and the blood vessels. Furthermore, these components can either belong to the systemic circulation and the pulmonary circulation. The systemic circulation is the main part of the circulatory system, while the pulmonary system oxygenates the blood.

SYSTEMIC CIRCULATION

Systemic circulation is the portion of the cardiovascular system which carries oxygenated blood away from the heart, to the body, and returns deoxygenated blood back to the heart. In the

STUDY–QUESTIONS

1. Explain the histology of alimentary canal.
2. Decribe the process of absorbtion.
3. Discuss the process of digestion.
4. Write short note on:
   (a) Faeces
   (b) Defecation
   (c) Enzymes
   (e) Bile and Bile juice.

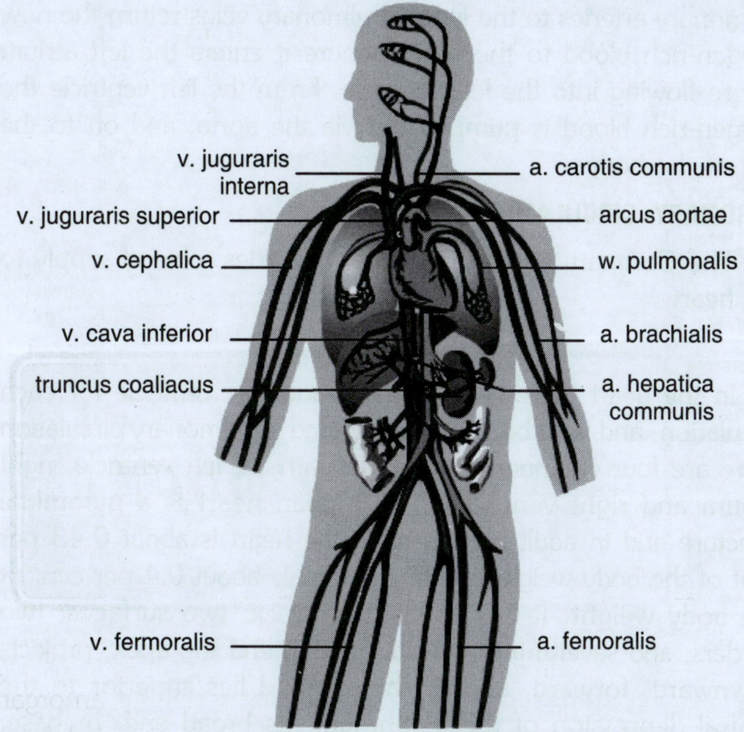

Fig. 11.1: *Circulatory system.*

systemic circulation, arteries bring oxygenated blood to the tissues. As blood circulates through the body, oxygen diffuses from the blood into cells surrounding the capillaries, and carbon dioxide diffuses into the blood from the capillary cells. Veins bring deoxygenated blood back to the heart.

The release of oxygen from red blood cells or erythrocytes is regulated in mammals. It increases with an increase of carbon dioxide in tissues, an increase in temperature, or a decrease in pH. Such characteristics are exhibited by tissues undergoing high metabolism, as they require increased levels of oxygen.

PULMONARY CIRCULATION

Pulmonary circulation is the portion of the cardiovascular system which carries oxygen-depleted blood away from the heart, to the lungs, and returns oxygenated blood back to the heart.

De-oxygenated blood enters the right atrium of the heart and flows into the right ventricle where it is pumped through the pulmonary arteries to the lungs. Pulmonary veins return the now oxygen-rich blood to the heart, where it enters the left atrium before flowing into the left ventricle. From the left ventricle the oxygen-rich blood is pumped out via the aorta, and on to the rest of the body.

CORONARY CIRCULATION

The Coronary circulatory system provides a blood supply to the heart.

HEART

In the heart there is one atrium and one ventricle for each circulation, and with both a systemic and a pulmonary circulation there are four chambers in total: left atrium, left ventricle, right atrium and right ventricle. The human heart is a pyramidal structure and in adult human male the heart is about 0.43 per cent of the body weight and in the female about 0.4 per cent of the body weight. It has a base, an apex, two surfaces, two borders, and several grooves. Its pointed end the apex, projects downward, forward, and to the left and lies superior to the central depression of the diaphragm. Its broad end, or base, projects upward, backward, and to the right and lies just inferior to the second rib. The atrioventricular (coronary) sulcus marks

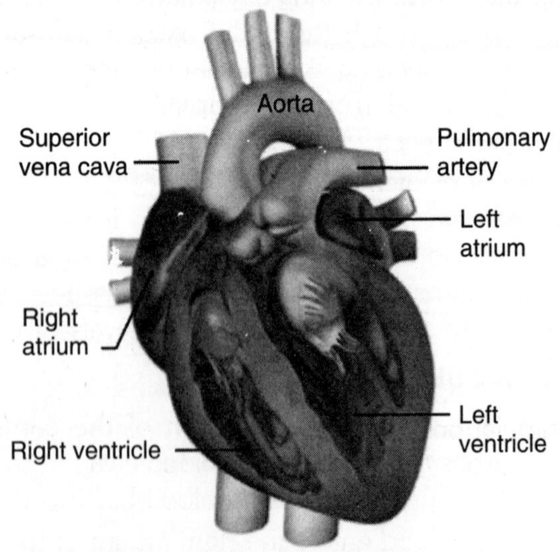

Fig. 11.2: *The Heart.*

the division between the atria and ventricles. The anterior and posterior interventricular sulci mark the division between the right and left ventricles.

The heart is composed of two chambers, upper small thin walled chamber is the auricle or atrium and receives blood from various parts of body that is why also known as *receiving chamber*, and lower large thick walled well muscularized ventricle that supplies blood to various body organs thus is also called the *distributing chamber*.

PHYSIOLOGY OF HEART BEAT

Cardiac cycle is the term referring to all or any of the events related to the flow of blood that occur from the beginning of one heartbeat to the beginning of the next. The frequency of the cardiac cycle is the heart rate. Every single 'beat' of the heart involves three major stages: atrial systole, ventricular systole and complete cardiac diastole. The term *diastole* is synonymous with relaxation of a muscle. Throughout the cardiac cycle, the blood pressure increases and decreases.

Cardiac muscle has automaticity, which means that it is self-exciting. This is in contrast with skeletal muscle, which requires either conscious or reflex nervous stimuli for excitation. The heart's rhythmic contractions occur spontaneously, although the rate of contraction can be changed by nervous or hormonal influences,exercise and emotions. For example, the sympathetic nerves to heart accelerate heart rate and the vagus nerve decelerates heart rate.

The rhythmic sequence of contractions is coordinated by the sinoatrial (SA) and atrioventricular (AV) nodes. The sinoatrial node, often known as the *cardiac pacemaker*, is located in the upper wall of the right atrium and is responsible for the wave of electrical stimulation that initiates atrial contraction by creating an action potential. Once the wave reaches the AV node, situated in the lower right atrium, it is delayed there before being conducted through the bundles of *His* and back up the Purkinje fibers, leading to a contraction of the ventricles. The delay at the AV node allows enough time for all of the blood in the atria to fill their respective ventricles. In the event of severe pathology, the AV node can also act as a pacemaker; this is usually not the case because their rate of spontaneous firing is considerably lower than that of the pacemaker cells in the SA node and hence is overridden.

Heart rate is a term used to describe the frequency of the cardiac cycle. It is considered one of the four vital signs. Usually it is calculated as the number of contractions (heart beats) of the heart in one minute and expressed as "beats per minute" (bpm). See "Heart" for information on embryofetal heart rates. The heart beats up to 120 times per minute in childhood.

When resting, the average adult human heart beats at about 70 bpm (males) and 75 bpm (females); however, this rate varies among people and can be significantly lower in athletes. The infant/neonatal rate of heartbeat is around 130-150 bpm, the toddler's about 100–130 bpm, the older child's about 90–110 bpm, and the adolescent's about 80–100 bpm.

The pulse is the most commonly used method of measuring the heart rate. This method may be inaccurate in cases of low cardiac output, as happens in some arrhythmias, where the heart rate may be considerably higher than the pulse rate. Listening to heart sounds using a stethescope, a process known as Auscultation, is a more accurate method of measuring the heart rate.

PULSE

Pulse varies in different individuals at different age groups:

At birth	140 per minute
7 years	85-90 per minute
Adult	70-80 per minute
Old age	60-70 per minute

Pulse increases during vigorous exercise, fever and nerve excitement.

HEART SOUNDS

These are described as 'lubb-dub' and are caused by closing of valves. Lubb is a long, long pitched sound caused by closing of AV valves while short-strap dub is produced by closure of semilunar valve

CIRCULATION OF BLOOD

Circulation of blood was first discovered by *William Harvey* in 1628. Blood is pumped by ventricles into arteries. The lesser circulation between right ventricle, the lungs and left atrium via pulmonary vein/pulmonary artery is called pulmonary circulation. While blood from left ventricle through body and back to the right atrium by veins is termed as systemic circulation.

BLOOD PRESSURE

Blood pressure (strictly speaking: vascular pressure) refers to the force exerted by circulating blood on the walls of blood vessels, and constitutes one of the principal vital signs. The pressure of the circulating blood decreases as blood moves through arteries, arterioles, capillaries, and veins; the term *blood pressure* generally refers to arterial pressure, i.e., the pressure in the larger arteries, arteries being the blood vessels which take blood away from the heart. Arterial pressure is most commonly measured via a sphygmomanometer, which uses the height of a column of mercury to reflect the circulating pressure. Although many modern vascular pressure devices no longer use mercury, vascular pressure values are still universally reported in millimetres of mercury (mmHg).

The systolic arterial pressure is defined as the peak pressure in the arteries, which occurs near the beginning of the cardiac cycle; the diastolic arterial pressure is the lowest pressure (at the resting phase of the cardiac cycle). The average pressure throughout the cardiac cycle is reported as mean arterial pressure; the pulse pressure reflects the difference between the maximum and minimum pressures measured.

Typical values for a resting, healthy adult human are approximately 120 mmHg (16 kPa) systolic and 80 mmHg (11 kPa) diastolic (written as 120/80 mmHg, and spoken as "one twenty over eighty") with large individual variations. These measures of arterial pressure are not static, but undergo natural variations from one heartbeat to another and throughout the day (in a circadian rhythm); they also change in response to stress, nutritional factors, drugs, or disease. Hypertension refers to arterial pressure being abnormally high, as opposed to hypotension, when it is abnormally low. Along with body temperature, blood pressure measurements are the most commonly measured physiological parameters.

ELECTROCARDIOGRAM

An electrocardiogram (ECG) is a graphic produced by an electrocardiograph, which records the electrical activity of the heart over time. Its name is made of different parts: *electro*, because it is related to electronics, *cardio*, Greek for heart, *gram*, a Greek root meaning "to write". Analysis of the various waves and normal vectors of depolarization and repolarization yields important diagnostic information. ECG shows both positive and negative deflection.

— P wave represents spread of excitation over two atria. During PQ segment atria whole is excited.

— QRS complex is second wave. It occurs 0.1 to 0.2 seconds after first wave. It is an expression of spread of excitation over both ventricles.

— T wave represents recovery in ventricles from excitation.

The ECG may be used to detect cardiac abnormalities Arrhythmias are disruptions of the normal heart rate; when the heart rate is below normal, the condition is brady cardia, when the heart rate is faster than normal, the condition is the tachycardia. In mitral stenosis enlargement of P-wave indicates the enlargement of the atrium. The P-R interval is the time required for an impulse to travel through the atria and atrioventricular node to the remaining, conducting tissues. The lengthening of this interval indicates the *arteriosclerotic heart* disease and *rheumatic fever*. An enlarged Q wave may indicate a myocardial infraction.

Most heart problems result from faulty coronary circulation. If a reduced oxygen supply weakens the cells but does not actually kill them, the condition is called ischemia. It is reflected by an alteration in the T-wave. *Angina pectoris* ('Chest pain') is ischemia of the myocardium. Stress, which produces vasoconstriction is a common cause. Equally common is strenuous exercise and a heavy meal. When any quantity of food enters the stomach, the body increases blood flow to the alimentary canal. As a result, some blood is diverted from other organs, including the heart. Doing heavy work while food is in the stomach can therefore lead to oxygen deficiency in the myocardium. When the interrupted blood supply results death of an area of tissue the stage brings about the *myocardial infraction* or coronary or heart attack.

TYPES OF BLOOD VESSELS

There are various kinds of blood vessels:

- Arteries
- Aorta (the largest artery, carries blood out of the heart) Branches of the aorta, such as the carotid artery, the subclavian artery, the celiac trunk, the mesenteric arteries, the renal artery and the iliac artery.
- Arterioles
- Capillaries (the smallest blood vessels)
- Venules
- Veins
- Large collecting vessels, such as the subclavian vein, the jugular vein, the renal vein and the iliac vein.
- Venae cavae (the 2 largest veins, carry blood into the heart)

They are roughly grouped as arterial and venous, determined by whether the blood in it is flowing away from (arterial) or toward (venous) the heart. The term "arterial blood" is nevertheless used to indicate blood high in oxygen, although the pulmonary artery carries "venous blood" and blood flowing in the pulmonary vein is rich in oxygen.

VENOUS SYSTEM

The venous system of human being is divided into four parts:

1. *Pulmonary Venous System*— It includes a pair of *pulmonary veins* which bring oxygenated blood in the left atrium of heart. Both the veins open into left auricle of heart by a single aperture.
2. *Venae Cavae System*—It consists of three caval veins and their branches. There are two anterior venae cavae a right and left and a posterior vena cava.
3. *Portal System*—A vein which collects blood from one organ and distributes it to another organ instead of sending it directly to the heart is known as the portal vein. In rabbit only hepatic portal system is seen which collects blood from the alimentary canal.
4. *Coronary System*—A number of coronary veins collect blood from heart and unite to form coronary sinus. The coronary sinus opens into the right auricle through an aperture guarded by the valve of Thebesius. Some veins independently open into the right auricle these are known as venae cordis minimae and their opening into right auricle is known as *foramina of Thebesius.*

LYMPHATIC SYSTEM

The lymphatic system is a complex network of lymphoid organs, lymph nodes, lymph ducts, lymphatic tissues, lymph capillaries and lymph vessels that produce and transport lymph fluid from tissues to the circulatory system. The lymphatic system is a major part of the immune system. The lymphatic system has three interrelated functions:

(i) removal of excess fluids from body tissues,

(ii) absorption of fatty acids and subsequent transport of fat, as chyle, to the circulatory system and,

(iii) production of immune cells such as lymphocytes (e.g. antibody producing plasma cells) and monocytes.

STUDY–QUESTIONS

1. Explain the structure of human heart. Describe the physiology of heart beat.
2. What do you mean by blood vessels? Explain the types of blood vessels.
3. Explain in detailedthe proces of the circulation of blood.
4. Write a breif note on hypertension.

12

CHAPTER
THE NERVOUS SYSTEM

NERVOUS SYSTEM

The nervous system is the system of all the nerves in the body. It is a highly specialized tissue network whose principal component are neurons. These cells, interconnecting to each other in a complex arrange, have the property of conducting, using electrochemical signals, a great variety of stimuli within the nervous tissue as well as from and towards most of the other tissues. Thus, neurons coordinate multiple functions in organisms.

The human nervous system can be studied both with gross anatomy, which describes the parts that are large enough to be seen with the plain eye, and microanatomy, which describes the system at a rather cellular level. At gross anatomy, the nervous system can be grouped in distinct organs, these being actually stations which the neural pathways cross through. Thus, with a didactical purpose, these organs can be divided in two parts: the central nervous system (CNS) and the peripheral nervous system (PNS).

BASIC STRUCTURE OF NEURONS

Neurons also known as neurones and nerve cells) are electrically excitable cells in the nervous system that process and transmit information. Yet most consist of three basic parts:

(i) a cell body,

(ii) an axon, and

(iii) one or more dendrites.

Neurons are usually considered amitotic; however, recent research shows that they do indeed undergo adult neurogenesis. Neurons are typically composed of a soma, or cell body, a dendritic tree and an axon. The majority of vertebrate neurons receive input on the cell body and dendritic tree, and transmit output via the axon. However, there is great heterogeneity throughout the nervous system and the animal kingdom, in the size, shape and function of neurons.

Neurons communicate via chemical and electrical synapses, in a process known as synaptic transmission. The fundamental process that triggers synaptic transmission is the action potential, a propagating electrical signal that is generated by exploiting the electrically excitable membrane of the neuron. This is also known as a wave of depolarization.

BASIC STRUCTURE AND FUNCTION OF NERVOUS SYSTEM

While the nervous system functions as an integrated whole, it is often divided into two major portions — the central nervous system and the peripheral nervous system.

1. The Central Nervous System

The central nervous system (CNS) represents the largest part of the nervous system, including the *brain* and the *spinal cord*. Together with the peripheral nervous system, it has a fundamental role in the control of behavior. The CNS is contained within the dorsal cavity, with the brain within the cranial cavity, and the spinal cord in the spinal cavity. The CNS is covered by the

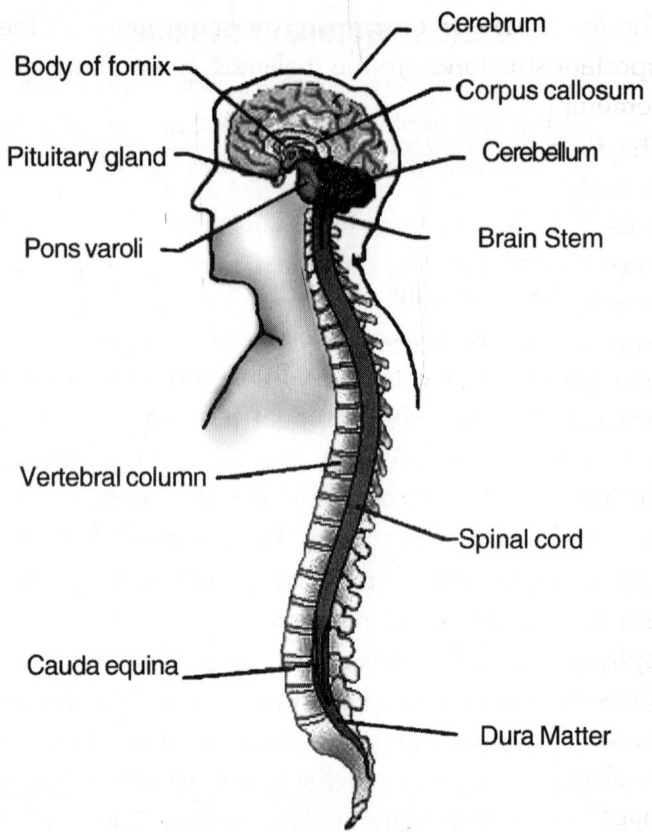

Fig. 12.1: *Central nervous system.*

meninges. The brain is also protected by the skull, and the spinal cord is also protected by the vertebrae

(a) The Brain

The brain is inside the head and it is the control center of the central nervous system, responsible for behavior. It is protected by the skull and close to the primary sensory apparatus of vision, hearing, equilibrioception (balance), sense of taste, and olfaction (smell). Brains can be extremely complex. For example, the human brain contains more than 100 billion neurons, each linked to as many as 10,000 other neurons. It is composed of three main divisions — the forebrain, the midbrain and the hindbrain.

The *forebrain*—The forebrain is at the very top of the brain. Its important structures are the thalamus, the hypothalamus and the cerebrum.

The *thalamus* consists of two egg-shaped structures situated in the central core of the forebrain just over the brainstem. The thalamus is a pair and symmetric part of the brain. It constitutes the main part of the diencephalon.The thalamus also plays an important role in regulating states of sleep and wakefulness. Thalamic nuclei have strong reciprocal connections with the cerebral cortex, forming thalamo-cortico-thalamic circuits that are believed to be involved with consciousness. The thalamus plays a major role in regulating arousal, the level of awareness and activity. Damage to the thalamus can lead to permanent coma.

The *hypothalamus*—The hypothalamus links the nervous system to the endocrine system via the pituitary gland (hypophysis). The hypothalamus is located below the thalamus, just above the brain stem. This gland occupies the major portion of the ventral region of the diencephalon. It is found in all mammalian brains. In humans, it is roughly the size of an almond. The hypothalamus regulates certain metabolic processes and other activities of the Autonomic Nervous System. It synthesizes and secretes neurohormones, often called hypothalamic-releasing hormones, and these in turn stimulate or inhibit the secretion of pituitary hormones. The hypothalamus controls body temperature, hunger, thirst, and circadian cycles.

The *cerebrum*—The telencephalon is the name for the forebrain, a large region within the brain to which many functions are attributed. Many people refer to it as the cerebrum; however, it is technically referred to as the telencephalon. As a more technical definition, the telencephalon refers to the cerebral hemispheres and other, smaller structures within the brain, although the telencephalon is one of the larger divisions (in terms of number). It is the anterior-most embryological division of the brain that develops from the prosencephalon.

The *midbrain*—The midbrain is a sort of bridge connecting the forebrain (at the top) and hindbrain (at the base). It is particularly concerned with the relaying of messages, particularly those related to hearing and sight to higher brain centres.

The *hindbrain*—The hindbrain is situated behind and beneath the forebrain. It is composed of three structures, the medulla, the pons and the cerebellum. The *medulla* and the *pons* are located just above the point where the spinal cord enters the brain.

Behind the medulla and pons is the *cerebellum*. The *Cerebellum* is composed of two circular hemispheres. It helps in performing many bodily functions. It is responsible for body balance and the coordination of body movements. Behaviours like dancing, typing and playing the piano depend on this structure.

(b) Spinal Cord

The spinal cord is a thin, tubular bundle of nerves that is an extension of the central nervous system from the brain and is enclosed in and protected by the bony vertebral column. The main function of the spinal cord is transmission of neural inputs between the periphery and the brain.

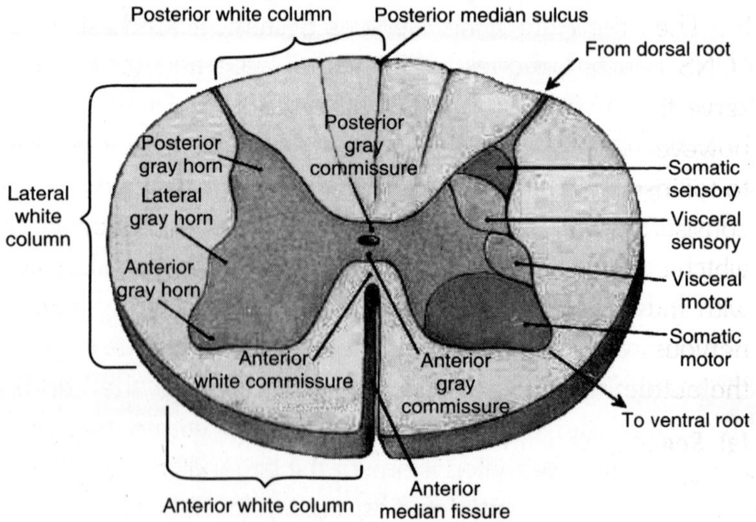

Fig. 12.2: *Spinal cord.*

The human spinal cord extends from the medulla oblongata in the brain and continues to the conus medullaris near the lumbar level at L1-2, terminating in a fibrous extension known as the filum terminale.

It is about 45 cm long in men and 42 cm long in women, ovoid-shaped, and is enlarged in the cervical and lumbar regions. The peripheral regions of the cord contains neuronal white matter tracts containing sensory and motor neurons. The central region is a four-leaf clover shape that surrounds the central canal (an anatomic extension of the fourth ventricle) and contains nerve cell bodies.

The three meninges that cover the spinal cord — the outer dura mater, the arachnoid membrane, and the innermost pia mater — are continuous with that in the brainstem and cerebral hemispheres, with cerebrospinal fluid found in the subarachnoid space. The cord within the pia mater is stabilized within the dura mater by the connecting denticulate ligaments which extends from the pia mater laterally between the dorsal and ventral roots. The dural sac ends at the vertebral level of S2.

2. The Peripheral Nervous System

The Peripheral nervous system resides or extends outside the "CNS" central nervous system (the brain and spinal cord) to serve the limbs and organs. Unlike the central nervous system, however, the PNS is not protected by bone, leaving it exposed to toxins and mechanical injuries. The peripheral nervous system consists primarily of *nerves,* bundles of axons from many neurons, which connect the central nervous system with sense organs and with muscles and glands throughout the body. The peripheral nervous system is divided into the somatic nervous system and the autonomic nervous system.

(a) Somatic Nervous System

The somatic nervous system is the part of the peripheral nervous system associated with the voluntary control of body movements through the action of skeletal muscles, and with reception of external stimuli, which helps keep the body in touch with its surroundings e.g., touch, hearing, and sight.

The system includes all the neurons connected with muscles, skin and sense organs. The somatic nervous system consists of afferent nerves that receive sensory information from external sources and transmit them to the brain, and efferent nerves responsible for receiving brain communications for, say, muscle contraction.

(b) The Autonomic Nervous System

The autonomic nervous system (ANS) (or visceral nervous system) is the part of the peripheral nervous system that acts as a control system, maintaining homeostasis in the body. These maintenance activities are primarily performed without conscious control or sensation. The ANS has far reaching effects, including: heart rate, digestion, respiration rate, salivation, perspiration, diameter of the pupils, micturition (the discharge of urine), and sexual arousal. Whereas most of its actions are involuntary, some ANS functions work in tandem with the conscious mind, such as breathing. Its main components are its sensory system, motor system (comprised of the parasympathetic nervous system and sympathetic nervous system), and the enteric nervous system.

STUDY–QUESTIONS

1. Explain the different parts of periphareal nervous system.
2. What is spinal cord?
3. Write short notes on:
   (a) Brain
   (b) Cranial nerve
   (c) Sacral nerve
   (d) Autonomic nervous system
   (e) Parasympathetic nervous system.

13

CHAPTER THE RESPIRATORY SYSTEM

RESPIRATORY SYSTEM

Our respiratory system is made up of the organs in our body that help us to breathe.

Remember, that Respiration = Breathing.

Deliver oxygen to the body and to take away carbon dioxide is the goal of breathing. In humans and other mammals, the respiratory system consists of the airways, the lungs, and the respiratory muscles that mediate the movement of air into and out of the body. Within the alveolar system of the lungs, molecules of oxygen and carbon dioxide are passively exchanged, by diffusion, between the gaseous environment and the blood.

Thus, the respiratory system facilitates oxygenation of the blood with a concomitant removal of carbon dioxide and other gaseous metabolic wastes from the circulation. The system also helps to maintain the acid-base balance of the body through the efficient removal of carbon dioxide from the blood.

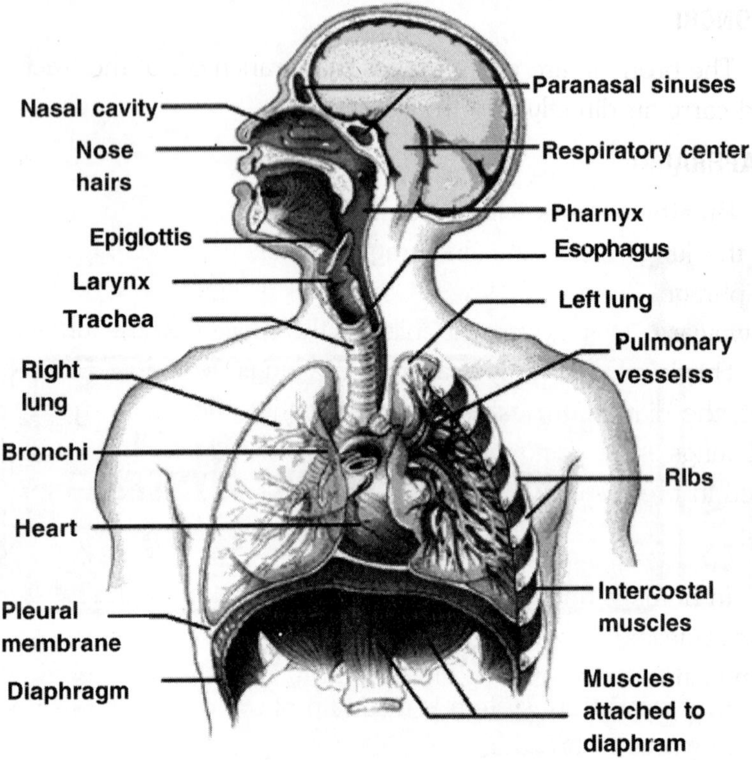

Fig. 13.1: *The respiratory system.*

PARTS OF THE RESPIRATORY SYSTEM

THE LUNGS

The main organs of the respiratory system are lungs in which oxygen is taken into the body and carbon dioxide is breathed out. The red blood cells are responsible for picking up the oxygen in the lungs and carrying the oxygen to all the body cells that need it. The red blood cells drop off the oxygen to the body cells, then pick up the carbon dioxide which is a waste gas product produced by our cells. The red blood cells transport the carbon dioxide back to the lungs and we breathe it out when we exhalents

THE TRACHEA

The trachea is sometimes called the windpipe. The trachea filters the air we breathe and branches into the bronchi.

BRONCHI

The bronchi are two air tubes that branch off of the trachea and carry air directly into the lungs.

DIAPHRAGM

Breathing starts with a dome-shaped muscle at the bottom of the lungs called the diaphragm. When you breathe in, the diaphragm contracts. When it contracts it flattens out and pulls downward. This movement enlarges the space that the lungs are in. This larger space pulls air into the lungs. When you breathe out, the diaphragm expands reducing the amount of space for the lungs and forcing air out. The diaphragm is the main muscle used in breathing.

ANATOMY

In humans and other animals, the respiratory system can be conveniently subdivided into an upper respiratory tract (or conducting zone) and lower respiratory tract (respiratory zone), trachea and lungs. Air moves through the body in the following order:

- Nostrils
- Nasal cavity
- Pharynx (naso-, oro-, laryngo-)
- Larynx (voice box)
- Trachea (wind pipe)
- Thoracic cavity (chest)
- Bronchi (right and left)
- Alveoli (site of gas exchange)

UPPER RESPIRATORY TRACT/CONDUCTING ZONE

The conducting zone begins with the nares (nostrils) of the nose, which open into the nasopharynx (nasal cavity). The primary functions of the nasal passages are to:

(i) filter,

(ii) warm,

(iii) moisten, and

(iv) provide resonance in speech.

The nasopharynx opens into the oropharynx (behind the oral cavity). The oropharynx leads to the laryngopharynx, and empties into the larynx (voicebox), which contains the vocal cords, passing through the glottis, connecting to the trachea (wind pipe).

LOWER RESPIRATORY TRACT/RESPIRATORY ZONE

The trachea leads down to the thoracic cavity (chest) where it divides into the right and left "main stem" bronchi. The subdivision of the bronchus are: primary, secondary, and tertiary divisions (first, second and third levels). In all, they divide 16 more times into even smaller bronchioles.

The bronchioles lead to the respiratory zone of the lungs which consists of respiratory bronchioles, alveolar ducts and the alveoli, the multi-lobulated sacs in which most of the gas exchange occurs.

BREATHING

INHALATION

Inhalation is initiated by the diaphragm and supported by the external intercostal muscles. Normal resting respirations are 10 to 18 breaths per minute. Its time period is 2 seconds. During vigorous inhalation (at rates exceeding 35 breaths per minute), or in approaching respiratory failure, accessory muscles of respiration are recruited for support. These consist of sternocleidomastoid, platysma, and the strap muscles of the neck.

Inhalation is driven primarily by the diaphragm. When the diaphragm contracts, the ribcage expands and the contents of the abdomen are moved downward. This results in a larger thoracic volume, which in turn causes a decrease in intrathoracic pressure. As the pressure in the chest falls, air moves into the conducting zone. Here, the air is filtered, warmed, and humidified as it flows to the lungs.

During forced inhalation, as when taking a deep breath, the external intercostal muscles and accessory muscles further expand the thoracic cavity.

EXHALATION

Exhalation is generally a passive process, however active or *forced* exhalation is achieved by the abdominal and the internal intercostal muscles. The lungs have a natural elasticity; as they recoil from the stretch of inhalation, air flows back out until the pressures in the chest and the atmosphere reach equilibrium.

During forced exhalation, as when blowing out a candle, expiratory muscles including the abdominal muscles and internal intercostal muscles, generate abdominal and thoracic pressure, which forces air out of the lungs.

CIRCULATION

The right side of the heart pumps blood from the right ventricle through the pulmonary semilunar valve into the pulmonary trunk. The trunk branches into right and left pulmonary arteries to the pulmonary blood vessels. The vessels generally accompany the airways and also undergo numerous branchings. Once the gas exchange process is complete in the pulmonary capillaries, blood is returned to the left side of the heart through four pulmonary veins, two from each side. The pulmonary circulation has a very low resistance, due to the short distance within the lungs, compared to the systemic circulation, and for this reason, all the pressures within the pulmonary blood vessels are normally low as compared to the pressure of the systemic circulation loop.

Virtually all the body's blood travels through the lungs every minute. The lungs add and remove many chemical messengers from the blood as it flows through pulmonary capillary bed . The fine capillaries also trap blood clots that have formed in systemic veins.

GAS EXCHANGE

The major function of the respiratory system is gas exchange. As gas exchange occurs, the acid-base balance of the body is maintained as part of homeostasis. If proper ventilation is not maintained two opposing conditions could occur:

(i) respiratory acidosis, a life threatening condition, and
(ii) respiratory alkalosis.

Upon inhalation, gas exchange occurs at the alveoli, the tiny sacs which are the basic functional component of the lungs. The alveolar walls are extremely thin (approx. 0.2 micrometres), and are permeable to gases. The alveoli are lined with pulmonary capillaries, the walls of which are also thin enough to permit gas exchange. All gases diffuse from the alveolar air to the blood in the pulmonary capillaries, as carbon dioxide diffuses in the opposite direction,. from capillary blood to alveolar air. At this point, the pulmonary blood is oxygen-rich, and the lungs are holding carbon dioxide. Exhalation follows, thereby ridding the body of the carbon dioxide and completing the cycle of respiration.

In an average resting adult, the lungs take up about 250 ml of oxygen every minute while excreting about 200 ml of carbon dioxide. During an average breath, an adult will exchange from 500 ml to 700 ml of air. This average breath capacity is called tidal volume.

Breathing by means of ribs is believed to be relatively more pronounced in human females than in males. This sexual difference in respiratory mechanism is merely an adaptation brought about by pregnancy during which period the presence of growing foetus interferes somewhat with the freedom of the movement of diaphragm.

TYPES OF BREATHING

Eupnea	—	normal quiet respiration.
Dyspnea	—	difficult breathing.
Apnea	—	no breathing.

Hyperpnea — increased depth or rate of breathing or both.

Polypnea — rapid, shallow breathing.

LUNG VOLUMES

Lung volumes refer to physical differences in lung volume, while lung capacities represent different combinations of lung volumes, usually in relation to respiration and exhalation. The average pair of human lungs can hold about 6 liters of air, but only a small amount of this capacity is used during normal breathing. Breathing mechanism in mammals is called "tidal breathing". Tidal breathing means that air goes into the lungs the same way that it comes out.

FACTORS AFFECTING LUNG VOLUMES

Several factors affect lung volumes, some that can be controlled and some that can not. These factors include:

Larger volumes	*Smaller volumes*
males	females
taller people	shorter people
non-smokers	heavy smokers
athletes	non-athletes
people living at high altitudes	people living at low altitudes

A person who is born and lives at sea level will develop a slightly smaller lung capacity than a person who spends their life at a high altitude. This is because the atmosphere is less dense at higher altitude, and therefore, the same volume of air contains fewer molecules of all gases, including oxygen. In response to higher altitude, the body's diffusing capacity increases in order to be able to process more air. The average healthy adult has 14 to 18 breaths a minute. During every breath the lungs exchange volumes of air with the atmosphere. The apparatus commonly used to measure the amount of air exchanged during breathing is referred to as a spirometer or respirometer.

YAWN

When you are sleepy or drowsy the lungs do not take enough oxygen from the air. This causes a shortage of oxygen in our bodies. The brain senses this shortage of oxygen and sends a message that causes you to take a deep long breath—a YAWN.

SNEEZE

Sneezing is like a cough in the upper breathing passages. It is the body's way of removing an irritant from the sensitive mucous membranes of the nose. Many things can irritate the mucous membranes. Dust, pollen, pepper or even a cold blast of air are just some of the many things that may cause you to sneeze.

HICCUPS

Hiccups are the sudden movements of the diaphragm. It is involuntary — you have no control over hiccups, as you well know. There are many causes of hiccups. The diaphragm may get irritated, you may have eaten to fast, or maybe some substance in the blood could even have brought on the hiccups.

DISEASES OF THE LUNGS

PNEUMONIA

Pneumonia is an infection of the alveoli. It can be caused by many kinds of both bacteria (e.g., Streptococcus pneumoniae) and viruses. Tissue fluids accumulate in the alveoli reducing the surface area exposed to air. If enough alveoli are affected, the patient may need supplemental oxygen.

ASTHMA

In asthma, periodic constriction of the bronchi and bronchioles makes it more difficult to breathe in and, especially, out. Attacks of asthma can be:

- triggered by airborne irritants such as chemical fumes and cigarette smoke
- airborne particles to which the patient is allergic.

EMPHYSEMA

In this disorder, the delicate walls of the alveoli break down, reducing the gas exchange area of the lungs. The condition develops slowly and is seldom a direct cause of death. However, the gradual loss of gas exchange area forces the heart to pump ever-larger volumes of blood to the lungs in order to satisfy the body's needs. The added strain can lead to heart failure.

The immediate cause of emphysema seems to be the release of proteolytic enzymes as part of the inflammatory process that follows irritation of the lungs. Most people avoid this kind of damage during infections, etc. by producing an enzyme inhibitor (a serpin) called alpha-1 antitrypsin. Those rare people who inherit two defective genes for alpha-1 antitrypsin are particularly susceptible to developing emphysema.

CHRONIC BRONCHITIS

Any irritant reaching the bronchi and bronchioles will stimulate an increased secretion of mucus. In chronic bronchitis the air passages become clogged with mucus, and this leads to a persistent cough. Chronic bronchitis is usually associated with cigarette smoking.

CHRONIC OBSTRUCTIVE PULMONARY DISEASE (COPD)

Irritation of the lungs can lead to asthma, emphysema, and chronic bronchitis. And, in fact, many people develop two or three of these together. This constellation is known as chronic obstructive pulmonary disease (COPD). Among the causes of COPD are:

- cigarette smoke (often)
- cystic fibrosis (rare)

Cystic fibrosis is a genetic disorder caused by inheriting two defective genes for the cystic fibrosis transmembrane conductance regulator (CFTR), a transmembrane protein needed for the transport of Cl^- ions out of the epithelial cells of the lung thus enabling water to follow by osmosis. Diminished CFTR function reduces the water content of the fluid in the lungs making it more viscous and difficult for the ciliated cells to move it up out of the lungs. The accumulation of mucus plugs the airways interfering with breathing and causing a persistent cough. Cystic fibrosis is the most common inherited disease in the U.S. white population.

LUNG CANCER

Lung cancer is the most common cancer and the most common cause of cancer deaths in U.S. males. Although more women develop breast cancer than lung cancer, since 1987 U.S. women have been dying in larger numbers from lung cancer than from breast cancer. Lung cancer, like all cancer, is an uncontrolled proliferation of cells. There are several forms of lung cancer, but the most common (and most rapidly increasing) types are those involving the epithelial cells lining the bronchi and bronchioles. Ordinarily, the lining of these airways consists of two layers of cells. Chronic exposure to irritants

- causes the number of layers to increase. This is especially apt to happen at forks where the bronchioles branch.
- The ciliated and mucus-secreting cells disappear and are replaced by a disorganized mass of cells with abnormal nuclei.
- If the process continues, the growing mass penetrates the underlying basement membrane.
- At this point, malignant cells can break away and be carried in lymph and blood to other parts of the body where they may lodge and continue to proliferate.
- It is this metastasis of the primary tumor that eventually kills the patient.

STUDY–QUESTIONS

1. What is respiration? Explain the breathing mechanism in human being.
2. Describe the various parts of respiratory system.

3. Explain the process of artificial breathing.
4. Write short notes on the following:
   (a) Lung Cancer
   (b) Chronic Obstructive Pulmonary Disease (COPD)
   (c) Chronic Bronchitis
   (d) Asthma.

14

CHAPTER

THE EXCRETORY SYSTEM

EXCRETION

Excretion is the process of eliminating waste products of metabolism and other non-useful materials. It is an essential process in all forms of life. In single-celled organisms, waste products are discharged directly through the surface of the cell. Multicellular organisms utilize more complex excretory methods. Higher plants eliminate gases through the stomata, or pores, on the surface of leaves. Animals have special excretory organs. The main organs of excretion in human body are the kidneys and accessory urinary organs, through which urine is eliminated, and the large intestines, from which solid wastes are expelled. The skin and lungs also have excretory functions: the skin eliminates water and salts in sweat, and the lungs expel water vapor and carbon dioxide.

STRUCTURE OF THE KIDNEY

The paired kidneys are reddish organs that resemble beans in shape. The kidneys are the organs that filter wastes (such as urea) from the blood and excrete them, along with water, as

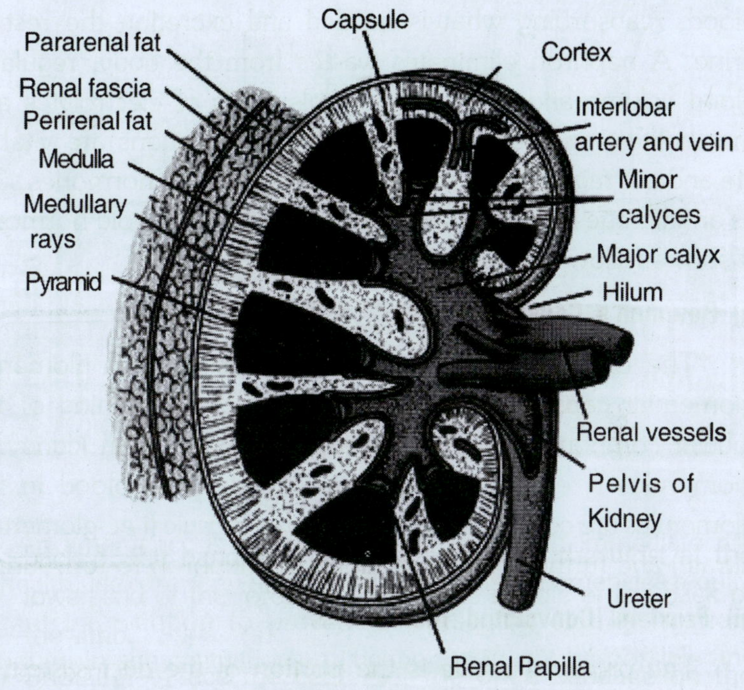

Fig. 14.1: *Structure of the kidney.*

urine. The medical field that studies the kidneys and diseases of the kidney is called nephrology. The weight of each kidney in the adult is about 150 gm, which is nearly 1% of the body weight. The medial border of the kidney is usually concave and has a marked depression, the *renal hilus* where blood vessels and nerves enter and the ureter and lymphatic vessels leave. The cortex is arbitrarily divided into an outer cortical zone and an inner juxtramedulary zone. Within the medulla, there are pyramids. In the renal sinus of the kidney is a large cavity called the renal pelvis.

NEPHRON

A nephron is the basic structural and functional unit of the kidney. Its chief function is to regulate the concentration of water and soluble substances like sodium salts by filtering the blood, reabsorbing what is needed and excreting the rest as urine. A nephron eliminates wastes from the body, regulates blood volume and pressure, controls levels of electrolytes and metabolites, and regulates blood pH. Its functions are vital to life and are regulated by the endocrine system by hormones such as antidiuretic hormone, aldosterone, and parathyroid hormone. It shows following parts :

(i) Bowman's Capsule

The Bowman's capsule (other names: capsula glomeruli, glomerular capsule) is a cup like sac at the beginning of the tubular component of a nephron in the mammalian kidney. A glomerulus is enclosed in the sac. Fluids from blood in the glomerulus are collected in the Bowman's capsule (i.e., glomerular filtrate) and further processed along the nephron to form urine.

(ii) Proximal Convoluted Tubule

The proximal tubule is the portion of the duct system of the nephron leading from Bowman's capsule to the loop of Henle.

(iii) Loop of Henle

In the kidney, the loop of Henle is the portion of the nephron that leads from the proximal convoluted tubule to the distal convoluted tubule. The loop has a hairpin bend in the renal medulla. The main function of this structure is to reabsorb water and ions from the urine. To do this, it uses a countercurrent multiplier mechanism in the medulla. It is named after its discoverer, *F. G. J. Henle.*

(iv) Distal Convoluted Tubule (DCT)

The distal convoluted tubule (DCT) is a portion of kidney nephron between the loop of Henle and the collecting duct system.

(v) The Collecting Tubules

In the kidney, the collecting tubule (CNT, or junctional tubule, or arcuate renal tubule) is a tubular segment of the renal collecting duct system that connects the distal convoluted tubule to the cortical collecting duct.

FUNCTIONS OF URINARY SYSTEM

The uriniferous tubules of the kidney form urine from the blood circulating in the glomerulus. Formation of urine by the kidneys is considered to be due to three types of activities — glomerular filtration, tubular secretion and selective reabsorption.

1. *Glomerular filteration or ultra filteration*—The initial stage of urine formation is the filteration of plasma and the accumulation of the ultra filterate in the lumen of Bowman's capsule.
2. *Tubular secretion*—Tubular reabsorption removes substances from the filterate into the blood. Tubular secretion adds material to the filterate into the blood. So these products of metabolism which are not at all required by the body, rather they are injurious to health, are secreted out by tubular epithelium in the tubular filterate. The secreted substances include potassium, hydrogen, ammonia, creatine, uric acid, and the drugs penicillin and para-amino hippuric acid. Tubular secretion has two principal effects, It rids the body of certain material, and it controls the blood pH.
3. *Selective Reabsorbtion (Counter current theory of urine concentration)*—The descending limb of loop of Henle is freely permeable to water and ions like Na^+ and Cl^-, but the ascending limb of the loop is absolutely impermeable for water. It has a mechanism that actively transport Cl^- from the filterate into the interstitial fluid of the medulla. The peculiarity of the loop is very important in relation to concentration of urine.

The normal osmality of the glomerular filterate as it enter the proximal tubules is about 300 milli-osmols/litre. The osmality of the interstitial fluid increases gradually. It is 300 milli-osmols/ litre in the cortex and 1200 milli-somols/litre at the pelvic tip of the medulla. This increase is due to the active transport of sodium out of the loop into the medullary interstitial fluid.

URINE

Urine formation helps to maintain the balance of minerals and other substances in the body. For example, excess of calcium is normally eliminated through the urine. Urine also excretes ammonia, the build-up of which is harmful to the body. In addition, urine is the result of a mechanism that maintains the appropriate amount of water in the body. A range of substances, including ethanol and artificial sweeteners, are also eliminated from the body through the urine. The amount of urine eliminated per 24 hours varies tremendously depending upon the water intake, state of mental and physical activity, environmental temperature and food intake. The volume of urine varies between 1000 to 1800 ml.

The colour of normal urine is transparent and pale yellow. The colour is due to the presence of pigment called *urochrome.* The intensity of the colour increases in the concentrated urine, and lightens in the dilute urine sample. The turbidity of the urine shows its alkaline nature which is due to the precipitation of calcium phosphate. The turbidity may result from mucin secreted by the lining of the urinary tract.

The odour of urine may vary. Fresh urine has a characteristic not pleasant odour. In case of diabetes, urine has a 'sweetish' odour because of the presence of acetone. Stale urine develops an ammonia like odour due to ammonium carbonate formation as a result of urea decomposition.

MICTURITION

It is the process of urination or the process by which the urinary bladder empties itself when it becomes filled. Basically the bladder (i) progressively fills until the tension in its walls rises above a threshold value, at which time (ii) a nervous reflex called the micturition reflex is elicited that (iii) greatly exacerbates the pressure in the bladder and simultaneously causes a conscious desire to urinate. The micturition reflex also initiates appropriate signals from the nervous system to relax the external sphincter of the bladder, thereby allowing micturition.

ABNORMAL INGREDIENTS OF URINE

Abnormal metabolism of the body results the excretion of abnormal ingredients in urine, like sugar, proteins, ketone bodies, bile and blood.

(i) *Sugar*—Under normal conditions, the blood sugar level remains within the normal limits. In diabetic person, it is excreted in urine. This is also called the glucosauria. Sometimes the fructose is also excreted causing fructosuria which is however, a rare abnormally. Galactose may also appear in the urine of infants and lactating woman. Here the condition is called galactosuria. The terms pentosuria is applied where pentose sugar is excreted.

(ii) *Proteins*—Proteins appear in the urine during nephrosis (kidney damage), or *nephritis* (kidney inflammation). Urine of patients suffering from nephroselerosis (a vascular form of renal disease) also contains proteins.

(iii) *Ketone bodies*—In diabetes millitus, acetone bodies frequently appear in the urine. The presence of ketone bodies in the urine indicates the state of starvation with respect to carbohydrates in the normal individual. In women during pregnancy, there might occur slightly raised level of ketone bodies in the urine. The abnormality is called ketosis.

(iv) *Bile*—Bile is given out through the gut but whenever bile duct is obstructed, obstructive jaundice results. Secondly, the jaundice may occur due to the over destruction of blood cells where it is called haemolytic jaundice. In hepatic jaundice the liver itself is diseased. Jaundice results in the rise of circulatory bile pigment level and its subsequent appearance in the urine.

(v) *Blood*—Whenever blood comes in the urine, the stage is called haematuria. This may be due to lesion in the kidney or renal tuberculosis, nephritis or malignancy. Sometimes only free haemoglobin appears in urine due to extensive haemolysis as occurs in severe burns, or after infusion of unmatched blood. Here, the liver fails to convert all the haemoglobin into bile pigments, that is why, it appears in the urine.

(vi) *Porphyrins*—Normally, it is excreted in a little amount but in polyphyria (metabolic disorder) it is excreted in higher proportions. Porphyria occurs commonly in cirrhosis, obstructive jaundice, and similar other disorders.

URINARY TRACT IN INFECTIONS

Urinary tract infections, or UTIs, result from the colonization of the urinary tract by bacterial or fungal invaders. The intestinal bacterium *Escheriochia coli* is most often involved and women are particularly susceptible to urinary tract infections because of the proximity of the urethral orifice to the anus. Sexual intercourse may also push bacteria into the urethra and - since the female urethra is relatively short - toward the bladder.

The condition may be asymptomatic (without symptoms), but it can be detected by the presence of bacteria and blood cells in the urine. If inflammation of the urethral wall occurs, the condition may be termed urethritis, while inflammation of the lining of the bladder represents cystitis. Many infections affect both regions to some degree. Urination becomes painful, a symptom known as dysuria and the bladder becomes tender and sensitive to pressure. Despite the discomfort produced, the individual feels the urge to urinate frequently. Urinary tract infections usually respond to antibiotic therapies, although subsequent reinfections may occur.

In untreated cases the bacteria may proceed along the ureters to the renal pelvis. The inflammation of the walls of the renal pelvis produces symptoms of pyelitis, and if the bacteria invade the renal cortex and medulla pyelonephritis results. Symptoms include a high fever, intense pain on the affected side, vomiting, diarrhoea, and the presence of blood cells and pus in the urine.

STUDY–QUESTIONS

1. Define the structure of the kidney. Also explain the different kinds of nephron.
2. Describe the functions of urinary system.
3. Explain the formation of urine.
4. Discuss the various disorders and abnormal ingredients of urine.
5. Write short note on micturition.

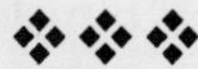

15 CHAPTER THE REPRODUCTIVE SYSTEM

INTRODUCTION

Human reproduction employs internal fertilization, and depends on the integrated action of hormones, the nervous system, and the reproductive system. Gonads are sex organs that produce gametes. Male gonads are the testes, which produce sperm and male sex hormones. Female gonads are the ovaries, which produce eggs (ova) and female sex hormones.

THE MALE REPRODUCTIVE SYSTEM

Testes are suspended outside the abdominal cavity by the scrotum, a pouch of skin that keeps the testes close or far from the body at an optimal temperature for sperm development. Seminiferous tubules are inside each testis, and are where sperm are produced by meiosis. About 250 meters (850 feet) of tubules are packed into each testis. Spermatocytes inside the tubules divide by meiosis to produce spermatids that in turn develop into mature sperm.

SPERMATOGENESIS

Sperm production begins at puberty at continues throughout life, with several hundred million sperm being produced each day. Once sperm form they move into the epididymis, where they mature and are stored.

MALE SEX HORMONES

The anterior pituitary produces follicle-stimulating hormone (FSH) and luteinizing hormone (LH). Action of LH is controlled by the gonadotropin-releasing hormone (GnRH). LH stimulates cells in the seminiferous tubules to secrete testosterone, which has a role in sperm production and developing male secondary sex characteristics. FSH acts on cells to help in sperm maturation. Negative feedback by testosterone controls the actions of GnRH.

SEXUAL STRUCTURES

Sperm pass through the vas deferens and connect to a short ejaculatory duct that connects to the urethra. The urethra passes

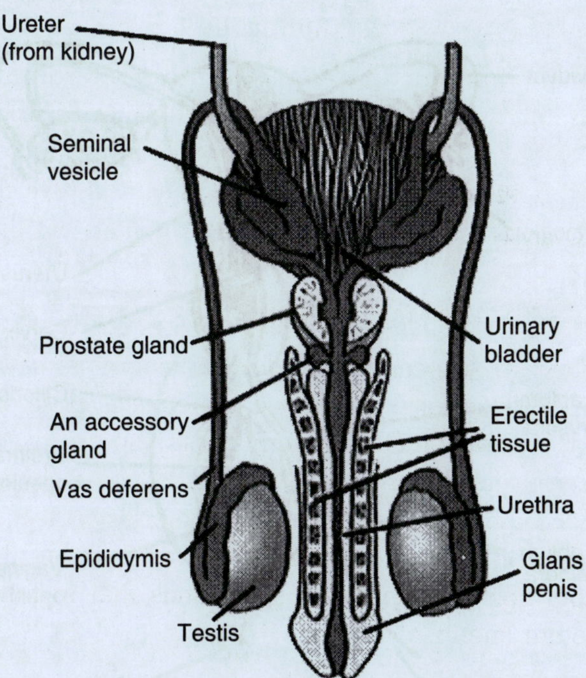

Fig. 15.1: *Male reproductive system.*

through the penis and opens to the outside. Secretions from the seminal vesicles add fructose and prostaglandins to sperm as they pass. The prostate gland secretes a milky alkaline fluid. The bulbourethral gland secretes a mucus-like fluid that provides lubrication for intercourse. Sperm and secretions make up semen.

THE FEMALE REPRODUCTIVE SYSTEM

The female gonads, ovaries, are located within the lower abdominal cavity. The ovary contains many follicles composed of a developing egg surrounded by an outer layer of follicle cells. Each egg begins oogenesis as a primary oocyte. At birth each female carries a lifetime supply of developing oocytes, each of which is in Prophase I. A developing egg (secondary oocyte) is released each month from puberty until menopause, a total of 400-500 eggs.

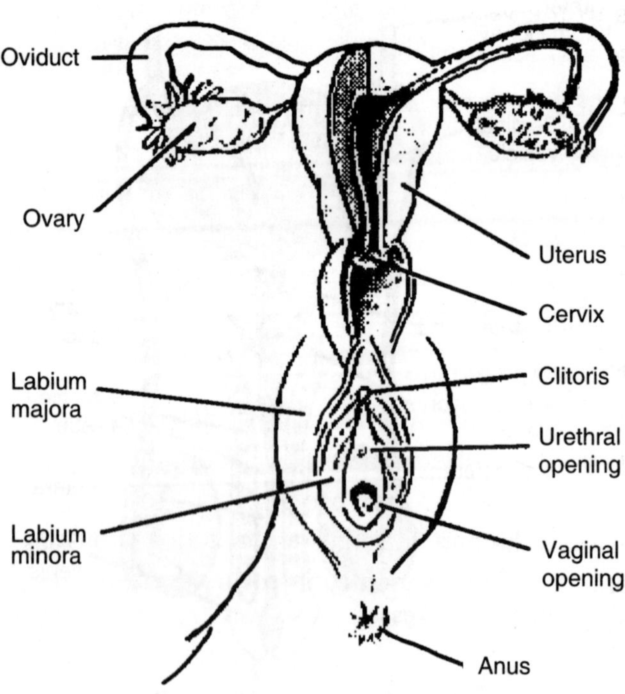

Fig. 15.2: *Female reproductive system*

OVARIAN CYCLES

After puberty the ovary cycles between a follicular phase (maturing follicles) and a luteal phase (presence of the corpus luteum). These cyclic phases are interrupted only by pregnancy and continue until menopause, when reproductive capability ends. The ovarian cycle lasts usually 28 days. During the first phase, the oocyte matures within a follicle. At midpoint of the cycle, the oocyte is released from the ovary in a process known as ovulation. Following ovulation the follicle forms a corpus luteum which synthesizes and prepares hormones to prepare the uterus for pregnancy.

The secondary oocyte passes into the oviduct (fallopian tube or uterine tube). The oviduct is connected to the uterus. The uterus has an inner layer, the endometrium, in which a fertilized egg implants. At the lower end of the uterus the cervix connects the uterus to the vagina. The vagina receives the penis during intercourse and serves as the birth canal.

EXTERNAL GENITALS

The female external genitals are collectively known as the vulva. The labia minora is a thin membrane of folded skin just outside the vaginal opening. The labia majora cover and protect the genital area. A clitoris, important in arousal, is a short shaft with a sensitive tip covered by a fold of skin.

HORMONES AND FEMALE CYCLES

The ovarian cycle is hormonally regulated in two phases. The follicle secretes estrogen before ovulation; the corpus luteum secretes both estrogen and progesterone after ovulation. Hormones from the hypothalamus and anterior pituitary control the ovarian cycle. The ovarian cycle covers events in the ovary; the menstrual cycle occurs in the uterus.

Menstrual cycles vary from between 15 and 31 days. The first day of the cycle is the first day of blood flow (day 0) known as menstruation. During menstruation the uterine lining is broken

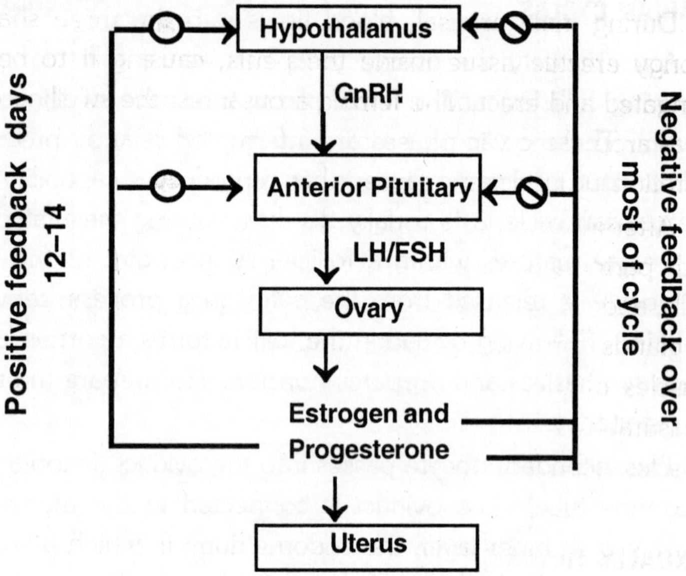

Fig. 15.3: *Hormones and Female Cycles.*

down and shed as menstrual flow. FSH and LH are secreted on day 0, beginning both the menstrual cycle and the ovarian cycle. Both FSH and LH stimulate the maturation of a single follicle in one of the ovaries and the secretion of estrogen. Rising levels of estrogen in the blood trigger secretion of LH, which stimulates follicle maturation and ovulation (day 14, or midcycle). LH stimulates the remaining follicle cells to form the corpus luteum, which produces both estrogen and progesterone.

Estrogen and progesterone stimulate the development of the endometrium and preparation of the uterine inner lining for implantation of a zygote. If pregnancy does not occur, the drop in FSH and LH cause the corpus luteum to disintegrate. The drop in hormones also causes the sloughing off of the inner lining of the uterus by a series of muscle contractions of the uterus.

SEXUAL RESPONSES

Humans do not have a mating season, females are sexually receptive to the male at all times of the year. There are *four* stages in mating: arousal, plateau, orgasm, and resolution.

During male arousal, blood flows into the three shafts of spongy erectile tissue inside the penis, causing it to become elongated and erect. The female arousal has the swelling of the areas around the vagina, erection of the clitoris and nipples, and secretion of lubricating fluids in the vagina.

After insertion of the penis into the vagina, pelvic thrusts by both partners stimulate sensory receptors in the penis, vaginal walls, and clitoris. The sperm leave the epididymis and secretions of glands form the semen. Orgasm involves contractions of muscles of the penis (male) or vagina (female) and waves of pleasurable sensations. Resolution reverses the previous phases: muscles relax, breathing slows, the penis returns to its normal size.

SEXUALLY TRANSMITTED DISEASES

Sexually transmitted diseases (STDs) cause over $7 billion to be expended for treatment. STDs can affect the sex partners, fetus, and newborn infants. STDs are grouped into three categories.

Category One

STDs that produce inflammation of the urethra, epididymis, cervix, or oviducts. Gonorrhea and chlamydia are the most common STDs in this category. Both diseases can be treated and cured with antibiotics, once diagnosed.

Category Two

STDs that produce sores on the external genitals. Genital herpes is the most common disease in this class, affecting more than 25 million individuals in the US. Symptoms of herpes can be treated by antiviral drugs, but the infection cannot be cured. Syphilis is a bacterially caused infection, and can, if left untreated, cause serious symptoms and death. However, the disease is curable with antibiotics.

Category Three

This class of STDs includes viral diseases that affect organ systems other than those of the reproductive system. AIDS and hepatitis B are in this category. Both can be spread by sexual contact or blood. Infectious individuals may appear symptom-free for years after infection.

NEW TECHNIQUES IN REPRODUCTION

New techniques have been developed to enhance or reduce the chances of conception. Social conventions and governing laws have developed far slower than this new technology, leading to controversy about moral, ethical, and legal grounds for the uses of such technologies. The separation of intercourse from pregnancy uses methods blocking one of the three stages of reproduction:

(i) release and transport of gametes

(ii) fertilization

(iii) implantation

EFFECTIVENESS

Various contraceptive methods have been developed; none of which is 100 per cent successful at preventing pregnancy or the transmission of STDs. Abstinence is the only completely effective method.

METHODS

Physical prevention (most effective) include *vasectomy* and tubal ligation. Vasectomy: the vas deferens connecting the testes with the urethra is cut and sealed to prevent the transport of sperm. Tubal ligation: the oviduct is cut and ends tied off to prevent eggs from reaching the uterus.

Oral contraceptives (birth control pills) usually contain a combination of hormones that prevent release of FSH and LH, inhibiting development of the follicle so that no oocytes are released. Time-release capsules (Norplant) can be implanted under

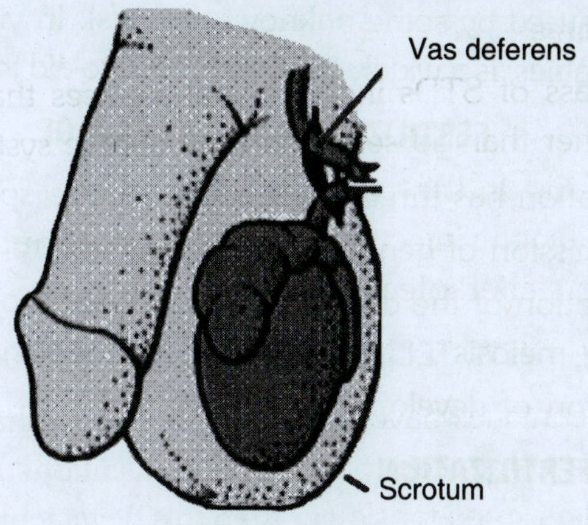

Fig. 15.4: *Penis.*

the skin and offer long-term suppression of ovulation. RU-486, the so-called morning after pill, interferes with implantation of the blastula into the uterine wall. Its use as a contraceptive is very controversial. Barrier methods employ physical (condom, diaphragm) or chemical (spermacides) means to separate the sperm from the egg. Male condoms are fitted over the erect penis; female condoms are placed inside the vagina. Only latex condoms prevent the spread of STDs. Diaphragms cap the cervix and block passage of the sperm into the uterus. Spermicidal jellies or foams kill sperm on contact and must be placed in the vagina prior to intercourse.

REPRODUCTIVE TECHNOLOGIES FOR ENHANCING FERTILITY

About 1 in 6 couples is infertile due to physical or physiological conditions preventing gamete production, implantation, or fertilization. Blocked oviducts (often from untreated STDs) are the leading cause of infertility in females. Low sperm count, low motility, or blocked ducts are common causes of male infertility.

Hormone therapy can cause increased egg production. Surgery can open blocked ducts. About 40 of the cases are due to male problems, 40 due to female problems and the remaining

20% are caused by some unknown agent(s). In vitro fertilization (test-tube babies) is a widely used technique to aid infertile couples.

FERTILIZATION AND CLEAVAGE

Fertilization has three functions:

(i) transmission of genes from both parents to offspring

(ii) restoration of the diploid number of chromosomes reduced during meiosis

(iii) initiation of development in offspring.

STEPS IN FERTILIZATION

(i) Contact between sperm and egg.

(ii) Entry of sperm into the egg.

(iii) Fusion of egg and sperm nuclei.

(iv) Activation of development.

Cleavage

Cleavage is the first step in development of all multicelled organisms. Cleavage converts a single-celled zygote into a multicelled embryo by mitosis. Usually, the zygotic cytoplasm is divided among the newly formed cells.

The blastula is produced by mitosis of the zygote, and is a ball of cells surrounding a fluid-filled cavity (the blastocoel). The decreasing size of cells increases their surface to volume ratio, allowing for more efficient oxygen exchange between cells and their environment. RNA and information carrying molecules are distributed to various parts of the blastula, and this molecular differentiation sets the stage for the layering of the body in the next phases of development.

Gastrulation

Gastrulation involves a series of cell migrations to positions where they will form the three primary cell layers.

- Ectoderm forms the outer layer.
- Endoderm forms the inner layer.
- Mesoderm forms the middle layer.

- Ectoderm— Ectoderm forms tissues associated with outer layers: skin, hair, sweat glands, epithelium. The brain and nervous system also develop from the ectoderm.
- Mesoderm— The mesoderm forms structures associated with movement and support: body muscles, cartilage, bone, blood, and all other connective tissues. Reproductive system organs and kidneys form from mesoderm.
- Endoderm—The endoderm forms tissues and organs associated with the digestive and respiratory systems. Many endocrine structures, such as the thyroid and parathyroid glands, are formed by the endoderm. The liver, pancreas, and gall bladder arise from endoderm.

INVAGINATION

Immediately after gastrulation, the body axis of the embryo begins to appear. Chordates have the cells that will form the nervous system fold into a neural tube (which will eventually form the spinal cord). The mesoderm forms the notochord (which will eventually form the vertebrae). The mesoderm at this time forms somites, which form segmented body parts, such as the muscles of the body wall.

PATTERN FORMATION AND INDUCTION

Blastulation and gastrulation establish the main body axis. Organ formation occurs in the next stage of the development of the embryo. During organ formation, cell division is accomplished by migration and aggregation.

Pattern formation is the result of cells "sensing" their position in the embryo relative to other cells and to form structures appropriate to that position. Gradients of informational molecules within the embryo have been suggested to provide the positional information to cells. Homeobox genes are pattern genes; they coordinate with gradients of information molecules to establish the body plan and development of organs.

Induction is the process in which one cell or tissue type affects the developmental fate of another cell or tissue. As a cell begins to form certain structures, certain genes are turned on, others are turned off. Induction affects patterns of gene expression through physical contact or chemical signals. Formation of the vertebrate eye is a well known example.

HUMAN DEVELOPMENT

Fertilization, the fusion of the sperm and egg, usually occurs in the upper third of the oviduct. Thirty minutes after ejaculation, sperm are present in the oviduct, having traveled from the vagina through the uterus and into the oviduct. Sperm traverse this distance by the beating of their flagellum. Of the several hundred million sperm released in the ejaculation, only a few thousand reach the egg.

Only one sperm will fertilize the egg. One sperm fuses with receptors on the surface of the secondary oocyte, triggering a series of chemical changes in the outer oocyte membrane that prevent any other sperm from entering the oocyte. The entry of the sperm initiates Meiosis II in the oocyte. Fusion of the egg and sperm nuclei forms the diploid zygote.

TRAVELS OF A YOUNG ZYGOTE

Cleavage of the zygote begins while it is still in the oviduct, producing a solid ball of cells (morula). The morula enters the uterus, continuing to divide and becomes a blastocyst.

IMPLANTATION

The uterine lining becomes enlarged and prepared for implantation of the embryo in the trophoblast layer. Twelve days after fertilization, the trophoblast has formed a two-layered chorion. Human chorionic gonadotropin (hCG) is secreted by the chorion, and prolongs the life of the corpus luteum until the placenta begins to secrete estrogen and progesterone. Home pregnancy tests work by detecting elevated hCG levels in the woman's urine.

Maternal and embryonic structures interlock to form the placenta, the nourishing boundary between the mother's and embryo's systems. The umbilical cord extends from the placenta to the embryo, and transports food to and wastes from the embryo.

STAGES

The period of time from fertilization to birth (usually 9 months) is divided into trimesters, each about three months long. During pregnancy the zygote undergoes 40 to 44 rounds of mitosis, producing an infant containing trillions of specialized cells organized into tissues and organs.

(i) *The First Trimester*—The three embryonic tissue layers form. Cellular differentiation begins to form organs during the third week. After one month the embryo is 5 mm long and composed mostly of paired somite segments. During the second month most of the major organ systems form, limb buds develop. The embryo becomes a fetus by the seventh week. Beginning the eighth week, the sexually neutral fetus activates gene pathways for sex determination, forming testes in XY fetuses and ovaries in XX fetuses. External genitalia develop.

(ii) *The Second Trimester*—The fetus increases in size during this trimester, and bony parts of the skeleton begin to form. Fetal movements can be felt by the mother.

(iii) *The Last Trimester*—During this trimester the fetus increases in size. Circulatory and respiratory systems mature in preparation for air breathing. Fetal growth during this time uses large parts of its mother's protein and calcium intake. Maternal antibodies pass to the fetus during the last month, conferring temporary immunity.

BIRTH

Birth is a positive feedback hormonal mechanism. During birth the cervix dilates to allow passage of the fetus. Uterine contractions propel the fetus through the birth canal, usually head first. Hormonal control of the birth process involves the release of oxytocin and prostaglandins, which are stimulated by uterine contractions, which stimulate more hormones that cause more contractions....etc.

(i) *First Stage*—The first stage of birth lasts from beginning of contractions to the full (10 cm) dilation of the cervix. Membranes of the amniotic fluid rupture, lubricating the vagina.

(ii) *Second Stage*—Strong uterine contractions of a minute in duration separated by two to three minute intervals propel the fetus down the birth canal. Abdominal muscles relax in synchrony with the uterine contractions.

(iii) *Third Stage*—After delivery of the baby, the umbilical cord is clipped and cut. The placenta (or afterbirth) in expelled through the vagina.

MILK PRODUCTION

Nursing mothers have their hormone levels and uterine size return to normal much faster than non-nursing mothers. Breasts develop the capability for milk secretion about the mid point of pregnancy. Secretion of milk does not occur until delivery, and the action of prolactin. Suckling by the infant causes production of oxytocin to promote release of milk into the ducts emptying into the nipple. The stages of life are noted by the acquisition of social, physical, and mental skills. Other signs of maturation include tattoos, body piercing, motorcycles, and backward-turned baseball caps.

INFANCY AND CHILDHOOD

Infancy lasts from birth until age two. Infant reflexes concern finding the nipple: suckling can occur minutes after birth, and the rooting reflex is a tactile clue for the infant to turn its head toward a touch. During the first year the infant passes through a series of developmental stages.

Childhood begins at two and lasts until puberty. Physical growth is accompanied by increasing development of motor and language skills. Play, make-believe, and increases in memory and attention span also occur.

ADOLESCENCE AND ADULTHOOD

Growth accelerates during puberty. Boys increase in height by 3-5 inches per year, girls 2-4 inches. The heart doubles in size, and hormones stimulate sexual maturity. Growth ends during the end of adolescence, and aging starts during the late twenties.

STUDY–QUESTIONS

1. Explain the male reproductive parts in male.
2. Discuss the female reproductive parts in female.
3. Write short notes on the following:
   (a) Milk Production
   (b) Adolescence and Adulthood
   (c) Human Development
   (d) Fetilization
   (e) Menstrual Cycle in female.

SECTION-III

Clinical Practice

Chapter: 16	Burns and Scalds	169–181
Chapter: 17	Injuries, Wounds and Haemorrhage	182–201
Chapter: 18	Head Injury	202–208
Chapter: 19	Accidents: Road, Air and Fire	209–228
Chapter: 20	Impaired Consciousness and Drowing	229–236
Chapter: 21	Poisoining, Bites and Stings	237–247
Chapter: 22	Fractures: Bones and Joints	248–268
Chapter: 23	Bandage and Dressing	269–276
Chapter: 24	Effects of Heat	277–283
Chapter: 25	Effects of Cold	284–291
Chapter: 26	Handling and Transporting of Casualty	292–302

16

CHAPTER

BURNS AND SCALDS

INTRODUCTION

Burns are injuries that are caused from corrosive substance, from dry heat (like fire, flame), friction or by lighting. *Scalds* are caused by moist heat due to boiling water, steam oil. The key factors in burn pathology are the area of the burn, the depth of the burn, and any special areas of the body, such as the respiratory tract, that are involved.

EXTENT OF BURN

Extent is the percentage of body's total surface area depending on the body surface burnt; percentage of burn can be calculated.

(i) Area of Burn

The burnt area will almost immediately begin to lose fluid which is very similar to plasma in its composition. If sufficient fluid is lost from the burn, hypovolaemic shock will develop. The area of the burn is, therefore, crucial as it determines the volume of fluid lost. Area may be estimated using *Wallace's Rule of Nine* (see Fig. 16.1).

As a rule of thumb it may be assumed that in burns of 15 per cent of surface area or greater in adults, and 10 per cent or greater in children, hypovolaemia will develop. In these cases, therefore, the patient will need an IVI. If such an infusion is not commenced and the hypovolaemia not vigorously treated, the outcome may be fatal.

In reading about burns, the nurse may be confused by the different statements that are made about the type of fluid that should be used to correct hypovolaemia from burns. This is because there is a marked difference of opinion among the various specialists in the field. The basic requirements in the burn patient are protein, salt and water in such a form as will stay in the circulation. Sodium chloride is lost in great quantities in the burn exudate, along with protein, and therefore must be replaced. However, the hypovolaemic patient also needs fluids that will

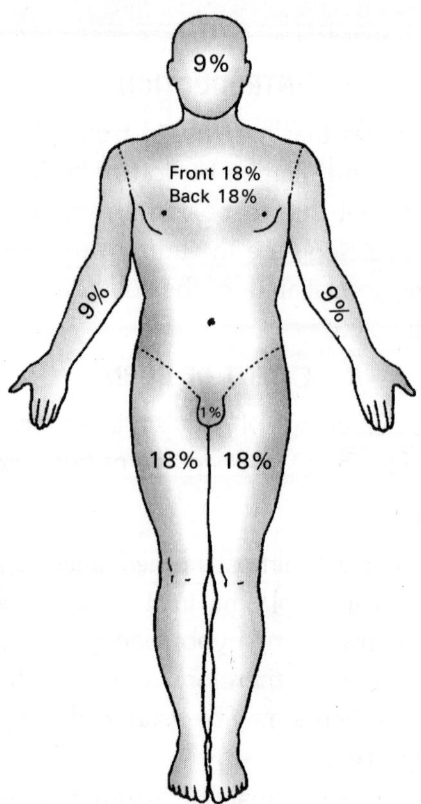

Fig. 16.1: *Wallace's Rule of Nine of estimating area of burns.*

stay in the circulation rather than those which rapidly escape into the various other fluid compartments of the body.

Thus, although normal saline contains the sodium chloride required, it will not effectively expand the circulation and, although Hemocoel is a plasma expander, it does not contain sodium chloride. Solutions such as Dextran 70 and Plasma Protein Faction (PPF), however, have both properties.

Fluid loss frum a burn continues for over 24 hours after injury. This is of significance in planning dressings for patients who are to be discharged home with relatively minor burns. For the major burn requiring in-patient treatment, the continual fluid loss has to be taken into account in working out an IVI regime. Various formulae are used in this connection, one of the best known being the *Mount Vernon* formula (*Wardrope* and *Smith*), which calculates a unit volume of fluid from the patient's size and the area burnt.

Unit volume = Area burnt (%) × Patient's weight (kg) 2. This unit volume of fluid is then administered in blocks of 4 hours, two blocks of 6 hours and one block of 12 hours, measured from the time of the burn and subject to adjustment in the light of the patient's condition.

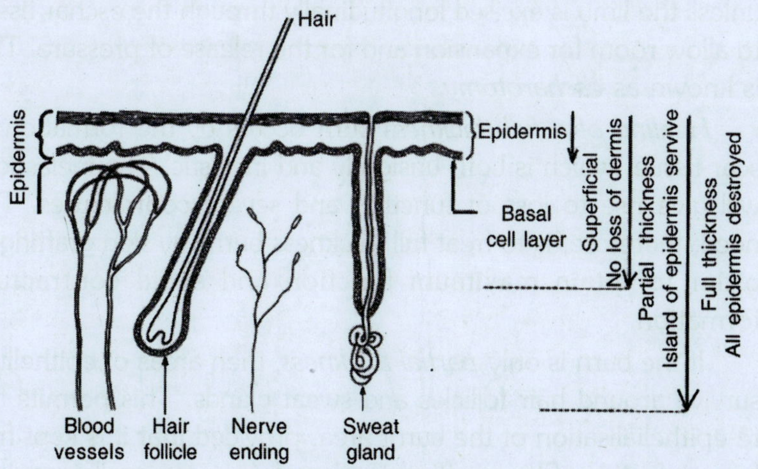

Fig. 16.2: *Depth of burns.*

(ii) Depth of Burns

The Ist, IInd and IIIrd degree burns classifications are to be avoided as they are imprecise terms that can mean different things to different people. It is more appropriate and precise to describe the depth of burns as either full thickness, partial thickness or superficial.

TYPES OF DEPTH OF BURNS

(I) Deep Burns

In deep burns epidermis and dermis both are burnt. It takes long time to heal and leaves a scar. There is little or no pain. It can be of two types: *full thickness burn* and *partial thickness burn.*

A *full thickness burn* is one in which the full thickness of the skin has been destroyed. The appearance is a typically dull grey area, or in flame burns, a dark brown or black. Because the nerve endings have been destroyed, there is usually a loss of sensation. The remaining tissue is hard and leathery. This poses a special problem in circumferential bums because the inelastic surface tissue will act as a touniquet around the limb, within which there will be swelling due to the burn oedema. The result is occlusion of the circulation, gangrene and loss of the limb, unless the limb is excised longitudinally through the eschar tissue to allow room for expansion and for the release of pressure. This is known as *escharotomy.*

Healing of a full thickness burn occurs by the formation of scar tissue, which is both unsightly and inelastic. The inelasticity will give rise to loss of function and severe contractures. The need, therefore, is to treat full thickness burns by skin grafting in order to retain maximum function and avoid contracture formation.

If the burn is only *partial thickness*, then areas of epithelium survive around hair follicles and sweat glands. This permits the re-epithelialisation of the burnt area, provided that it is kept free from infection. Skin grafting is, therefore, not usually required and healing should occur with a full range of movement. Partial thickness burns usually leave the nerve endings intact; therefore, they may be differentiated from full thickness burns by a pin prick sensation test. Scalds and flash burns are typically partial thickness.

(ii) Superficial Burns

Superficial burns involve a reddening only of the most superficial layers. This is known as *erythema* and is of minor importance compared to the other two types so far discussed. In estimating burn areas, erythema should be excluded.

CAUSES OF BURNS

(i) Burn due to Electricity

It is characterised by a small surface wound where the current entered the body, but within there may be major damage with burns extending down to the bone and involving structures such as tendons, muscles and nerves. The potential effect of the electric current on the heart, lungs should be the first focus of nursing and medical attention.

(ii) Burn due to Chemicals

Certain chemicals may irritate or damage the skin, e.g., strong acid, sulphuric acid, strong alkalies, e.g., caustic soda and strong ammonia. To protect from these firstly remove immediately any clothing which is wet by the chemicals. Wash thoroughly the burn area with cold water. If more than 10 per cent body surface is affected send the casualty to the nearest medical centre.

(iii) Burn due to Severe Body Area

In severe burn body area more than 30 per cent burnt. In this case first remove the cause if the victim is still on fire. Remove quickly rings, shoes, bangles, belt etc. If limb starts swelling, it will be difficult to remove them. Don't give anything by mouth. Don't try to remove the burnt clothing which sticks to the body surface. Send the casualty to the nearest hospital as soon as possible.

SPECIAL AREAS AFFECTED BY BURNS

Oedema of the face and neck can have serious implications for the airway. Inhalation of flames or hot gases will cause burn oedema in the respiratory tract itself. The threat of an occluded airway is very real in such cases and an early tracheotomy or intubation, if possible, is indicated.

Facial oedema will quickly make it impossible for the patient to open their eyes. This has two implications; first, if the eyes are to be examined properly, they must be examined immediately, and second, the patient may fear that their sight has been lost altogether, when the problem is simply that they cannot open their eyes.

Immobilization of hands in bulky dressings will lead to long-term problems of joint stiffness. For this reason, the 'Flamazine bag' dressing is recommended for burnt hands rather than more traditional methods. Flamazine is silver sulphadiazine, a very effective antibacterial agent.

MINOR BURNS AND SCALDS

In the case of minor burns, firstly clean the area gently with clean water, submerge the burnt area in cold water, cover with dry dressing, do not apply cotton wool direct to the burnt area, give warm drinks, for example, sweetened tea or coffee.

The effects of both burns and scalds are the same. The skin may be reddened or blister formed or destruction of the skin, or the deeper tissues. There will be severe pain. There is immediate danger from shock which may be severe and made worse by the intense pain and by loss of plasma into the burnt area. Later, there is danger from septic infection.

The areas of burns and scalds, including the clothing involved are all intents and purposes sterile for a short period and try your best to keep them so, until medical aid is available. Always use prepared dry sterile dressings and great care must be taken in handling and applying them.

The dangers of a burn increase with its surface area (even if it is only superficial) and if one-third or more of the skin area is involved, the patient may become dangerously ill. In small children and infants even small burns should be considered as serious injuries and medical aid sought without delay.

When a person's clothing catches fire, approach him holding a rug, blanket, coat or table cover, in front of yourself for protection, wrap it round him, lay him flat and so smother the flames. If a person's clothing catches fire when he is alone, he should roll on the floor, smothering the flames with the nearest available wrap and call for help. Under any circumstances, he should not run into the open air.

PSYCHOLOGICAL EFFECTS

The nurse should realize that there are profound psychological effects from a burn which affect not only the patient but also their relatives. There is the fear of disfigurement and altered body image on the one hand, and on the other, there are the inevitable feelings of guilt associated with the parent of a young child that has been burnt.

INFECTION

If a partial thickness burn becomes infected, healing will be delayed until the infection is cleared up. In the case of a full thickness burn, infection will make skin grafting impossible. In severe cases, infection from burns can cause death. The risk of tetanus should not be forgotten.

OTHER LATER EFFECTS

After the patient has moved to the ward, complications can develop. These include renal failure, toxaemia, anaemia, paralytic ileus, and in the case of children 'burn encephalopathy'. These complications can combine to make the burns victim an extremely challenging person to care for.

ASSESSMENT

Assessment of the burns victim starts with the airway. The nurse should note whether the burns involve the face and neck areas, and whether there is any evidence of the patient having inhaled flames or hot gas. Such evidence would include soot in the nasal passages or blistering around the mouth and lips.

It is important to obtain a history of the accident–what caused the burn, the time the burn occurred and what, if any, first aid has been applied. The next point to determine is how much pain the patient is feeling. Some burns cause remarkably little pain; ironically they are usually the more severe full thickness burns as the actual nerve endings have been destroyed, but other burns can be extremely painful.

The area of the burn should be estimated, using *Wallace's Rule of nine*. This rule divides the body area up into multiples of 9 per cent. For small areas, the area of the patient's hand can be taken as 1 per cent of the body area. Areas of superficial erythema and redness should not be included in this calculation.

The last point to estimate is the depth of the burn. The appearance will give some clue: a full thickness bum is typically a dull grey colour with tough leathery eschar tissue; a partial thickness burn is usually red or pink in colour. Sensation is absent in the full thickness burn but present in a partial thickness burn. This may be tested for with the pin prick method.

A sketch of the burn is a useful means of recording its extent; areas of suspected full thickness burn can be shaded in and labelled as such.

Baseline observations are important to monitor the circulatory status of the patient and to detect any signs of hypovolaemic shock at the earliest stage. They should be repeated as frequently as the patient's condition indicates.

The psychological effects of the burn on the patient and on the family should be assessed, especially where young children are involved. Is the mother hostile and defensive, or anxious and expressing feelings of guilt? One important aspect that has to be assessed is whether the child's injuries match the story of the parent, as burns constitute a common form of child abuse.

In electrical burns, it is important to take an ECG and to monitor the patient's heart rhythm continually on a cardiac monitor. Function should be assessed together with sensation in view of the risk of damage to deep structures such as tendons and nerves.

INTERVENTION

First Aid — The appropriate first aid for burns is irrigation with copious amounts of cold water. This will retard the process of tissue destruction due to heat and also afford the patient considerable pain relief.

Airway— The first priority for the burns patient is to safeguard the airway, and if assessment reveals problems *due to oedema, tracheotomy* or *intubation* will be considered. The nursing team must be able to respond at once to the need for emergency tracheotomy or intubation in such a situation. Upper airway oedema peaks at 24–48 hours after injury. Treatment in less severe cases consists of administering humidified oxygen, maintaining close observation, an upright position and chest physiotherapy aimed at preventing atelectasis.

Pain Relief— The application of cold soaks (gauze dressing pads and sterile water for irrigation) to the burnt area will usually reduce the pain felt by the patient though the risk of hypothermia should not be overlooked. The generous administration of Entonox gas will further relieve pain.

In major burns, the administration of intravenous morphine is recommended by many authorities. The best method is to dilute 10 mg of morphine in 10 ml of water for injection, and then to give, slowly, sufficient of the drug to achieve the desired degree of sedation and pain relief.

In dealing with young children, sedation is very important as it is impossible to dress properly limbs that are flailing in all directions at once. Furthermore, the more distressed the child, the more distressed will be the parents who are already probably feeling desperately guilty and blaming themselves for their young child's misfortune. A child may be sedated with oral trimeprazine syrup, but it must be remembered that the child can still feel the pain and that therefore some other analgesic agent is required in addition. Wherever possible, when dressing burns on young children, nurses should allow them to sit on their parent's lap as being held by a parent will be a source of comfort in what the child is currently experiencing as a very frightening experience.

Psychological Support — From the nurse's very first encounter with the patient, psychological support will be essential. Reference has already been made to the likely guilt feelings that parents of young children will be experiencing. In addition, adults will be fearing disfigurement as a result of their injuries.

It is very difficult at this early stage in A & E to deal with a straight 'Will I be scarred for life?' question. But this is precisely what is in the mind of the burn victim, and may even be on their lips. If asked, the nurse should try to answer the question fairly and frankly, pointing out that at this early stage it is very difficult to say with any degree of certainty what the outcome will be. Such an answer is better than bland reassurances about the wonders of modern plastic surgery. On the other hand, the question may remain unasked; if this is the case, the nurse should try to get the patient to verbalize their fears and to get the matter out in the open for realistic discussion.

The degree of distress displayed by the patient may be markedly reduced by simply talking about the problem and offering support as appropriate.

The IVI and Fluid Balance — If the burn is over 15 per cent of the body surface area, an IVI will be required to prevent hypovolaemia. Apart from nursing assistance in siting the infusion, it will be a key part of the resuscitation effort that an accurate fluid balance be kept. Catheterization, with hourly urine measurements, is essential due to the risk of renal failure. The kidneys should be able to produce a minimum of 0.5 ml of urine per kg body weight per hour; failure to do so indicates that they are being underperfused and that, therefore, inadequate IV fluids are being given to deal with the burn shock. For an average adult, the hourly urine output should not drop below about 35 ml.

BURNS DRESSINGS

The aim of the dressing is to provide an aseptic environment in which, depending on the depth of the burn, either healing can occur or the wound can be readied for successful grafting.

The first step is to debride the wound. Contaminants such as charred clothing and soot should be washed away using copious amounts of sterile water for irrigation. After cleansing, a pair of non-toothed McIndoe's dissecting forceps should be used to remove all dead tissue and blisters. Alternatively, clean blister tissues may be left and the blister fluid aspirated with a needle and syringe. Little pain should be felt by the patient as the tissue is dead; once pain is felt, it is a signal to stop as that tissue is obviously alive!

The wound dressing should be occlusive and secure, in order to preserve the aimed–for aseptic environment, yet at the same time it should be easy to remove the redressing. These criteria are best met with the Flamazine and Melolin dressing technique which consists of spreading Flamazine cream over an appropriate sized sheet of Melolin with a sterile spatula to a thickness of 3-4 mm and then applying this to the burn. The Flamazine will act as a powerful prophylactic agent in preventing infection of the burn, and yet it can also be used for treating infected burns as well; the Melolin will ensure that the dressing is easily removed without sticking.

Because bums will ooze exudate for at least 24 hours, there is a need for a considerable thickness of gauze backing up the Melolin, possibly two large dressing pads thick. The whole dressing should be secured with tape and then by an elasticated tubular bandage rather than crepe.

Elevation of the burnt limb is essential because of the volume of oedema that is to be expected. If the patient is going home, this must be one of the key points made in discharge instructions.

The problems associated with finger stiffness after prolonged immobilisation necessitate the special technique used for burns involving the hands-the 'Flamazine bag dressing'. Debridement and cleaning are carried out as normal. Then the hand is smeared generously with Flamazine and inserted in a plastic bag which is securely taped to the wrist. A large dressing pad should be taped around the wrist inside the bag to soak up the oedema and the whole arm should be placed in a high arm sling.

The key point about this dressing is that the fingers are unrestricted and therefore, provided that the patient remembers to exercise them, stiffness will not be a problem. Instruction about finger exercises is essential prior to discharge, in addition to warning the patient that the appearance of the hand may be alarming due to maceration of the skin. Daily bag change may be necessary initially due to the volume of tissue exudate produced.

The same technique may be used for burns to the foot and toes. The nurse will find it a great deal quicker than the traditional burns dressings which would involve separate dressings for each finger in addition to dressings for the rest of the hand. If the patient has suffered a major burn, he or she is best treated in a regional centre and an immediate transfer should be arranged.

Self-care of Burns Dressings

The majority of burns patients seen in an A & E department are usually discharged home and followed up on an out-patient basis. Therefore, the patient must fully understand how to look after the dressing if best results are to be obtained and complications such as infection are to be avoided.

Key points are the need to keep the limb elevated in fresh burns, the importance of exercising the fingers in hand burns, and for any bum, the need to keep the dressing clean and dry. The patient needs to know when he or she has to return to hospital, i.e., at an arranged time such as a burns clinic held in A & E, or if the dressing has soaked through, started to disintegrate or emit an unpleasant smell, or if there is another indication of infection.

The ability of the patient or the patient's family to care for the dressing, and the effect that dressing will have on the patient's universal self-care demands should be carefully thought about by the nurse before discharge. Failure to do so can have serious implications for the patient and make for a much more prolonged and painful period of ill health because of the problems that may arise if the burn becomes infected.

EVALUATION

The psychological state of the patient, together with the degree of pain being felt, should be closely watched in order to determine the effectiveness of intervention in these two areas. It is also important to check that an elevated limb remains elevated as it may easily slip.

The effectiveness of the other main area of nursing intervention, the dressing, is usually measured at the patient's next attendance. It is important that senior nursing staff check the state dressings are in upon return to ensure that staff within the unit are carrying out effective burns dressings, i.e., dressings that will last, with a minimum infection rate and which can be easily removed without causing the patient undue distress. It is only by monitoring dressing standards that steps, such as teaching, can be taken to improve dressings to the standard required should there be a shortfall.

Finally, it remains to check that the information that has been taught has been learnt, i.e., does the patient understand the self-care instructions that have been given? Only questioning of the patient will allow nurses to discover whether he or she has truly learnt what has been taught.

STUDY–QUESTIONS

1. Discuss the various types of depth of burns in brief.
2. Write a short note on minor burns and scalds.
3. Describe the various types of burns.

***

17

CHAPTER

Injuries, Wounds and Haemorrhage

INJURIES

Soft tissue injuries can either be closed, as in bruising or a ligament sprain, sprain, or open, in which case some sort of wound will be developed. Wounds and other injuries to muscles and joints make up a large proportion of an A & E department's workload, some of which are old infected wounds rather than acute injuries.

Crush injury — The most commonly involved parts of the body are fingers and toes. There may be a fracture of the bone underneath which will, therefore, be an open fracture. The force of the impact causes the soft tissue to burst open; a very painful injury with much swelling involved. Crush injuries carry a high risk of infection due to the damaged and devitalised tissue present.

Strain is overstretching of a muscle while rupture is tearing of partial or entire muscle bundle. Rupture is a serious condition. Strain generally happen due to twist or sudden effort to lift heavy weight or suddenly getting up and moving briskly. So, motion is an important activity of the body which is made possible by special development of the functions of contractibility in muscle tissue. Muscles are fleshy part of the body. There are over 650 muscles in the human body. Mainly there are three types of muscles, i.e., voluntary, involuntary and cardiac muscles.

Voluntary muscles—These are under the control of will. They are attached to the bones either directly or indirectly by means of white fibrous bonds called *tendons*. Movement of the body part take place by contractions and relaxations of these muscles. These are found in head, neck, limbs and wall of the trunk.

Involuntary muscles—These are not under the control of will. They work under the effect of the set of nerves called autonomic nerves. They are found on the walls of the stomach, intestine, air passage, blood vessels etc.

Cardiac muscles—These are not under the control of will. Their main function is to eject blood from heart to great blood vessels. They constitute that the heart structure of these muscles is mixed, i.e., partly resemble voluntary and partly involuntary muscles.

WOUNDS

A wound is break in the skin or mucous membrane or other body structure, resulting from physical means. It may be involving blood vessels, muscles, nerve and bones.

The wounds seen in A & E are rather different from surgical incisions that the nurse will have encountered elsewhere: A & E wounds can be in all shapes and sizes, and are all caused by nonsterile agents, with an accompanying high risk infection.

COMPLICATIONS OF WOUNDS

Wounds get many complications but two of them are important, i.e., bleeding and infection. Bleeding is the immediate danger and should be treated immediately. Normally a wound is not initially infected though it may be contaminated by dirt, germs and other infected material. Infection occurs after sometime when the micro-organism get time to multiply.

TYPES OF WOUNDS

The following summary of wounds commonly seen in A & E will be of use as an introduction:

1. *Laceration or lacerated wound*—A linear cut in the skin, usually superficial but may involve deep structures.
2. *Incised wound or surgical wound*—It is a clean, smooth cut made with a sharp cutting instrument such as surgical blade or scalpel. It has lean cut edges.
3. *Penetrating wound*—A narrow but deeply penetrating track is involved. The cause can be anything from treading on a nail to a stabbing or gunshot wound.
4. *Abrasions or abrasive wound*—A superficial but very painful injury. Dirt and grit is commonly ingrained or tattooed into the skin and has to be removed by scrubbing.
5. *Bites wounds*—Ragged wounds are produced by bites and have a high risk of infection. Human bites carry a very high risk of infection as the mouth is heavily contaminated with bacteria, whilst the risk of hepatitis B or HIV transmission also exists. Such wounds should not be sutured due to the risk of infection.
6. *Degloving injury*—If a force is involved that is parallel to the skin, layers of tissue may be torn away, exposing a whole area of deeper structures.
7. Burns—Already explained in a separate chapter.
8. *Contused wound*—It is wound made by blunt instruments or heavy sacks or boxes falling on the body parts. The surface tissue may or may not be broken. Bruising of the surface tissues results in extravasation of blood into the skin or mucous membranes resulting in bluish discolouration. The swelling resulting from haemorrhage into the tissues is known as *haematoma.*

The normal healing process will produce fresh epithelial cover within 48 hours if the wound has been closed, although the healing process below the surface will take much longer. An impaired blood supply, infection or the presence of foreign material will all delay or prevent healing. The aim in A & E, therefore, is to clean the wound thoroughly, removing foreign material and reducing the risk of infection, and then to close the wound so as to promote rapid healing with the minimum of scar formation and infection risk.

The most feared pathogens are the anaerobic Clostridium family. Clostridium tetani gives rise to tetanus, and Clostridium welchii and Clostridium sporagenes are involved in gas gangrene. The spores of these organisms are found in the soil, and the fact that they are anaerobic means that they can live without free atmospheric oxygen. Therefore, if they are present in a wound that is closed over, they will thrive.

Tetanus is characterised by the toxins which are released by the Clostridium tetani attacking the nervous system. The result is severe muscle spasm which could be fatal once the muscles of respiration become involved. In established cases, therefore, the treatment involves long-term ventilatory support.

In gas gangrene, putrefactive changes occur within damaged or dead tissue. The clostridia are responsible for forming various hydrogen gases which escape into the tissue planes, giving the characteristic odour. The gas increases the pressure in the tissues surrounding the wound. This further impairs blood supply. Meanwhile, the toxins released by the bacteria cause a severe toxaemia. The condition is extremely painful and carries a high mortality rate.

A wide variety of other pathogens cause *wound sepsis*. As the patient in most cases is going home after treatment, it is important that the signs of infection be carefully explained. The patient should be given instructions to return should there be any signs of infection, such as pain, swelling, redness or inflammation tracking up the limb along the line of a vein.

The elderly have very fragile skin, and suturing is not necessarily the best means of closing wounds in this case as sutures may simply cut through the skin. The pre-tibial flap laceration is a common injury seen in elderly ladies and is best treated by the use of steristrips rather than sutures. If it is proximally based there is a good chance of healing. The distally based flap, however, has a very poor blood supply and often necroses, and a skin grafting operation is needed.

In dealing with gunshot or shrapnel injuries, it is important to consider the velocity and hence energy of the projectile. If the velocity exceeds that of sound, the particle is supersonic and is defined as a high energy missile. It will behave in a very different way from a subsonic particle (a particle travelling below the speed of sound). For example, the muzzle velocity of the average handgun is some 550 feet per second. The velocity of sound is 1100 feet per second. A modem military rifle, on the other hand, has a muzzle velocity of about 2500 feet per second and the Colt Armalite exceeds 3000 feet per second. At these supersonic speeds, there is a high pressure shock wave preceding the projectile and, in its wake, there is a vacuum.

The result on hitting the human body is an instantaneous pressure wave, causing *catastrophic damage.* This is followed by the vacuum which sucks gross contamination deep into the wound. A volume of tissue roughly equal to that of a football may be destroyed by a single bullet, with only a tiny entrance and exit wound to show for it. Bone is shattered, muscle and soft tissue infracted and blood vessels destroyed, simply due to the pressure wave and without any physical contact with the projectile.

SPRAINS

Sprains consist of ligament injury where the ligament is grossly intact, but some individual fibres have been torn. The result is painful and associated with a lot of swelling, but the joint is stable. Bruising can have serious consequences because in areas such as the foot and calf there may be little room for expansion to accommodate the extra tissue fluid. Pressure levels can rise to such a point that the microcirculation is impaired and serious neurovascular complications can develop.

Signs and Symptoms

— Pain at the joints
— Swelling
— Inability to move the joint

— At the times, it is difficult to diagnose whether the casualty has a sprain, dislocation or fracture. When in doubt, treat as a case of fracture.

TRAUMA TO CARTILAGE AND BURSAE

Other commonly seen injuries include trauma to cartilage and bursae. In the knee, a tear of one of the semilunar cartilages is commonly associated with a twisting movement when the knee is flexed, resulting in the patient's knee locking in a flexed position.

Repeated wear and tear on the bursae of the elbow or knee can lead to inflammation, swelling and pain, the so-called housemaid's knee or tennis elbow. Although not traumatic in origin, the A & E department is commonly visited by patients with a wide variety of skin lesions.

HAEMORRHAGE OR BLEEDING

Haemorrhage or bleeding is the expulsion of blood due to injury or rupture of blood vessels. Blood from an artery in the systemic circulation is bright red in colour and tends to spurt out in jets corresponding with pulsations of the heart. Blood from a *vein* is dark red in colour and flows in a brisk continuous stream. Bleeding from injured capillaries is slight and flows in a continuous stream.

Blood is an important biological fluid which circulates constantly throughout the body. It carries oxygen from the lung to all parts of the body and brings back deoxygenated blood to the lungs for purification. Blood consists of red blood cells, white blood cells and plasma. In an adult, blood volume has been estimated to be 1/12th or 1/13th of body weight. This means that in an individual weighing 70 kg, there would be 6 litres of blood. If more than one litre of blood is lost, then person's life is in great danger. Hence bleeding must be stopped and the victim taken to the nearest hospital for blood transfusion.

It is important to remember that infection may occur due to the invasion of disease producing bacteria into the body through the broken skin. The bacteria multiply in a wound and make it septic. Cleanliness is essential to prevent infection and everything which comes in contact with a wound such as hands and dressings must be thoroughly cleaned.

TYPES OF HAEMORRHAGE OR BLEEDING

Haemorrhage is classified in many ways.

A. According to the Blood Vessel Broken

1. Arterial Bleeding—An artery which carries oxygenated blood is broken. The blood comes out in jets because it corresponds to the beats of the heart in action. Blood is bright red in colour.
2. Venous Bleeding—Blood is dark red in colour being deoxygenated blood and it flows in continuous stream.
3. Capillary Bleeding—Blood oozes out from capillaries and is very slow in flow. If it is on the surface of skin, it is not serious and stops without any first aid/medical treatment.

B. According to the Surface of the Body

1. External Bleeding (revealed haemorrhage)—If it is on the surface of the body, it is called External Bleeding.
2. Internal Bleeding (concealed haemorrhage)—It is within the body cavities and can not be seen immediately, but gradually the blood pressure drops and pulse rate increases. In some cases blood may ooze out from nose, ear, mouth or coughed up, passed in urine depending upon the body organ involved.

C. Bleeding from Special Sites

Like bleeding from nose, ear, eye, in urine, in stool or in vomitus.

Signs and Symptoms of Bleeding:

1. Casualty feels light headedness and may even collapse.
2. Casualty is anxious and trembling.
3. There may be blueness of the lips and paleness of skin.

4. Skin is cold and clammy.
5. Dryness of the mouth.
6. Fast pulse.
7. Eyesight may feel blurred and concentration poor.
8. There is profuse sweating.
9. The casualty feels exhausted and may become unconscious.

Natural/Physiological Arrest of Bleeding

When the skin is broken and blood vessels are injured, bleeding starts. When bleeding starts, blood vessels contract and from injured tissues, and blood cells thromboplastin is released which forms a clot (soft jelly like substance) and prevents further bleeding. Blood clots only when tissues are injured and not inside the blood vessels. The time taken for blood to clot is usually about four to six minutes.

Minor Bleeding—Minor bleeding on the surface of the skin is from capillaries in minor wounds (Mostly abrasions). This bleeding stops by itself or by firm pressure with bandaging.

Major Bleeding—Major bleeding could be external or internal. It results from injury to a large blood vessel or from diseases of blood and blood vessels.

Arrest of Severe External Bleeding

1. Inspect the wound, if any foreign body is visible and can be removed easily without further injury to the wound, remove it and press the edges of the wound together.
2. Apply a clean/sterilised dressing bigger than the wound and press it firmly with palm and when bleeding stops, bandage it tightly.
3. Press on the pressure points firmly for 10 minutes if bleeding does not stop.
4. Place the casualty in comfortable position and raise the injured part on a pillow.
5. Reassure the casualty and give sips of water.

6. If bleeding continues, do not take off the original dressing but keep on adding more pads.
7. Reach the casualty to the nearest hospital as soon as possible.

PRESSURE POINTS TO ARREST HAEMORRHAGE

This is indirect method of stopping bleeding. Pressure is applied on a particular point in an area where an artery can be pressed against an underlying bone, so as to prevent the flow of blood beyond that point. Following pressure points are easily palpable and pressure can be applied on them depending upon the body part bleeding.

1. *Femoral Pressure Points*—Femoral arteries run in the thighs. They supply oxygenated blood to lower limbs. To apply pressure on femoral pressure points, grasp the thigh with both hands, so that each thumb is in the centre of the groin. Femoral artery can be palpated before pressing it. Place one thumb on the other and apply pressure directly backwards and downwards against the pelvic bone.
2. *Popliteal Pressure Point*—Popliteal artery is the continuation of the femoral artery and runs behind the knee joint. Pressure on this point can be applied by asking the casualty to bend his knees tightly, touching the abdomen. Ensure that there is no fracture.
3. *Carotid Pressure Point*—Carotid artery is located at the point of the triangle between the shaded muscle which runs from the ear to the collar bone and the muscles covering the voice box and the windpipe. Pressure is applied by the thumb placed in the shadow beneath the voice box and the prominent muscle nearby. It is pressed against the vertebral column behind it.
4. *Facial Pressure Point*—The facial artery, as the name suggests supplies blood to the face and runs along the lower jaw. Pressure is applied by placing the palm on the upper part of the neck in such a way that the thumb is on the lower portion of the lower jaw and fingers on the back of the head and neck. Apply pressure at the site of the thumb.

5. *Temporal Pressure Point*—Pressure is applied on the temporal artery which runs in the temporal region (sides and base of skull). Pressure is applied about an inch in front of the upper part of the ear backwards against the temporal bone.
6. *Arm or Brachial Pressure Point*—Brachial artery runs along the inner border of the biceps muscle (upper arm). Pressure is applied on the middle third of the arm by compressing the artery against humerus bone.
7. *Radial or Ulnar Pressure Point*—These arteries are at the level of wrist and are commonly used for recording pulse rate. Pressure is applied against radius or ulna just above the wrist.
8. *Palmar Arch Pressure Point*—Ulnar and radial arteries which further extend to the palm and in middle of the hand/palm form an arch called as *palmar arch*. Pressure is applied by a single thumb which is placed flat in the centre of the palm and rest of the palm and fingers are on the back of the injured palm.

MANAGEMENT OF INTERNAL BLEEDING

Since the bleeding is not visible, main aim of giving first aid is to prevent the condition from getting worse.

1. Put the casualty to bed at once. Raise his legs by use of pillows.
2. Reassure him. Do not allow him to move.
3. Keep the body warm with thin blankets or a quilt depending on the weather. Do not over warm.
4. Do not give anything to eat or drink, as he may require anaesthesia and operation at the hospital.
5. Take him to the hospital as soon as possible. Transportation should be gentle and preferably in lying position.

ASSESSMENT

In order to assign the correct priority to the patient (triage) an accurate assessment of the wound and its effects on the whole patient is essential. The patient may be very distressed as the effect of the sight of blood can be very dramatic for some people. Therefore, the nurse needs a calm, reassuring manner in order to obtain a history. The nurse needs to find out what caused the injury, how and when and how much blood loss there has been. It is worth remembering, however, that the lay person is prone to exaggerate blood loss.

Taking a pad of gauze, the next thing the nurse should do is to examine the wound itself, carefully removing the patient's own first aid dressing. The nurse should look for the depth and extent of the wound, see if any deep structures such as tendons are visible and if so whether they are damaged, note any contamination and, if bleeding occurs, note whether it is pulsatile and therefore arterial in nature. Finally the degree of pain felt by the patient should be assessed. Universal precautions against the transmission of blood-borne disease should be taken at all times.

The assessment should then move on to the area distal to the wound to see if there is any evidence of damage to structures such as tendons and nerves. The nurse should test sensation and movement with this consideration in mind and also note the colour and warmth of the skin.

The psychological state of the patient should be assessed as the sight of blood can be a very frightening experience; the possibility of either the patient or relative fainting as a result should always be kept in mind. When there has been significant blood loss, or a penetrating injury, it is essential to record vital signs and then monitor them as necessary, as hypovolaemia can develop very quickly. Remember that a small entry wound in the case of a penetrating wound can conceal devastating injury within.

The patient's antitetanus status should also be ascertained, together with any other information relevant to wound healing, such as whether the patient is a diabetic or on steroid therapy. In assessing closed soft tissue injuries, a history should first be obtained. Then the nurse should move on to look at the injury. It needs examining for localized bony tenderness, which would raise the possibility of a fracture, and for swelling, pain and degree of function. It is important to know how rapidly the existing amount of swelling occurred so that a reasonable estimate can be made of future swelling and, therefore, whether there is a significant risk of neurovascular compromise.

A common type of lesion that is presented at A & E is the wound that has become infected because the person did not seek treatment at the time. In addition, people present with a wide range of abscesses, some of which can be extremely painful. In assessing the patient, the nurse should obtain a history of how long the problem has existed and of any likely precipitating factor. The area should be examined for signs of the infection spreading such as a red prominent track along the line of a vein or the swelling of lymph nodes. Due to the association of infective lesions with diabetes, the patient should have a routine stix test performed for blood glucose. Temperature and pulse should also be recorded to assess the degree of systemic involvement.

INTERVENTION

(i) Control Bleeding

To stop and check any bleeding is the first intervention. This may be done by direct pressure over the wound with a firm dressing-initially this can be held by hand, remembering to use universal precautions, but a firm bandage will suffice once the bleeding has been stopped and by elevating the injury, for example, by using a roller towel and a drip stand for a hand or arm injury. Injuries as extreme as traumatic amputations of limbs may be dealt with in this way. There is no indication for the use of a tourniquet in A & E other than to provide a temporary bloodless field for a brief examination of the wound.

(ii) Cleaning the Wound

Whether it is a major wound that will require repair in theatre or a minor wound that can be dealt with in A & E, it will need cleaning out thoroughly. If the wound is major, irrigation with a litre of normal saline in A & E is recommended. This can be followed by a dressing of saline soaks and iodine to keep the tissue in the best condition possible for theatre, where a formal toilet and debridement will take place. The aim is, in addition to a thorough toilet of the wound to wash out all contamination, to remove surgically any dead or dubious tissue which may act as a focus for infection (e.g., gas gangrene). The surgeon may leave badly contaminated wounds open for 3 days after surgery, covering them with only a light dressing. Only when absolutely sure that there is no evidence of sepsis, will the surgeon proceed to a delayed primary suture. This procedure is mandatory for all high velocity missile wounds.

In dealing with smaller wounds, research indicates that cleaning with antiseptics is of little value in preventing infection because the solution is not in contact with micro-organisms long enough and resistant strains are increasingly common. A further major problem is that naturally occurring body fluids can make most antiseptics ineffective. A thorough cleansing with a sterile saline solution (e.g., Normasol) is therefore recommended and if the wound is very contaminated, hydrogen peroxide may be used as its effervescent effect may help loosen debris. It should be noted, though, that it has little if any antiseptic action, and there have been reports of tissue damage and near fatal air embolism associated with its use.

Abrasions demand special attention as grit may be tattooed into the wound. If left there, it will cause infection and possibly a permanent disfiguring mark. The use of a scrubbing brush or toothbrush may be the only effective way to remove such grit. Needless to say this is a very painful procedure and the patient should have the benefit of either a general anaesthetic, Entonox and local anaesthesia, or IV pethidine.

WOUND CLOSURE

The main techniques used in A & E for wound closure are suturing and steristripping, although the use of tissue glue is a recent development which may have much to commend it. The suture or steristrip should always be applied at right angles to the wound, skin edges should never be inverted (turned under) as this delays healing, and the tension in the skin around the wound should be evenly distributed. If there is too much tension in the skin the wound will breakdown. The nurse should therefore resist the temptation to pull skin edges together tightly. They should only be placed in opposition.

If more than one stitch is required, the area should first be infiltrated with local anaesthetic which should be introduced via a needle inserted parallel to the wound and injected as the needle and syringe are gradually withdrawn. Lignocaine 2 per cent is the agent of choice. However, in a very vascular area, such as the scalp, where bleeding often proves a problem, lignocaine with adrenaline may be used. Such a solution should never be used on a finger or toe as the vasoconstrictor effects of adrenaline are so great that peripheral gangrene may result.

The needle should be firmly gripped half-way to one-third along its length by the needle holders. When the needle is introduced into the skin, it is important that the wrist be rotated in alignment with the curvature of the needle, otherwise the needle will be bent. The needle should enter some 4 mm from the wound edge and exit the same distance from the opposite side of the wound. Dissecting forceps may be used to hold the wound edge to facilitate passing the needle through.

The knot is tied some three turns being needed, each in the opposite direction from its predecessor. Each stitch needs to be about 3 mm from its neighbour. In cutting the stitch, the nurse should remember that a colleague will have to remove that stitch in a few days time 3 days for faces, 5 days for scalps, 7 days for elsewhere. For faces, 5-0 size suture material is usually used; 4-0 is used elsewhere although if considerable force is involved (e.g., over a knee), 3-0 may be used. Scalps are also often sutured with 3-0.

Steristrips are simply thin strips of adhesive paper. They are suitable for many wounds, do not require local anaesthetic and leave less scar than sutures. They cannot, however, be applied

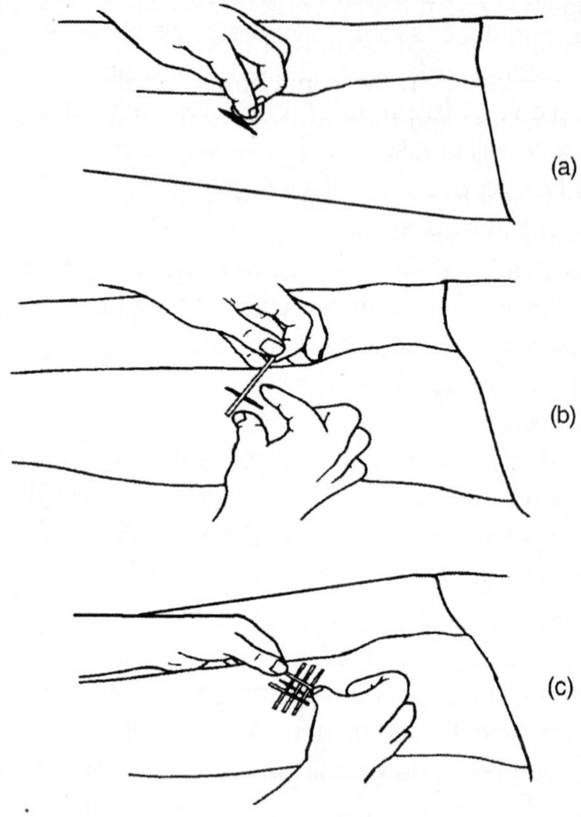

Fig. 17.1: *Steristripping technique. (a) After a thorough cleaning of the wound, wipe the skin on either side of the wound with techt. benzene. (b) Pinch the edges together and lay the strips across it. (c) Leave gaps between the strips and finish by lying two anchor strips a parallel to the wound.*

to hairy areas such as the scalp, and if the wound is over a joint, they will probably be pulled apart by tension in the skin as movement occurs.

The skin on either side of a wound should be prepared by having tinct benzene spray wiped over it to improve its adhesive properties. For most wounds 3 mm strips will suffice; 6 mm or 12 mm are available for bigger wounds. The strip should be attached first to one side of the wound. The wound is then pulled together and the strip stuck down onto the skin the other side. In large or ragged wounds, it may be necessary to perform a two-stage closure, using some strips initially to approximate the wound edges, and then proceeding to close the wound fully with further strips, removing the first strips in the process. A gap should be left between strips to allow for drainage of any fluid from the wound. Finally, anchoring strips should be applied parallel to the wound to distribute skin tension evenly.

If tissue glue is used (Histoacryl) it should be remembered that it is only suitable for simple lacerations less than 3 cm long and should not be used around the eyes or mouth. *Cockerill and Sweeting* recommend the use of forceps to oppose the two skin edges and suggest one nurse should apply gentle lateral pressure to elongate the wound while the other brings the skin edges together with finger pressure which should be maintained for a minute or until the glue becomes opaque to ensure bonding has occurred. As with steristrips there is the advantage of not requiring infiltration with local anaesthesia. It is therefore very useful in treating children with minor lacerations. Minor scalp lacerations can be effectively dealt with by simply tying together strands of hair from either side of the wound.

DRESSING THE WOUND

The optimum dressing should produce a moist, sterile environment with minimum trauma to newly forming tissue. Dressings which shed loose fibres into the wound will significantly delay healing. They should therefore be free from toxic or particulate material. Additionally, they should cause the minimum interference to the patient's normal activity, remain in place as long as required and be easily removed.

Plain dry gauze should not be in direct contact with the wound itself because it absorbs blood and exudate to form a hard, adherent mass that can be very difficult and painful to remove. One of the non-adherent proprietary dressings should be used in contact with the wound itself. *Eyre* has argued strongly against the use of the traditional paraffin impregnated gauze dressing for abrasions and other wounds, as there are many superior dressings now available which have far less of a problem with regard to adherence and 'strike through', i.e., the dressing soaking through to the outside with wound exudate. *James* is equally critical of these traditional dressings in A & E. Antibiotic impregnated gauze should never be used as it is expensive, ineffective and contributes to the development of resistant strains of bacteria.

The dressing may be secured to the skin with a hypoallergenic tape (e.g., Micropore) applied longitudinally as any swelling may give rise to circulatory impairment if there is a circumferential constriction around the limb or digit. Many modern dressings though are self-adhesive. The use of an elasticated tube type of bandage (e.g., Tubigrip) is recommended, rather than the traditional crape bandage, to complete the dressing. It is cheaper, easier to apply, gives a more even pressure over the limb with no risk of the wrinkles that can cause skin problems, and will stay in place far more effectively than a crape bandage.

Finger dressings can be retained with a tubular bandage (e.g., Tubinette), the important point being to tie the bandage at the wrist, and not at the base of the digit, in order to avoid the risk of circulatory impairment. If swelling is anticipated, the hand should be placed in a high arm sling. The use of Flamazine cream or Granuflex for finger tip injuries is highly effective compared to traditional dressings.

Head wounds may need a pressure bandage even after suture. A size F Tubigrip, 10 cm long, worn as a headband provides a very simple and effective solution to the problem, rather than the intricacies of head bandaging so beloved of the first aid manuals. Similarly, the elasticated tube bandages (e.g., Netelast) provide a better means of securing dressings to the trunk than does the traditional body bandage.

TETANUS VACCINATION

The effectiveness of the anti-tetanus immunization programme in the UK can be judged from the fact that there are no more than one or two dozen cases per year compared to the death toll from tetanus of approximately a million per year in developing countries.

The adsorbed tetanus toxoid that is given to patients in A & E units is a form of active immunization in that it stimulates the patient to manufacture their own antibodies. *Wardrope* and *Smith* recommend that a full course be completed by two subsequent injections at monthly intervals and that the average adult needs a booster at ten-yearly intervals thereafter. Anti-tetanus injections are a normal part of the childhood injections received in the UK. Therefore, any child that has had its triple injections as an infant will have received anti-tetanus cover.

If the patient states that they have never received any anti-tetanus immunization, it is possible to give passive immunity in the form of the appropriate human immunoglobulin if the medical staff assess the risk as being significant.

CLOSED SOFT TISSUE INJURY

The usual aim is to treat closed soft tissue injury conservatively by rest and support. Swelling can be reduced by elevation and ice packs if necessary. Gradually the area can be mobilized as pain and swelling ease off. A tubular support bandage should be used to lend support to the injury in this stage. If a sprain of the ankle is so severe as to prevent full weight-bearing, consideration should be given to plaster of Paris to immobilise the injury. Crape bandage is of little effective use.

ABSCESSES AND INFECTED WOUNDS

Abscesses are commonly treated by surgical incision and drainage, under general or local anaesthesia. The appropriate preparation of the patient is, therefore, required in line with hospital procedure, together with a full *explanation* of what is *to happen and how long* the procedure will take.

In dressing an old infected wound or a recently drained abscess, the principles of providing a sterile moist environment which can heal from the bottom up remain. In a review of the research,

Walsh and *Ford* have shown that traditional solutions such as mercurichrome and the chlorine-based antiseptics (Eusol, Chloramine T) are ineffective and potentially very harmful. The authors conclude that they should be withdrawn from use and point out that there are many far superior new products on the market to debride and dress infected wounds (e.g., Iodosorb and Granuflex). Although more expensive per dressing, they are cheaper in the long run since they achieve healing much more quickly and safely, requiring far fewer dressings and much less nursing time.

The patient will usually be discharged with a course of antibiotics and analgesics. The nurse should ensure that the patient understands the labels on the bottles and knows which are the analgesics and which are the antibiotics. The patient also must understand the need to complete the full course of antibiotics even if the infection appears to clear up before completion. The nurse can remember that the patient's care from now on will be self-care until they return for their next appointment when the nurse will be able to check progress on the healing of the abscess. The use of a wound assessment chart to monitor progress is essential for professional nursing care, although the change involved in introducing such a chart needs careful management. If necessary, patients may be given dressings to take home and may change the dressing themselves, provided that correct instruction is given in A & E first. The value of developing a self-care approach to nursing in the mode of Orem is evident from just this one common example of A & E care.

SELF-CARE

It is important that the patient be instructed in self-care of the injury before discharge. Key points include the need for elevation, keeping the dressing dry and clean, the length of time until dressing or suture removal, and instructions about how to remove the dressings or where to go to get the sutures removed. The patient should be alerted about the signs of infection and instructed to return immediately if there is any suspicion of infection. If a full course of tetanus is required, the patient should be given a card with the dates of the next two injections and the nurse should emphasise the importance of the follow-up injections. In this case, the nurse is filling the educative/supportive role of *Orem* after the partly compensatory role which kill have been filled at an earlier stage during treatment.

EVALUATION

All dressings performed by junior staff should be checked before the patient is discharged, for if they are done incorrectly, they go home wrong and remain wrong.

In many respects, the only real evaluation of treatment is if the patient returns or not. If the patient does not return, the assumption is that the nursing interventions have been successful. If the patient does return with a problem, however, the nursing staff should try to see how nursing care could have been better carried out. This will benefit other patients in the future. In order to evaluate the effectiveness of self-care instruction, it is essential to question the patient to see that they fully understand what has been taught.

STUDY–QUESTIONS

1. What do you mean by injuries?
2. Elaborate the wounds and its various types.
3. Discuss the different types of haemorrhage or bleeding.
4. Describe the sprains in brief.

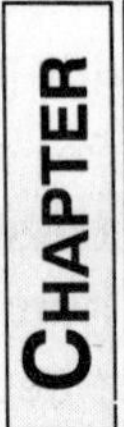

18

CHAPTER

HEAD INJURY

INTRODUCTION

The most important part of the body the brain has relatively incompressible tissues. Therefore, any force applied to it will be immediately transmitted through the tissue. This means that a blow delivered to one side of the head can produce brain injury on the opposite side, as the brain, which is independent of the skull, impinges on the inner surface of the skull.

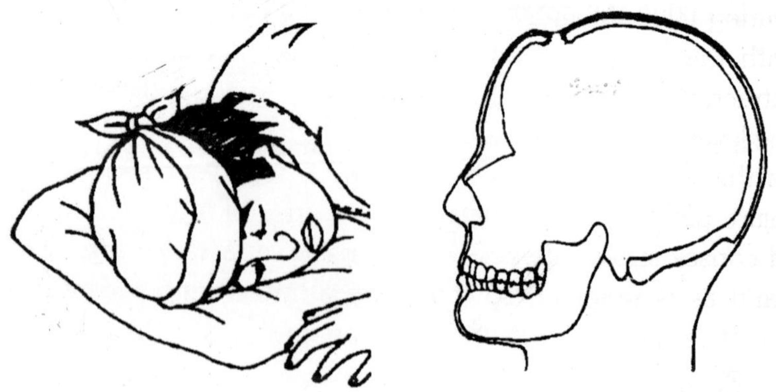

Fig. 18.1: *Head Injury.*

The skull forms a closed box. The clinical implication of this is that if any bleeding occurs within the skull, raised intracranial pressure will result as there is nowhere for the haematoma to expand, other than to force the brainstem through the tentorial notch or foramen magnum. This condition is known as brainstem herniation.

Bullock and *Teasdale,* estimate that the patients having head injury account for 10 per cent of the workload of the A & E service. Despite this, the majority of head injuries seen in A & E are simple concussions. In concussion, after impacting on the inner surface of the skull, the brain suffers a brief interruption to the reticular activating system. This causes a short period of unconsciousness and amnesia. Bruising or contusion of the brain surface leads to more significant injury and neurological disturbance.

A much more serious injury occurs when a blood vessel is torn, leading to haemorrhage and haematoma formation in either an epidural (between dura and skull) or subdural (below the dura) location, or within the brain itself. North American studies have shown mortality rates for epidural haematoma of 25-50 per cent and for subdural haematoma 70 per cent, indicating the seriousness of these injuries.

In such major injuries, there is often a short period of unconsciousness after which the patient regains consciousness. During this period of consciousness, the haematoma associated with the bleeding blood vessel develops, leading to a rise in intracranial pressure which will cause a gradual diminishing in the level of consciousness. This period of consciousness is known as the 'lucid interval', and the reason for observation of head injury patients is to try to detect evidence of a diminishing level of consciousness, associated with rising intracranial pressure, as early as is possible, so that surgical intervention (burr holes) might relieve the pressure and improve the outcome.

Raised intracranial pressure or haematoma formation may manifest itself by compression of the third cranial nerve (oculomotor) which controls the iris and hence the size of the pupil. A sluggishly reacting or dilated pupil is evidence of compression of the *oculo-motor* nerve if it is associated with diminished level of consciousness. There are a variety of other causes of unequal or nonreactive pupils unassociated with head injury. It must be emphasized that this is a late sign that will develop after a fall in the level of consciousness.

Skull fracture is not a very reliable guide to the seriousness of the injury, as many patients with a fractured skull have no significant neurological deficit, while other patients sustain serious brain damage without a fracture.

Two types of skull fracture are important, however. First, if the fracture is an open one, there is the risk of infection which may involve the skull itself (osteomyelitis) or the meninges surrounding the brain leading to meningitis. For an *open fracture* of the skull, there does not need to be a scalp wound as the fracture may be through the base of the skull, communication with the fracture occurring via one of the Eustachian tubes, the mouth or one of the ears. Secondly, if the skull fracture is depressed, the piece of bone pressing on the brain may act as an irritable focus and may cause fitting. A CSF leak may occur due to a tear in the meninges and as a consequence there is the risk of intracranial infection.

ASSESSMENT

To measure the level of consciousness and changes that occur in that level as this will give the first warning of rising intracranial pressure. It is essential to establish a baseline level of consciousness, and the nearer that baseline is to the time of the accident the better. Witnesses, relatives, ambulance crew and policemen are all key personnel who can help nurses to estimate what the patient's level of consciousness was before arrival in A & E. The importance of level of consciousness as a guide to head injury progress cannot be overemphasized.

Such an assessment must avoid subjective terms like 'semi-conscious' or 'drowsy' which mean different things to different people. The objective *Glasgow coma scale* is, therefore, recommended. On this scale, consciousness is assessed in terms of motor response, verbal response and minimum stimulus required to produce eye opening.

In assessing motor response to painful stimuli, the nurse is recommended to apply pressure to the nail bed of one of the patient's fingers with a pen or similar object and his/her own thumb. Note whether the arm is withdrawn towards the patient's body (flexion to pain) or extended away from the body (extension to pain). This latter extensor response indicates brainstem compression, a very serious condition.

In order to determine if the patient lost consciousness, in the absence of witnesses, the nurse should ask the patient to recall the accident. A gap in recall indicates the strong likelihood of unconsciousness, although this period may not be as long as the period of amnesia. Retrograde amnesia refers to a period of amnesia before the accident, while post-traumatic amnesia refers to amnesia after the accident.

In assessing pupil size and response, light of the same intensity should be used in each eye. The nurse should also be checking that when light is shone in one eye, the other responds as well. Unequal pupils in an alert, orientated patient are highly unlikely to indicate any head injury pathology as unequal pupils are a late sign following diminished level of consciousness due to raised intracranial pressure.

Physical signs that should be looked for include scalp wounds. Scalp wounds should alert the A & E team to the possibility of open fractures of the skull and of hypovolaemic shock which can be greatly exacerbated by profusely bleeding scalp wounds, if not primarily caused by such wounds, especially in the elderly. An important sign to look out for is bruising around the eyes (periorbital ecchymosis)—often called 'raccoon eyes'; this indicates an intraorbital fracture or basilar skull fracture. Bruising appearing 12 to 24 hours after injury, behind the ears in the mastoid area, is known as Battle's sign and also indicates basilar skull fracture.

Further evidence of a fracture of the base of the skull is provided by CSF leakage from the nose (rhinorrhoea) or the ear (otorrhoea). Bleeding from within the ear also indicates a fracture of the base of the skull. If there is fluid leaking from the nose, the patient should not be allowed to blow the nose as this could cause contamination of the meninges.

The development of any obvious limb weakness should be reported as this suggests damage to the motor centres in the brain. The nature and duration of any fits must be carefully documented, and medical attention drawn to their presence immediately.

In monitoring the vital signs, respiratory rate is vital, as brain damage may involve the respiratory centre leading to disturbance of both depth and rate of breathing. Respirations may become progressively more shallow and gradually fade away. The temperature regulating centre is thought to be adjacent to the hypothalamus and damage in this region can lead to hyperthermia (temperatures over 40°C). The patient may however be hypothermic as a result of lying still for a period of time after the injury in a cold environment. An accurate baseline temperature is therefore required, taken rectally where appropriate.

A late sign of serious head injury is a rising BP and a slowing pulse. This is explained in terms of the raised intracranial pressure making the heart beat more strongly as blood has to be forced into the brain in order to overcome capillary resistance. Baroreceptors that are situated in the carotid arteries monitor blood pressure and in response to a rising blood pressure act via the cardiac centre in the brain to slow the heart rate. This is the same mechanism responsible for increasing the heart rate when the blood pressure falls.

Assessment of children after head injury requires the nurse to allow for the varying stages of cognitive development. Information from the parent about normal behaviour is invaluable if the nurse is to observe abnormal behaviour. As *Harrison* (1991) states, the normal observation of adult head injured patients requires adaptation to suit the needs of children and her paper gives a good account of such procedure.

INTERVENTION

Administration of high concentration oxygen to head injury patients is beneficial because it reduces cerebral CO_2 levels, and high levels of CO_2 in the brain cause cerebral oedema, thereby raising intracranial pressure further.

In handling and moving head injury patients, the nurse must realize the possibility of spinal injury. Unconscious patients must be assumed to have a spinal injury until proven otherwise, and great care should be taken even if the patient is conscious. The absolutely vital role of the nurse is the scrupulous monitoring of the level of consciousness, and the maintenance of the patient's airway and respiration.

One final word of caution concerning the nursing management of head injury–many apparently unconscious patients have surprisingly accurate recall of events that occurred and of words that were spoken while they were 'unconscious' in hospital. Perhaps a more accurate description is to say they are 'unresponsive' but possibly aware or 'conscious' of what is said in their presence. Nursing staff should bear this in mind while looking after such patients and talk and behave at all times as if their patient can hear every word they say, because they just might.

Medical interventions that will require nursing support include intubation and ventilation of the patient in order to ensure adequate oxygenation of the brain and airway management, a detailed neurological exam, X-rays, possibly CAT (Computerised Axial Tomography) scanning to define areas of bleeding in the brain accurately (this may be done under general anaesthetic), anticonvulsant or antibiotic therapy as required, and possibly in extreme cases, burr holes which will be drilled in the skull to relieve intracranial pressure and allow clot evacuation. An osmotic diuretic, mannitol, may be given to try to shrink the brain by reducing oedema. This requires 'catheterization but may help as a temporary measure pending transfer to specialist neurosurgical care.

The administration of powerful opioid analgesics in multiply-injured patients is not advisable if there has been head injury, as they have a depressing effect on the level of consciousness. The mistake may be made of assigning a decreased level of consciousness to the effect of the drug, when in fact it is due to rising intracranial pressure. Entonox should also not be used with confused patients or where a serious head injury has occurred.

The vast majority of patients seen in A & E will fortunately have only suffered minor head injury and will be discharged home. Medical criteria for admission or neurosurgical consultation may be found in Sinclair. Symptoms such as dizziness, headaches, irritability, poor concentration and memory loss may last for days afterwards and a study by *Lowdon et al.*, reported that among a sample of 114 such patients, 90% reported these symptoms lasting up to two weeks after injury. It is important that the nurse discuss these symptoms with the patient and a friend or relative, and also stress the need for the patient to be brought back to hospital if they persist or worsen.

EVALUATION

It is essential that senior nursing staff ensure that junior staff understand fully the reasons why they are performing the repeated observations that they are carrying out on the head injury patient. If junior staff do not understand fully, the observations will not be performed accurately and the significance of some vital change will go unreported. Senior staff should monitor the accuracy of their juniors' observations, doing so discreetly and using such a process as a teaching tool.

STUDY–QUESTION

Write a short note on head injury.

***

19

CHAPTER

Accidents: Road, Air and Fire

INTRODUCTION

An accident is a specific, identifiable, unexpected, unusual and unintented external event which occurs in a particular time and place, without apparent cause but with marked effect. It implies a generally negative probabilistic outcome which may have been avoided or prevented had circumstances leading up to the accident been recognized, and acted upon, prior to its occurrence.

Narrowly defined, the designation may refer only to the event, while not including the circumstances or results of the event; i.e., 'accident' is constrained to an immediate incident, the occurrence of which results in an unplanned outcome. In common use, however, 'accident' may include the entire interacting circumstantial framework (chance, pre-existing, or uncontrolled dynamically developing conditions; commonplace actions; random time and place; participants; etc.) leading up to, including, and resulting from, the accident's immediate occurrence.

Accidents of particularly common types (auto, fire, etc.) are investigated to identify how to avoid them in the future. This is sometimes called root cause analysis, but does not generally apply to accidents that cannot be deterministically predicted.

For example, a root cause of an uncommon and purely random accident may never be identified, and thus future similar accidents remain "accidental."

Physical examples include unintended collisions or falls, being injured by touching something sharp, hot, or electric, or ingesting poison. Non-physical examples are unintentionally revealing a secret or otherwise saying something incorrectly, forgetting an appointment, etc.

The word accident conveys a sense that the losses are due exclusively to fate. Perhaps this is what gives accident its most potent appeal – the sense that it exonerates participants from responsibility. Accident also conveys a sense that losses are devoid of predictability. Yet the purpose of studying safety is to examine factors that influence crashes. Some crashes are purposeful acts for which the term accident would be inappropriate even in popular use. At least a few percent (perhaps as much as 5 per cent of driver fatalities are suicides, while a lesser number are homicides. Very few of the deaths that are suicides or homicides can be identified as such. When a severely damaged vehicle with a dead driver is observed, saying the driver was killed in a traffic crash describes in simple terms what is observed; calling it an accident implies you know more than you do.The problem of red light running and speeding has galvanized a broad range of professional communities interested in reducing deaths and injuries caused by red light runners.

ROAD TRAFFIC ACCIDENTS

Road traffic accidents are increasing in number and in severity. With the development of high-speed motorways, multiple collisions and involvements are becoming more common, particularly in times of reduced visibility, fog, or torrential rain. Cars rapidly lose control by skidding on smooth surfaces such as ice and by aquaplaning on water.

When confronted with a road traffic accident you must first carefully assess the situation to make sure that you and your car are visible and not at risk of being hit by another vehicle. Pull well away from the traffic stream if possible, as many 'samaritans' have been killed or severely injured.

Assess the position of the cars in the accident, turn off ignition and ensure no smoking, particularly if there is a smell of fuel. Detach the batteries if necessary. Check the airway of any people who are injured, unconscious or trapped. Blood, vomit, or dentures may need to be cleared, and the position of the patient's head should he adjusted carefully to improve air entry. Quickly examine the patient, assessing fractures, shock and wounds. If there is excessive bleeding, treat this by the application of a firm pad and bandage, with supplementary splintage if necessary.

If the patient is trapped in the scat, leave him alone unless he is in danger from fire or further damage. Send for assistance rapidly to the fire and ambulance services. It is important to inform the ambulance service that the casualties are trapped or there is some other serious hazard, because in some areas of the UK the ambulance service can call on appropriately equipped and trained doctors to attend the scenes of accidents. This may be a hospital-based flying squad or volunteer immediate care doctors belonging to Schemes Affiliated to the British Association for Immediate Care (BASICS). This saves time and improves the patients' chance of recovery.

Attempts should be made to count the passengers, as quite often passengers are thrown from the car and may travel several yards landing behind hedges or in ditches. Children may be lying on the floor of the car and should be looked for. On the whole, it is better to leave trapped patients in the vehicle until the emergency services arrive unless there is considerable risk, in which case swift action should be taken with as many people as possible to move the patient rapidly and steadily, preferably after applying splints. In this situation be careful of the cervical and thoracic spine; move the patient 'in one piece', using as many of the bystanders as possible. He should then be placed in a position of safety; if unconscious in the recovery position, otherwise on his back. If he has a chest injury, he may be more comfortable sitting up.

What Happened

History:

From the patient

From bystanders

Note damage to vehicles which may give clues to the type of injury to be expected. Count all casualties. Is anyone known to be missing?

What does the Casualty Feel? (Symptoms)

- Pain
- Breathlessness
- Loss of normal sensation
- Nausea
- Faintness
- Disorientation
- Loss of memory
  - *For events before the incident*
  - *For events after the incident*
- Thirst
- Palpitations
- Cold, clammy skin

Information Gained by Examination (Signs)

- Adequacy of:
  - *Airway*
  - *Breathing*
  - *Circulation (and control of bleeding)*
  - *Colour*
  - *Conscious level*
  - *Eyelash reflex*
- Swelling

— Deformity
— Bruising
— Tenderness
— Incontinence
— Temperature

ROAD-TRAFFIC SAFETY

Road-traffic safety aims to reduce the harm (deaths, injuries, and property damage) resulting from crashes of road vehicles traveling on public roads. Harm from road-traffic crashes is greater than that from all other transportation modes (air, sea, space, off-terrain, etc.) combined.

ROAD-TRAFFIC CRASH

Road-traffic crashes are one of the world's largest public health and injury prevention problems. The problem is all the more acute because the victims are overwhelmingly young and healthy prior to their crashes. According to the World Health Organization more than a million people are killed on the world's roads each year.

Road-traffic safety deals exclusively with road-traffic crashes – how to reduce their number and their consequences. A road-traffic crash is an event starting on a public road involving a road vehicle that results in harm. For reasons of clear data collection, only harm involving a road vehicle is included. A person tripping with fatal consequences on a public road is not included as a road-traffic fatality. To be counted a pedestrian fatality, the victim must be struck by a road vehicle.

CAR ACCIDENT

In an accident resulting from excessive speed, this concrete truck rolled over into the front garden of a house. There were no injuries, but significant damage was caused.Minor collisions such as this one are the most common type of crash.

A car accidentor car crash is an incident in which an automobile collides with anything that causes damage to the automobile, including other automobiles, telephone poles, buildings or trees, or in which the driver loses control of the vehicle and damages it in some other way, such as driving into a ditch or rolling over. Sometimes a car accident may also refer to an automobile striking a human or animal. Car crashes — also called road traffic accidents (RTAs), traffic collisions, auto accidents, road accidents, personal injury collisions, motor vehicle accidents (MVAs), — kill an estimated 1.2 million people worldwide each year, and injure about forty times this number (WHO, 2004).

LEGAL CONSEQUENCES

Car collisions usually carry legal consequences in proportion to the severity of the crash. Nearly all common law jurisdictions impose some kind of requirement that parties involved in a collision (even with only stationary property) must stop at the scene, and exchange insurance or identification information or summon the police. Failing to obey this requirement is referred to as hit and run and is generally a criminal offence. Most car claims are settled without using an attorney.

Parties involved in an incident may face criminal liability, civil liability, or both. Usually, the state starts a prosecution only if someone is severely injured or killed, or if one of the drivers involved was clearly grossly negligent or intoxicated or otherwise impaired at the time the accident occurred. Charges might include driving under the influence of alcohol or drugs, assault with a deadly weapon, manslaughter, or murder; penalties range from fines to jail time to prison time to death (although the death penalty is not applicable in many jurisdictions). It is notable that the penalties for killing and injuring with motor vehicles are often very much less than for other actions with similar outcomes.

As for civil liability, automobile accident personal injury lawsuits have become the most common type of tort. Because these cases have been litigated often in the developed First World nations, the legal questions usually have been answered in prior judgments. So, the courts usually need to decide only the factual questions of who is at fault, and their percentage of fault, as well as how much must be paid out in damages to the injured plaintiff by the defendant's insurer.

Another element of liability involves the administrative fines or license suspension/revocation that may be imposed by civil or criminal authorities when a driver has violated the rules of the road and thus the terms of a driver's license. Such complaint may be filed by a police officer or sometimes by other witnesses of an incident. In some jurisdictions such administrative penalties, may be imposed through quasi-criminal infractions; other jurisdictions do *not* recognize infractions and charge all violations, at a minimum, as misdemeanors or felonies.

BACKUP COLLISIONS

Backup collisions happen when a driver reverses the car into an object, person, or other car. Although most cars come equipped with rear view mirrors which are adequate for detecting vehicles behind a car, they are inadequate on many vehicles for detecting small children or objects close to the ground, which fall in the car's blind spot. Large trucks have much larger blind spots that can hide entire vehicles and large adults.

The National Highway Traffic Safety Administration found that back-up collisions most often:

- Occur in residential driveways and parking lots.
- Involve sport utility vehicles (SUVs) or small trucks.
- Occur when a parent, relative or someone known to the family is driving.
- Particularly affect children less than five years old.

The driver of the car backing up and hitting an object, a person, or another car is usually considered to be at fault. Prevention organizations suggest that parents use common sense, and also take safety measures such as installing cross view mirrors, audible collision detectors, rear view video camera and/or some type of reverse backup sensors.

COLLISION PREVENTION

Although many crashes are caused by behavior that is difficult to alter, by mechanical failure, or by road conditions, some technical solutions would automatically detect how close the driver is to the car in front and automatically adjust the car's acceleration to prevent the car from getting closer than the distance in which it can safely stop.

- *Sobriety detectors*—These locks prevent the ignition key from working if the driver breathes into one and is shown to have consumed alcohol.
- *Drifting monitors*—These devices monitor how close a vehicle is traveling to lane markers and, if it starts to drift toward or over the markers without the turn signal being activated, sounds an alarm.

The young and inexperienced drivers are by far the most likely to be involved in a car crash, and this has become an area of focus. Reasons suggested for this include inexperience combined with over-confidence, peer pressure, a desire to show off, and even neurological development arguments. In addition most serious collisions occur at night and when the car has multiple occupants. This has led to the following proposals:

- A "curfew" imposed on young drivers to prevent them driving at night.
- Requiring an experienced supervisor to chaperone the less experienced driver.
- Forbidding the carrying of passengers.
- Zero alcohol tolerance.
- Compulsory advanced driving courses.
- Vehicle restrictions (e.g., 'high performance' vehicles)
- Vehicle restrictions, not to flat windshield and pillar (car) for the best driver visibility angle.
- Requiring a sign placed on the back of the vehicle to notify other drivers of a less-experienced individual in the driver's seat.

AIR SAFETY

Air safety is a broad term encompassing the theory, investigation and categorization of flight failures, and the prevention of such failures through appropriate regulation, as well as through education and training. It can also be applied in the context of campaigns that inform the public as to the safety of air travel. No matter the speed and economy of any mode of transportation, if it is not perceived and demonstrated as safe, it will find few customers and, with few customers, unless it can still be priced to make a profit, the transportation mode will fail and fade from the scene.

Balanced against the speed of travel and the convenience of schedule, transportation by air must overcome various phobias of much of the traveling public: fear of heights, enclosed spaces, surrender of control. Human phobias are not a factor with cargo shipments. If the shipment does not arrive safely, the air carrier will find few customers seeking its service.

Air accidents tend to make national, even international, news. In major airliner accidents, hundreds of passengers may be affected. Add to this the number of family members who will be available at the airports at either end of the flight, ready for interviews, providing pictures of anguish on television news and the task before the industry becomes plain.

Therefore, the entire industry and the government bodies who regulate and support it put a great deal of effort into making air transportation not only appear safe, but demonstrating that it is the safest mode of transportation available.

Safety improvements have resulted from a wide variety of factors, including improved aircraft design, engineering and maintenance, the evolution of navigation aids, and safety protocols and procedures. It is often reported that air travel is the safest in terms of deaths per passenger mile.

With the spread of radio technology, several experimental radio based navigation aids were developed from the late 1920s onwards. These were most successfully used in conjunction with instruments in the cockpit in the form of Instrument landing systems (ILS), first used by a scheduled flight to make a landing in a snowstorm at Pittsburgh in 1938.

All of the ground-based navigation aids are rapidly being supplemented by satellite-based aids like Global Positioning System (GPS), which make it possible for aircrews to know their position with great precision anywhere in the world. With the arrival of Wide Area Augmentation System (WAAS), GPS navigation has become accurate enough for vertical (altitude) as well as horizontal use, and is being used increasingly for instrument approaches as well as en-route navigation. However, since the GPS constellation is a single-point of failure that can be switched off by the U.S. military in time of crisis, onboard Inertial Navigation System (INS) or ground-based navigation aids are still required for backup.

The effects of normal lightning on traditional metal-covered aircraft are well understood and serious damage from a lightning strike on an airplane is rare. However, as more and more aircraft, like the upcoming Boeing 787, whose whole exterior is made of non-conducting composite materials take to the skies, additional design effort and testing must be made before certification authorities will permit these aircraft in commercial service.

AIRBORNE WEATHER RADAR

Snowy and icy conditions are frequent contributors to airline accidents. The December 8, 2005 accident where Southwest Airlines Flight 1248 slid off the end of the runway in heavy snow conditions is just one of many examples. Just as on a road, ice and snow buildup can make braking and steering difficult or impossible if severe enough.

The icing of wings is another common problem that is well known and measures have been developed to combat it. The greatest concern regarding icing is that even a small amount of ice or coarse frost can greatly decrease the ability of a wing to develop lift. This could prevent an otherwise capable aircraft from safely taking off.

Airlines and airports expend considerable effort to ensure that aircraft are properly de-iced before takeoff whenever the weather threatens to create icing conditions. Modern airliners are designed to prevent ice buildup on wings, engines, and tails (empennage) by either routing heated air from jet engines through the leading edges of the wing, tail, and inlets, or on slower aircraft, by use of inflatable rubber "boots" that expand and break off any accumulated ice. Finally, airline dispatch offices keep close watch on weather along the routes of their flights, helping the pilots avoid the worst of possible inflight icing conditions. Pilots can also be equipped with an ice detector in order to leave icy areas they have inadvertently flown into.

ENGINE FAILURE

Although aircraft are now designed to fly even after the failure of one or more aircraft engines, the failure of the second engine on one side for example is obviously serious. Losing all engine power is even more serious, as illustrated by the 1970 Dominicana DC-9 air disaster, when fuel contamination caused the failure of both engines. To have an emergency landing site is then very important.

In the 1983 Gimli Glider incident, an Air Canada flight suffered fuel exhaustion during cruise flight, forcing the pilot to glide the plane to an emergency deadstick landing. The automatic deployment of the ram air turbine maintained the necessary hydraulic pressure to the flight controls, so that the pilot was able to land with only a minimal amount of damage to the plane, and minor (evacuation) injuries to a few passengers.

The ultimate form of engine failure, physical separation, occurred in 1979 when a complete engine detached from American Airlines Flight 191, causing damage to the aircraft that contributed significantly to the loss of control shortly afterwards.

METAL FATIGUE

Metal fatigue has occasionally caused failure either of the engine for example in the January 8, 1989 Kegworth air disaster, or of the aircraft body, for example the De Havilland Comets in 1953 and 1954 and Aloha Airlines Flight 243 in 1988. Now that the subject is better understood, rigorous inspection and nondestructive testing procedures are in place to attempt to identify potential problems.

DELAMINATION

Composite materials consist of layers of fibers embedded in a resin matrix. In some cases, especially when subjected to cyclic stress, the fibers may tear off the matrix, the layers of the material then separate from each other - a process called delamination, and form a mica-like structure which then falls apart. As the failure develops inside the material, nothing is shown on the surface; instrument methods (often ultrasound-based) have to be used.

Numerous modern aircraft have developed delamination problems, but most were discovered before they caused a catastrophic failure. Delamination risk is as old as composite material. Even in the 1940s, several Yakovlev Yak-9s experienced delamination of plywood in their construction.

STALLING

Stalling an aircraft (increasing the angle of attack to a point at which the wings fail to produce enough lift) is a potential danger, but is normally recoverable. Certain devices have been developed to warn the pilot as stall approaches. These include stall warning horns (now standard on virtually all powered aircraft), stick shakers and voice warnings. Two well known stall-related airline accidents, were British European Airways Flight 548 in 1972, and the United Airlines Flight 553 crash, while on approach to Chicago Midway International Airport, also in 1972.

FLY BY WIRE

Safety regulations control aircraft materials and the requirements for automated fire safety systems. Usually these requirements take the form of required tests. The tests measure flammability and the toxicity of smoke. When the tests fail, they fail on a prototype in an engineering laboratory, rather than in an aircraft.

Fire on board the aircraft, and more especially the toxic smoke generated, have been the cause of several incidents. An electrical fire on Air Canada Flight 797 in 1983 caused the deaths of 23 of the 46 passengers, resulting in the introduction of floor level lighting to assist people to evacuate a smoke-filled aircraft. Two years later a fire on the runway caused the loss of 53 lives, 48 from the effects of smoke, in the 1985 British Airtours Flight 28M. This incident raised serious concerns over the standard aircraft emergency evacuation time of ninety seconds, and calls for the introduction of smoke hoods or misting systems although both were rejected. It did result in the introduction of revised overwing emergency exit doors on certain new aircraft, and a small increase in the spacing between seats next to the emergency exit.

The cargo holds of most airliners are equipped with "fire bottles" (essentially remote-controlled fire extinguishers) to combat a fire that might occur in with the baggage and freight below the passenger cabin. This was due to a terrible accident in 1996. In May of that year ValuJet Airlines Flight 592 crashed into the Florida Everglades a few minutes after takeoff after a fire broke out in the forward cargo hold. All 110 aboard were killed.

The investigation determined that improperly packaged chemical oxygen generators (used for the drop-down oxygen masks in the aircraft cabin) had been loaded into the cargo hold. Oxygen generators produce oxygen through a chemical reaction that also generates hundreds of degrees of heat. When installed for use in the ceiling above the passenger seats they are surrounded by heat-resistant shielding and present no fire hazard. On this flight they had been put loosely into a cardboard box for shipment from a maintenance facility.

It is likely that one or more of the generators ignited, during or immediately after takeoff, producing an oxygen-rich environment. The cardboard box containing the generators would have quickly caught fire from the heat of the ignited generator. The fire spread to an aircraft tire that was also carried in the hold. Ordinarily the fire would have smothered itself, because of the airtight design of that cargo compartment. But the oxygen generators kept feeding oxygen to the fire, defeating the smothering design of the McDonnell Douglas DC-9 cargo hold. The fire rapidly burned through the passenger cabin floor, incapacitating all aboard with smoke and poisonous gases very quickly. The pilots, although having smoke masks and separate oxygen supplies, had no hope of maintaining control as control cables and electrical wiring burned through.

The maintenance facility (SabreTech) was subjected to large fines and ValuJet, due to this accident and other irregularities, was grounded. The airline reemerged as a smaller airline and eventually merged with AirTran Airways, a smaller carrier. Adopting the acquired airline's name, the airline has since provided safe service. For the airline industry, rules for the shipment of oxygen generators was severely restricted and cargo holds on larger airliners were required to have "fire bottles" installed.

BIRD STRIKE

Bird strike is an aviation term for a collision between a bird and an aircraft. It is a common threat to aircraft safety and has caused a number of fatal accidents. In 1988 an Ethiopian Airlines Boeing 737 sucked pigeons into both engines during take-off and then crashed in an attempt to return to the Bahir Dar airport; of the 104 people aboard, 35 died and 21 were injured. In another incident in 1995, a Dassault Falcon 20 crashed at a Paris airport during an emergency landing attempt after sucking lapwings into an engine, which caused an engine failure and a fire in the airplane fuselage; all 10 people on board were killed.

Modern jet engines have the capability of surviving an ingestion of a bird. Small fast planes, such as military jet fighters, are at higher risk than big heavy multi-engine ones. This is due to the fact that the fan of a high-bypass turbofan engine, typical on transport aircraft, acts as a centrifugal separator to force ingested materials (birds, ice, etc.) to the outside of the fan's disc. As a result, such materials go through the relatively unobstructed bypass duct, rather than through the core of the engine, which contains the smaller and more delicate compressor blades. Military aircraft designed for high-speed flight typically have pure turbojet, or low-bypass turbofan engines, increasing the risk that ingested materials will get into the core of the engine to cause damage.

The highest risk of the bird strike is during the takeoff and landing, in low altitudes, which is in the vicinity of the airports. Some airports use active countermeasures, ranging from a person with a shotgun through recorded sounds of predators to employing falconers. Poisonous grass can be planted that is not palatable to birds, nor to insects that attract insectivorous birds. Passive countermeasures involve sensible land-use management, avoiding conditions attracting flocks of birds to the area (eg. landfills). Another tactic found effective is to let the grass at the airfield grow taller (approximately 12 inches (30 centimetres)) as some species of birds won't land if they cannot see one another.

GROUND DAMAGE

Aircraft are occasionally damaged by ground equipment at the airport. In the act of servicing the aircraft between flights a great deal of ground equipment must operate in close proximity to the fuselage and wings. Occasionally the aircraft gets bumped or worse.

Damage may be in the form of simple scratches in the paint or small dents in the skin. However, because aircraft structures (including the outer skin) play such a critical role in the safe operation of a flight, all damage is inspected, measured and possibly tested to ensure that any damage is within safe tolerances. A dent that may look no worse than common "parking lot damage" to an automobile can be serious enough to ground an airplane until a repair can be made.

VOLCANIC ASH

Plumes of volcanic ash near active volcanoes present a risk especially for night flights. The ash is hard and abrasive and can quickly cause significant wear on the propellers and turbocompressor blades, and scratch the cabin windows, impairing visibility. It contaminates fuel and water systems, can jam gears, and can cause a flameout of the engines. Its particles have low melting point, so they melt in the combustion chamber and the ceramic mass then sticks on the turbine blades, fuel nozzles, and the combustors, which can lead to a total engine failure. It can get inside the cabin and contaminate everything there, and can damage the airplane electronics.

With the growing density of air traffic, encounters like this are becoming more common. In 1991 the aviation industry decided to set up Volcanic Ash Advisory Centers (VAACs), one for each of 9 regions of the world, acting as liaisons between meteorologists, volcanologists, and the aviation industry.

HUMAN FACTORS

Human factors including pilot error are another potential danger, and currently the most common factor of aviation crashes. Much progress in applying human factors to improving aviation safety was made around the time of World War II by people such as Paul Fitts and Alphonse Chapanis. However, there has been progress in safety throughout the history of aviation, such as the development of the pilot's checklist in 1937. Pilot error and improper communication are often factors in the collision of aircraft. This can take place in the air (1978 Pacific Southwest Airlines Flight 182) (TCAS) or on the ground (1977 Tenerife disaster) (RAAS). The ability of the flight crew to maintain situational awareness is a critical human factor in air safety. Failure of the pilots to properly monitor the flight instruments resulted in the crash of Eastern Air Lines Flight 40 in 1972 (CFIT), and error during take-off and landing can have catastrophic consequences, for example cause the crash of Prinair Flight 191 on landing, which also in 1972.

TERRORISM

Terrorism can also be considered a human factor. Crews are normally trained to handle hijack situations. Prior to the September 11, 2001 attacks, hijackings involved hostage negotiations. After the September 11, 2001 attacks, stricter airport security measures are in place to prevent terrorism using a Computer Assisted Passenger Prescreening System, Air Marshals, and precautionary policies. In addition, counter-terrorist organizations monitor potential terrorist activity.

Although most air crews are screened for psychological fitness, some may take suicidal actions. In the case of:

Egypt Air Flight 990, it appears that the first officer (co-pilot) deliberately dove his aircraft into the Atlantic Ocean while the captain was away from his station, in 1999 off Nantucket, Massachusetts. Motivations are unclear, but recorded inputs from the black boxes showed no mechanical problem, no other aircraft in the area, and was corroborated by the cockpit voice recorder.

AIRPORT DESIGN

Airport design and location can have a big impact on air safety, especially since some airports such as Chicago Midway International Airport were originally built for propeller planes and many airports are in congested areas where it is difficult to meet newer safety standards. For instance, the FAA issued rules in 1999 calling for a runway safety area, usually extending 500 feet (152 m) to each side and 1,000 feet (305 m) beyond the end of a runway. This is intended to cover ninety per cent of the cases of an aircraft leaving the runway by providing a buffer space free of obstacles. Since this is a recent rule, many airports do not meet it. One method of substituting for the 1,000 feet (305 m) at the end of a runway for airports in congested areas is to install an Engineered materials arrestor system, or EMAS. These systems are usually made of a lightweight, crushable concrete that absorbs the energy of the aircraft to bring it to a rapid stop. They have stopped three aircraft (as of 2005) at JFK Airport.

There is very limited research done on contagious diseases on aircraft. The two most common respiratory pathogens to which air passengers are exposed are parainfluenza and influenza. Certainly, the flight ban imposed following the attacks of September 11, 2001 restricted the ability of influenza to spread around the globe, resulting in a much milder influenza season that year, and the ability of influenza to spread on aircraft has been well documented. There is no data on the relative contributions of large droplets, small particles, close contact, surface contamination, and certainly no data on the relative importance of any of these methods of transmission for specific diseases, and therefore very little information on how to control the risk of infection. There is no standardisation of air handling by aircraft, installation of HEPA filters or of hand washing by air crew, and no published information on the relative efficacy of any of these interventions in reducing the spread of infection.

FIRE

Fire spreads very quickly, so warn any people at risk and alert the fire service immediately. Without putting yourself at risk, do your best to help everyone if fire occurs in a building or house. Shut the doors behind you look for the notices giving the location of the fire exits and assembly points. Familiarize yourself with guidelines at your work place.

A fire needs three components to start it and keep it going. They are ignition (an electric spark or naked flame), a source of

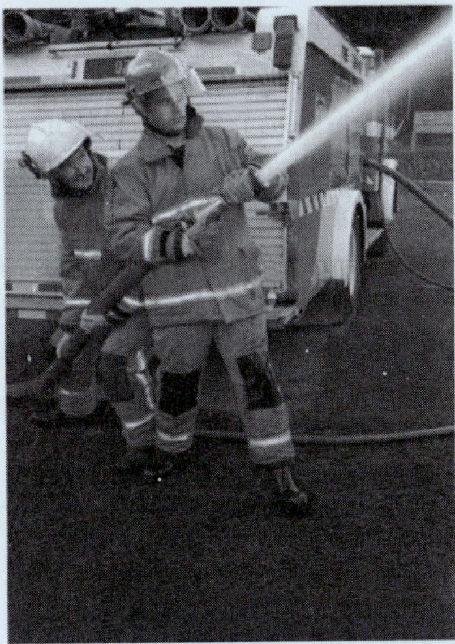

Fig. 19.1: *Fire.*

fuel such as petrol, wood, or fabrics, and oxygen (air). Remove any one of these and you break this triangle of fire. For example, switch off electricity, remove combustible materials and shut door on a fire, smoother flames with an impervious substance such as blanket or wood.

Treatment: The casualty must be prevented from panicking and rushing outside. Any movement or breeze will fan the flames. Quickly lay the casualty down with the burning side uppermost and put off the flames by dousing the victim with water, or other non-inflammable liquid. Wrap the casualty tightly in a coat, curtain blanket, rug or other heavy fabric. Then lay him on the ground. This starves the flames of oxygen (air) and puts them out.

FIREARM INJURY

These are the injuries that are caused by the high velocity bullets or pellets. In such cases note the following:

1. Nature of injury weather homicidal, suicidal. Or accidental most of these injuries are homicidal.

2. Time, place of the incidence and name of the accused and the weapon used.
3. Note the site of entry and exit, look for any discoloration around the entry site that could be due to the gunpowder, dirt, grease, or smoke.
4. Keep any pellets, or bullets that you find during examining the patient, seal it and send to the police.
5. Take off the clothes covering the site of injury and mark on it the bullet entry or exit point, seal it and send it to the police.
6. Always do the X-ray of the site.

STUDY–QUESTIONS

Write a short note on:

(a) Road accident.

(b) Air accident.

(c) Fire.

20

CHAPTER

IMPAIRED CONSCIOUSNESS AND DROWNING

INTRODUCTION

Unconsciousness is a serious state, so the patient's condition may cause anxiety and worry to the first aider. However, prompt, efficient action which secures a good airway and removes any obstruction such as blood, vomit or dentures may prevent complications and save the life of the patient. The primary cause of unconsciousness the patient becomes unconscious as the immediate result of any injury or a disease affecting the central nervous system. In psychogenic hysteria etc., the patients are not truly unconscious but appear unconscious.

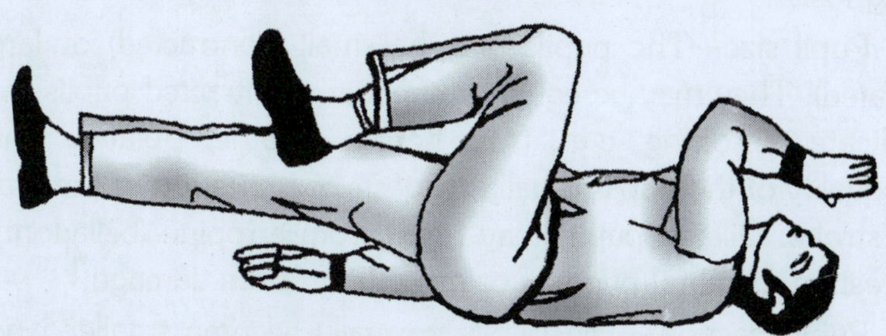

Fig. 20.1: *Unconsciousness*

DEPTH OF UNCONSCIOUSNESS

It is important that the level of consciousness is noted and timed. If there is any change in the level of consciousness, this must be noted and the time recorded. The levels described merge one into the other and there may be slow or rapid movement from one level to another. All these are of significance in establishing a diagnosis or assessing progress of the patient.

1. *Lucid*—The patient is cooperative and conscious.
2. *Confusion*—He is disorganized but will obey commands.
3. *Semi-coma*—The patient will only react to painful stimuli but not voice commands; unconscious.
4. *Coma*—There is no response to stimuli; deeply unconscious.

Glasgow coma Scale —This scale is widely accepted in hospitals and is an easily understood description of the level of consciousness. It gets rid of the vague expressions which have been used for many years to describe unconscious people.

Respiration—The breathing may be quick, shallow, stertorous (snoring) or irregular. Stertorous breathing tends to occur in deeper unconsciousness (coma) and may also be seen in stroke, epilepsy or severe head injuries, and in some cases of poisoning. Irregular breathing, particularly if there are short periods when breathing stops, is a bad sign. It may occur after severe head injury, poisoning or uraema.

Eyes—Examination of the eyes and the pupils and their reaction to light is always of great value in establishing the diagnosis.

Pupil size—The pupils may be small (contracted) or large (dilated). They may be equal or unequal. Contracted pupils may indicate poisoning, e.g., from heroin or other opiates, while inequality of the pupils usually suggests compression of the brain or stroke. Dilated pupils may result from atropine (belladonna) ingestion, cerebral hypoxia or other brain stem damage.

Pupil reaction—The pupils normally become smaller when exposed to light. This reaction is seen when raising the eyelids or shining a light into the eyes, when the pupils will become smaller. The light response may be absent in coma or poisoning from narcotics.

The pulse rate must be noted—A rapid pulse occurs in shock, fainting, collapse and sometimes concussion of the brain. A slow pulse may result from stroke or cerebral compression. Irregularity of the pulse occurs in diseases affecting the heart, and also in the later stages of poisoning.

Odour of breath—The odour of the breath should be carefully noted, as it may supply a clue in a lease of poisoning. The smell of alcohol should be noted but does not always indicate a diagnosis of drunkenness. The patient may in unconscious patients. Other factors, most notably a low blood sugar rather like urine, whilst in diabetes a faint aroma of acetone or nail may be noticed.

REASONS OF IMPAIRED CONSCIOUSNESS

There are many reasons why a person's level of consciousness might be diminished. The following section concentrates on some of the more common causes of patients presenting at A & E with impaired consciousness with the exception of head injury and the effects of drugs and alcohol.

1. *Cerebrovascular accident (CVA)*—The cause may be bleeding from a cerebral blood vessel leading to either a subarachnoid haemorrhage or intracerebral haemorrhage. The onset will be sudden in most cases. Alternatively, there may be occlusion of a blood vessel due to a thrombus (a more gradual onset) or an embolus (a sudden onset).
2. *Fits*—Fitting may be a sign of a range of pathological conditions although there may also be no apparent cause of the fitting behaviour (idiopathic epilepsy).

   In grand mal epilepsy, the problem is an abnormal discharge of electricity within the brain which first produces a characteristic aura if it is located near one of the sensory centres (e.g., smell, visual disturbance) and then goes on to produce a tonic period of some 30 seconds or so when the patient's musculature goes into spasm and the patient is, as a result, unable to breathe. This is followed by the clonic stage of convulsions which passes into a deep coma from which the patient gradually wakes up. At this stage, often referred to as the 'postictal stage', confusion is likely.

3. *Diabetes* — In hyperglycaemic states, the metabolism of fats leads to the formation of ketones whose effects on the brain lead to unconsciousness and brain damage if the ketotic state is not reversed. The body's efforts to excrete the excess glucose in the urine lead to dehydration, hypovolaemic shock and electrolyte imbalance. Ketone formation leads to acidosis which the body seeks to correct by reducing CO_2 levels in the blood (CO_2 dissolves in water to form a weak acid). Hence the deep, sighing respirations characteristic of the hyperglycaemic state.

   In hypoglycaemic states, the lack of blood glucose affects the brain to produce drowsiness, confusion and unconsciousness. As urine output has been normal, the patient will not be dehydrated or hypovolaemic.

4. *Acute infections and toxaemic states* — Any acute infection involving the brain, for example, meningitis or encephalitis, will obviously affect the level of consciousness. Furthermore, any infection that leads to hypoxia (e.g., chest infections) will diminish consciousness as will toxaemic states e.g., uraemia.

ASSESSMENT

The first step must always be to assess airway, breathing and circulation, before moving on to assessing level of consciousness. A history of the event together with any relevant medical history should be obtained.

An epileptic fit may be described or the patient may be known as a *diabetic.* In undressing the patient, clues such as Medic-Alert bracelets, sugar lumps, out-patient cards and injection sites should be searched for. Identification of the patient is essential, not only so that next of kin can be informed, but also so that hospital notes can be obtained.

In assessing vital signs, the nurse will find further evidence of the cause of the patient's problem. The person in a hyperglycaemic diabetic condition will be dehydrated and hypovolaemic. The CVA patient will often be hypertensive. Rapid respiratory rate will indicate hypoxia and a pyrexia an infection. The patient may also be hypothermia if they have been in a cold environment for several hours with impaired consciousness. A rectal temperature below 35°C indicates hypothermia.

Blood sugar should always be tested, using a needle prick stix test. Limb weakness should be assessed for evidence of hemiplegia (or monoplegia). Plantar reflexes should be tested by stroking the outer soles of the feet with a sharp object. An abnormal upward curling of the toes indicates an upper motor neurone lesion such as a CVA or a post-epileptic state. Extensor response to pain indicates a brain stem CVA.

A urine specimen should be tested, the hyperglycaemic patient's urine revealing glucose and probably ketones. A uraemic state will cause protein to appear in the urine. An unconscious diabetic patient may be catheterised to obtain a specimen as the presence of ketones in the urine is a very important medical sign.

INTERVENTION

If the patient is conscious but confused, steps must be taken to protect the patient from potential harm. Cot sides should be set up and carefully checked. There should be continual nursing observation and, if necessary, the patient can be nursed on a mattress on the floor. Reality orientation is required with the nurse telling the patient what has happened, what time it is and where the patient is, in order that the patient may make some sense out of the situation. The information should be kept simple as consciousness is impaired.

By providing reality orientation, nurses can help the patient hang on to reality. Try to imagine waking up in totally unfamiliar surroundings, with complete strangers standing around, a gap of maybe several hours in your consciousness and your mental processes impaired by illness. You will then appreciate the importance of reality orientation as a major nursing intervention.

Specific problems revealed by the assessment should be dealt with on their merits. Therefore, if the patient has had a fit, along with care of the patient in a confused *postictal state*, the possibility of the patient having a further fit should be considered. Observation is essential, with the aim of preventing accidental self-harm should a further fit occur. In such a situation, the patient is best left to get on with their fit, intervention being restricted to protecting the head if possible by using a blanket or pillow and by removing any objects that may harm the patient.

The nurse should not attempt to restrain the patient or to force an airway into the mouth during either the tonic or clonic stages. This is dangerous and can lead to either the patient's teeth being knocked out or the nurse accidentally being bitten. Once the patient has stopped convulsing, he or she should be turned into the recovery position. The nurse should only then consider the use of an airway and then only if the patient tolerates it. Incontinence may occur due to relaxation of muscle sphincters at this stage. Therefore, the nurse must be prepared to clean the patient accordingly.

If fitting is continuous and does not resolve after one attack, status epilepticus is said to be present. This serious condition requires medical intervention to control the fitting (to prevent anoxic brain damage). This intervention usually consists of intravenous diazepam or if needed a general anaesthetic and muscle relaxants to facilitate airway management and prevent further anoxic cerebral damage.

If assessment reveals that the patient is hypoglycaemic, and if the patient is able to drink, a glucose drink should be given immediately. If the patient cannot drink, IV dextrose 50 per cent is given via a butterfly needle; 50 ml is usually sufficient to restore the patient to a normal level of consciousness.

In a hyperglycaemic state, the medical staff will need to correct the dehydration rapidly with an IV infusion. The first litre is usually given as quickly as possible, together with a stat dose of intravenous insulin (one of the rapid-acting varieties). Nursing assistance will be required, together with accurate fluid balance and vital signs monitoring, and usually catheterization to test for ketones and manage the urine output.

If a pyrexia of over 39°C is present, active steps, such as fanning and tepid sponging, must be taken to reduce the temperature. This is because if it rises to 40°C or above, fitting will often develop. A space blanket should be used if the rectal temperature is below 35°C.

The possibility of an infection that could be transmitted to other patients in the department should be considered and the appropriate steps taken in line with hospital policy e.g., disposal of waste and linen.

Pressure area care does not begin on the wards. It begins in A & E, and this fact is particularly important for patients with impaired consciousness. The trolleys in most A & E departments are very hard, and delays in moving patients to the wards are common, therefore, patient care should include full pressure area care. Nurses should also check for incontinence which must be cleaned up at once to protect the skin and the patient's own self-image and pride. Nurses should make sure that the patient understands how to summon help if needed for the toilet or any other purpose. The phrase 'basic nursing care' is easily paid lip service to, but this should not be the case in A & E where with the help of Orem's model of nursing the patient's self-care demands should all be met.

EVALUATION

Frequent checks should be made of level of consciousness and orientation to assess progress and the effectiveness of reality orientation. Temperature monitoring will reveal the effectiveness of measures such as tepid sponging and the use of a fan. Finger prick tests allow capillary blood sugar to be checked frequently so the effectiveness of care of the patient with a diabetic problem can be evaluated. Regular examination of the patient is needed, to ensure intervention as frequently as required, if there is a risk of incontinence and pressure sores. After a patient has had a fit, it is important to check that there is no evidence of a head injury and to monitor level of consciousness subsequently during the postictal period.

DROWNING

Drowning is the result of complete immerse of the nose and mouth in water. Water enters the wind-pipe and lungs, clogging the lungs completely. The aim is to get the casualty on to dry land with minimum danger to yourself.

Treatment—Choose the safest way to rescue the casualty. If possible stay on land and reach with your hand a stick or a branch or throw a rope or float. Swim to the casualty and tow him only if you are a trained life-saver, or if the casualty is unconscious, it is safer to wade, if you can, than to swim.

The aim of first aid is to draw out water from lungs and to give artificial respiration, turn the victim face down with head to one side and arms stretched beyond his head. Infants or children could be held upside down for a short period, raise the middle part of the body with your hands round the belly. This is to cause water to draw out of the lungs and give artificial respiration until breathing comes back to normal. This may have to go on for as long as two hours.

STUDY–QUESTIONS

1. Describe the various causes of impaired consciousness.
2. How would you make a assessment in case of impaired consciousness?
3. Write a short note on drowning.

***

21 CHAPTER

POISONING, BITES AND STINGS

POISONING

Poisons are any harmful substances which when taken into the body in large quantities can damage the organ of digestion or, if absorbed into the blood may affect the vital organs cause harmful action on the human body, injuring health and even causing death. The majority of medicines if taken in excessive doses act as poison.

Poison enters the body through the mouth due to by eating or drinking poisonous substances. It may enter through lungs by inhaling household or industrial gases. It may enter the body by injection into the skin as a result of bites and stings. It is always best to shift the patient to the nearest hospital, as quickly as possible.

Routs of Poisoning

Poisons get into the body by

(a) Ingestion, i.e, swallowing.

(b) Inhalation, i.e., inhaling of gases.

(c) Injection by means of syringe and needle.

CAUSES OF POISONING

(i) Accidental poisoning—Due to contaminated food, poisonous fungi berries, clinical substance, overdoses and sleeping pills etc.

(ii) Suicidal poisoning—When a person ingests any harmful substance intentionally with a purpose to commit suicide.

(iii) Homicidal poisoning—It may be administered intentionally for killing enemies.

SOURCE OF POISONING

(i) Swallowed Poisons

Sometimes acids, alkalies, disinfectants etc., are swallowed by mistake. They burn the lips, tongue, throat, food passage and stomach and cause great pain. Other swallowed poisons cause vomiting, pain and later on diarrhoea. Poisonous fungi-berries, metallic poisons and stale food belong to the latter group. Some swallowed poisons affect the nervous system. To this group belong.

(a) Alcoholic drink when taken in large quantities.

(b) Tablets for sleeping, tranquillizers and pain killing drugs. All these victims must be considered as seriously ill. The symptoms are either fits or coma. Some poisons act on nervous system.

(ii) Inhaled Poisons

Fumes or gases from charcoal stoves, household gas, motor exhausts and smoke from explosions etc., cause choking which may result in unconsciousness in addition to difficulty in breathing.

(iii) Injected Poisons

Poisons get into the body through injection, bites of poisonous snakes and rabis dogs or stings by scorpions and insects. Danger to life is again by choking and coma.

(iv) Household Poisons

Many substances found in and about the home can be poisonous. These include liquid soap, some cosmetics, white spirit, rat poison etc. Children who are not aware of the consequences of eating these substances, fall an easy prey to these poisons. The symptoms and signs vary according to the nature of these poisons. In most cases, vomiting and abdominal pain are common symptoms. Children take medicines, found in medicine cabinets without knowing the consequences.

Even though most of them are not poisonous, if taken as per the directions of the doctor. If taken in larger doses than suggested, they act as poisons. So, always make sure that all bottles and jars containing substances are kept out of reach of children. It is important to distinguish between those poisons which are corrosive and burn the mouth and those which are not.

While giving first aid the first thing to do is to ensure that respiration and circulation of air are maintained. Then, it is necessary to decide as to what type of poison has been used. If a corrosive which will cause burning of lips, mouth and tongue or if paraffin or petroleum product which, though harmless in the stomach, would cause grave damage if inhaled, send quickly to the hospital. With all other poisons, the patient should be made to vomit by giving two table spoonfuls of salt in a glass of warm water or two teaspoonfuls of mustard in a glass of warm water, then send the patient to the hospital as quickly as possible.

SIGNS AND SYMPTOMS OF POISONING

Signs and symptoms of poisoning will depend on the poison consumed. General signs and symptoms are : Burning pain in alimentary canal, feeling of thirst, blood stained vomiting, extreme diarrhoea, diminished urine output, cyanosis, cold skin, pulse rate fast and feeble, difficulty in breathing, perspiration, convulsions and many casualties fall unconscious.

FIRST AID IN POISONING

1. Poisoning is a serious condition, which threatens life. Casualty must be taken to the hospital at once or doctor be sent for, with findings and if possible the name of the poison must be written on a chit and sent to the doctor.

2. Preserve all packets or bottles which first aider suspects to be poison and also preserve any vomitus, sputum and stool for doctor to examine.

Proceed as follows when the casualty is conscious

3. Aid vomiting by tickling the back of throat by inserting two fingers in throat or make him drink tepid water mixed with two tablespoons of common salt to a glass of water.
4. Do not induce vomiting if the poison was corrosive in nature. Corrosives are those chemicals which destroy or burn the tissues. These include strong acids or alkalies such as sulphuric acid, nitric acid and sodium hydroxide (caustic soda). Signs of corrosive poisoning are lips, mouth and skin show grey white or yellow patches. If the victim's mouth is burnt dilute the poison with water or milk to neutralize its corrosive effect. Treat any pain caused by corrosion with something soothing such as icecream or olive oil.
5. If the casualty is unconscious (i) do not induce vomiting. (ii) Make the casualty lie on his back on a flat hard bed without any pillow and turn the head to one side. As there is no pressure on the stomach and oesophagus (gullet) is horizontal, the vomited matter will not get into the air passages and tongue will not fall back closing the air passage. This positioning is also suitable for giving artificial respiration in case the casualty needs it. (iii) Sometime there is excess of vomiting. Under such conditions put the casualty in three quarter prone position.
6. Factories which use certain poisons should have the respective antidotes ready and displayed in an easily available place. The personnel should be taught about the use of antidotes, so that anyone can render assistance in case of emergency.

SPECIFIC POISONS

(i) Food Poisoning

This is due to the contamination of food by bacteria. It may also be due to incorrect cooking and storing. The most common bacteria present is staphylococci. This multiplies in food and produces a poisonous substance which causes dysentery like illness. Symptoms of food poisoning depend upon the type of poisoning. The patient feels nauseated and may already be vomiting. The patient may be suffering from abdominal pain and may have headache. At a later stage, diarrhoea may develop. There may appear symptoms of shock. Seek immediate medical aid. Follow the general treatment for poisoning. Make sure, the patient rests. Give him plenty of fluids to drink. If you have any doubt, arrange removal to hospital.

(ii) Drug Poisoning

This is caused by an accidental over dose of drug abuse. Drug abuse may be defined as the self-administration of a drug in a manner that is not according to approved medical or social patterns. Drugs can be inhaled, swallowed or injected into the body. Drugs commonly abused are narcotics, depressants, stimulants and hallucinogens. The symptoms depend on the drug and the quantity taken. The pupils of the eye may be abnormally dilated or contracted.

Narcotics are injected or taken in tablet form or inhaled. Breathing becomes difficult and, eventually, stops. The patient may have injection marks on the front of one or both the arms. When depressants are taken, breathing will be shallow. Patient's skin feels cold and clammy. Pulse will be weak and rapid. The patient may be unconscious.

When stimulants are taken, the patient will be excitable and sweating profusely. The patient may be suffering from tremors and hallucinations. If the patient has taken hallucinogens, he will be anxious and sweating. The patient may be behaving strangely. When an over dose of aspirin has been taken, the patient has abdominal pain and may be vomiting. He may be depressed and drowsy. He may complain of ringing in the ears. There will be difficulty in breathing. He may be sweating profusely. His pulse will be full.

While treating such patients, follow the general treatment for poisoning. Arrange for urgent removal to the hospital. You must be prepared to resuscitate.

(iii) Barbiturates

This is usually suicidal, though it may be accidental in children. They may eat sleeping tablets carelessly left around by the parents. The patient goes in to a deep sleep and then into coma with respiratory depression, low blood pressure, a quick and feeble pulse and a cold clammy skin emetic, given soon after the tablets are taken, will be effective as the drug has sedative action on the stomach. Early admission to the hospital should be arranged. In the meanwhile, the first aider must be on the look out for respiratory failure and be prepared to give artificial respiration.

(iv) Aspirin

It is used in large doses as a suicidal attempt. Its repeated and prolonged usage for the treatment of pain may irritate the lining of the stomach and produce haemorrhage. If taken in large doses, it may produce vomiting and its effect on the central nervous system is to produce confusion, convulsions, sweating, over breathing etc. Extensive gastric bleeding may also occur. The emetic is effective because of the slow rate of absorption. So, a doctor may wash out the stomach with good results.

(v) Carbon Monoxide

Common sources are, domestic gas, exhaust fumes from petrol engines etc. It may be accidental or suicidal. Giddiness, headache and tightness of the chest, loss of use of lower limbs and unconsciousness are common symptoms. The patient will have a characteristic pink appearance and may have stopped breathing.

(vi) Poisonous Plants

Certain plants grown in our garden as well as in the forest are dangerous if eaten or if one comes into contact with them. Laburnum, deadly night shade and death cap fungus are more common examples of plants which can poison the system. The severity of the condition will depend on how much is consumed.

If it is found that the patient has consumed poisonous plant, you must maintain an open air way and remove the patient to the hospital.

(vii) Alcohol Poisoning

Alcohol depresses the central nervous system. It affects different people in different ways. The drug affects the areas of higher reasoning within the brain. As the concentration of alcohol in blood increases, the behaviour of the patient becomes exaggerated and coordination will be affected.

Patient's breath may smell of alcohol. Patient may be vomiting. The patient may be partly conscious or fully unconscious. The patient may breathing deeply. Face will be moist and flushed. Pulse will be full and bounding. In later stages of unconsciousness, pulse may become rapid but weak. Breathing will be shallow. The patient's face will appears dry and look bloated. Eyes will be blood shot and pupils may be dilated.

Maintain a open air way. If the patient becomes unconscious or vomiting is likely, place her in the recovery position. If necessary, complete resuscitation. If there is any doubt about the condition of the patient make arrangements to remove the patient to the hospital.

(viii) Industrial Poisons

As a result of failure of a chemical plant, the workers may come in contact with dangerous chemicals or gases. Most common industrial poisons are gases. There are so many different poisonous substances that, it is impossible to give a list. Always remember that any patient suffering from the effects of gas or toxic fumes, needs air. While giving first aid, be sure that you yourself are not trapped in any fumes that remain in the area. Do not try to rescue a patient trapped in an enclosed space, if you are not equipped with and are not trained in the use of breathing apparatus and life lines.

BITES AND STINGS

1. Snake Bite

In countries where there are many venomous snakes, identification of the snake is important to enable appropriate treatment to be given. If the snake has been killed, it should be taken with the casualty to hospital. If in a zoo, it can be identified on the spot. Most people will not die because of the venom but from fear. There are more than 3,500 different kinds of snakes. Only about 250 of them are venomous. All snake bites are not fatal. Only a very small quantity of the venom might have been injected.

Symptoms and Signs—These depend to some extent on the particular venom, but general malaise, nausea, vomiting, confusion and difficulty with breathing and vision may be experienced. A shock state may develop. Small puncture wounds, usually two, may be visible at the site of the bite. As time passes, severe drooling of saliva may occur.

First Aid Treatment

1. Reassurance. Lay the casualty down.
2. If a limb is affected, immobilize it.
3. Call an ambulance immediately, stating that the casualty is a victim of snake bite.
4. Observe pulse, respiration and level of consciousness.
5. The bite is on the arm or leg, apply a constrictive bandage on the heart side of the bite, tight enough to obstruct and stop the flow of the venom to all the parts of the body. Do not tie it too firmly.
6. Wash the wound with soap and water, flush the wound with a lot of water.

2. Dog Bite

Dog bites are sometimes very serious. They may cause infection. If the animal is suffering from rabies, it will be transmitted to the casualty. The condition is known as *Hydrophobia*. Therefore, the dog must be chained and kept under observation for seven to ten days. If the dog is healthy after this period, there is no danger of rabies.

First Aid Treatment

All dog bites must be treated as potentially as bite by a rabies dog.

(a) To prevent rabies or other infections.

(b) To get medical aid.

(c) Wipe the saliva away from the wound.

(d) Wash the wound thoroughly, with plenty of soap and water.

(e) Cover the wound with a dry, sterile dressing. Do not put carbolic acid, nitric acid etc., on the wound within 1/2 hour of bite.

(f) Get medical aid or send the patient to the hospital for proper treatment of the wound and also the casualty.

3. Insect and Spider Bites

Mites, ticks and leeches are found in marshes and jungles. These animals do not bite but attach themselves firmly to the skin. Mites and ticks may carry Typhus and may transmit it to the person. Leeches are normally harmless, but they suck blood from the victim.

First Aid Treatment

(a) Don't try to remove the insects normally, their mouth parts may remain in the skin, due to that skin may get inflamed and infected.

(b) Put the burning end of a cigarette to the body of the ticks and leeches, they will fall off.

(c) Apply weak ammonia or bicarbonate of soda or antihistamine content. This will relieve irritation.

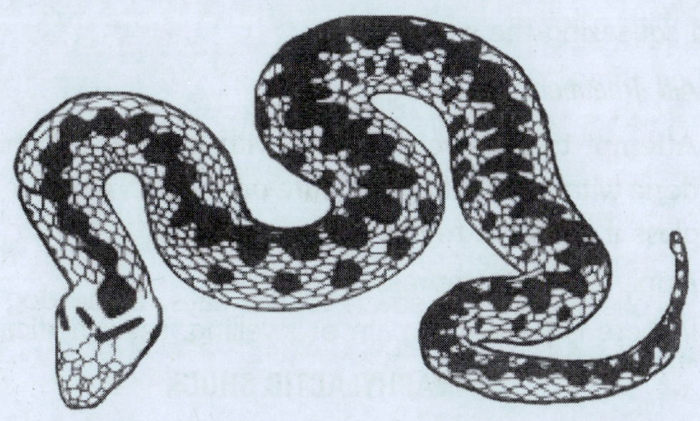

Fig. 21.1: *Vipera berus.*

(d) Mites are so small that they cannot be easily seen to be removed.

(e) Clean the suspected area of mite infestationand clean the area with methylated spirit.

(f) Application of salt results in leech dropping off.

4. Stings of Bees, Rasps, Fleas and Hornets

The stings of bees, rasps etc., can cause a lot of pain. The area may swell. Sometimes, the person may suffer from shock. Stings, including those of jellyfish and certain fish such as the weaver, may be very painful but are not usually a threat to life unless:

1. The individual is allergic to the venom.
2. Many stings are suffered.
3. The sting is in the mouth or throat causing swelling which may obstruct the airway, causing asphyxia.

First Aid Treatment

(a) A sting should be removed with forceps or with the tip of a sterilised needle.

(b) Apply weak ammonia or bicarbonate of soda or antihistamine ointment to the area. This will relieve the pain.

5. Bee and Wasp Stings

Following a sting, the poison sac and, in the case of bee stings, the sting itself will he left in the skin. It is essential to avoid squeezing the sac.

First Aid Treatment

1. Attempt to remove the sting with tweezers, if this can be done without exerting pressure on the sac. Use a magnifying glass if available to get a close up view.
2. Apply a cold compress.
3. If there is persistent pain or swelling, seek medical aid.

ANAPHYLACTIC SHOCK

Some individuals are so sensitive to foreign substances, such as the from an insect sting or a certain drug, that large amounts of the histamine are released in the body. This causes swelling around eyes as well as at the site of the sting, difficulty with breathing and — development of a shock state. This situation may occur within minutes

First Aid Treatment

1. Call for an ambulance immediately.
2. Maintain an open airway.
3. Lay the casualty down; treat for shock.
4. Cardiopulmonary resuscitation may be required; monitor pulse and respiration frequently.

STUDY–QUESTIONS

1. Describe the various sources of poisoning.
2. Write short notes on the following:
   (a) Food poisoning;
   (b) Anaphylactic shock;
   (c) Alcohol poisoning;
   (d) Snake bite; and
   (e) Insect and spider bites.

22 CHAPTER

FRACTURES: BONES AND JOINTS

INTRODUCTION

Fracture is the breaking or discontinuity of a bone. It could be either a crack or complete fracture but both are technically termed as a fracture. Fractures are usually thought of as being due to trauma. This is not always the case, however, as repeated stress on a bone can lead to its fracture by a process similar to mental fatigue. Such a fracture is logically known as a stress fracture and is commonly seen in the foot (metatarsal) or the lower limb (fibula). Alternatively, bone can be so weakened by disease that it fails with little or no force involved. This is known as a *pathological fracture* and is seen, for example, where a tumour has led to secondary deposits in the bone (bony metastases).

The vast majority of fractures are due to trauma, and these are described as direct or indirect.

In an *indirect fracture,* the break occurs at some point other than that where the force impacted against the bone. For example, a fall on an outstretched hand may lead to a fracture of the clavicle or wrist.

Conversely, a *direct fracture* occurs when the bone breaks at the point of impact; thus, an over-the-ball-tackle in football leads to a fractured lower third of tibia and fibula.

VARIOUS TYPES OF FRACTURE

If the fracture site is in direct contact with the outside environment, no matter how small the wound, it is an *open or compound fracture*. The importance of this consideration stems from the risk of infection which can involve the bone, leading to the very serious condition of osteomyelitis.

Closed or simple fracture in which a bone has been broken, but there is no serious injury to other important tissues in the vicinity. They are further classified as:

(a) Transverse fracture—In these the bone is broken almost straight across due to direct violence.

(b) Spiral fracture—In this the bone is obliquely broken due to indirect violence.

(c) Fissured fracture—In this the bone is cracked but not completely broken.

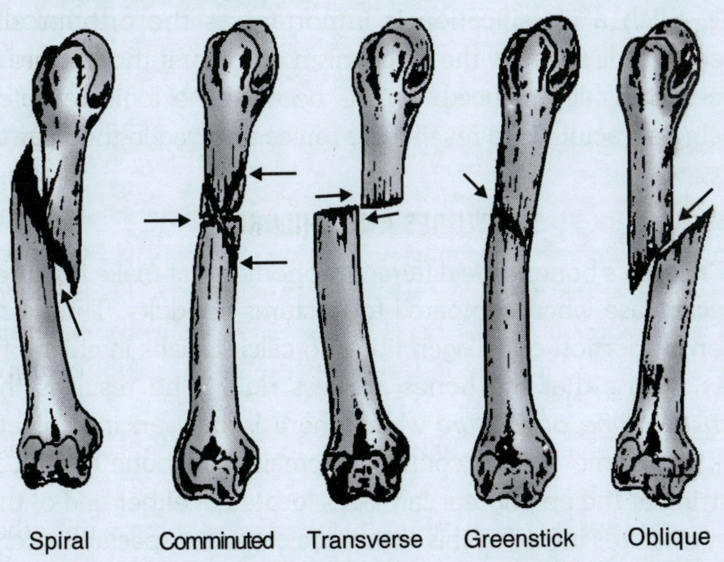

Fig. 22.1: *Different types of fracture.*

Complicated fracture is one when there is associated injury to some important internal structure, e.g., brain, spinal cord, lung, spleen etc., and when a fracture at a joint is associated with dislocation.

A *comminuted fracture* is one in which a bone is broken and there are more than two fragments, e.g., fracture of patella due to direct violence.

An *impacted fracture* is one when the fragments of a fracture are driven into one another and wedged firmly together. This kind of fracture occurs usually at the ends of long bones, e.g., upper end of humerus.

The *green stick fracture* occurs in children under the age of twelve. In this bone may be cracked and bent without breaking completely across.

A *depressed fracture* is one in which the broken part of the bone is driven inwards, e.g., when the vault of the skull has been fractured and a piece of the bone is pressed inwards. This may cause the signs and symptoms of compression.

Fracture types may be described according to the diagram in Fig.1. Such a classification is important as the orthopaedic surgeon needs to know the mechanism of injury if the fracture is to be successfully reduced. This is because the logical way of reducing a fracture is to reverse the forces involved in the original injury.

FRACTURES AND CHILDREN

Children's bones have different properties that make fractures a special case when compared to fractures in adults. The much higher proportion of collagen fibres to calcium salts in children's bones means that the bones are less rigid. The result is the *greenstick type of fracture* where there is only an incomplete break and some cortical continuity remains. As bone growth is occurring at the epiphyceal cartilages located at either end of the bone, fractures involving this region are cause for special concern due to the risk of deformity from damage to the growing area. Such fractures are known as *Salter's fractures* and are graded I through V in order of seriousness.

FRACTURE HEALING

Fracture healing is a complex process that requires an infection-free environment, fracture immobilization and a good blood supply. Where possible the aim of management is to provide such a situation, so that healing can occur conservatively. However, if it is felt that the nature of the fracture is such that this will not occur or that the hazards of lengthy immobilization are too great e.g., in the cases of a pathological fracture or a fracture of the femur in an elderly person, then the surgeon may opt to fix the fracture internally by an operation.

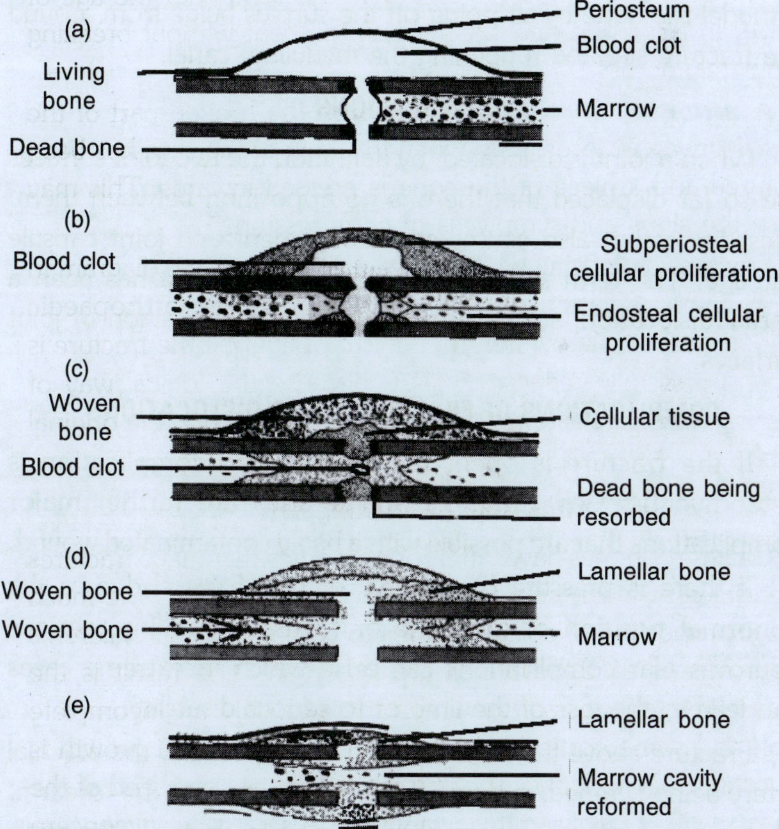

Fig. 22.2: *Pathology of fracture~ and the healing of fractures.*

The first step in healing is the formation of a haematoma at the fracture site. The haematoma takes little active part in the healing process and is quickly absorbed as cells from the deep surface of the periosteum divide and invade the haematoma. These cells are precursors of the osteoblasts, the cells that play an active part in the construction of new bone. The osteoblasts are responsible initially for the formation of callus which is an immature matrix of collagen and polysaccharides that becomes impregnated with calcium salts and as a result is visible on X-rays. As the callus matures into bone, the final stage of healing occurs with another type of cell, the osteociasts, helping to remodel the bone by stripping off the surplus bulge from around the fracture site and reopening the medullary canal.

DISLOCATIONS

When a joint is dislocated, by definition the two joint surfaces are so far displaced that there is no apposition between them. This dislocation also causes serious ligament and joint capsule damage. The term subluxation is used when there has been a partial dislocation, so that there is still some apposition of joint surfaces.

COMPLICATIONS OF FRACTURES AND DISLOCATIONS

If the fracture is open, the most feared complication is osteomyelitis. Gas gangrene and tetanus are further major complications that are possible with a badly contaminated wound.

If there is pressure on a nerve or blood vessel due to the abnormal position of the bone or to tissue swelling, serious neurovascular complications can arise which in extreme cases can lead to the loss of the limb or to serious disability.

Fracture above the humeral condyles can lead to the brachial artery being trapped, cutting off the blood supply to the forearm. This is most often seen in children and leads to *Volkmann's ischaemic contracture*, a flexion deformity of the hand and wrist. Arterial damage in leg fractures can lead to amputation.

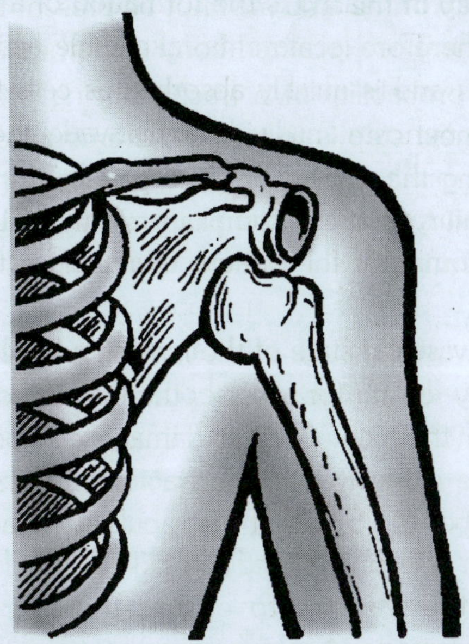

Fig. 22.3: *Dislocated shoulder joint.*

Bleeding from a fractured bone can cause *hypovolaemic shock*. One litre of blood may be lost from a mid-shaft fracture of the femur and two litres may be lost from fractures of the pelvis.

In joint injuries, bleeding into a joint cavity is called a *haemarthrosis*; such is the limited space within a joint capsule that the result can be a very tense painful joint indeed.

If a fracture enters a joint, it is essential for the surgeon to seek as anatomically perfect a reduction as possible as any irregularity left in the joint will lead to the rapid development of osteoarthritis.

ASSESSMENT

The triage nurse will have to carry out a rapid assessment of the injured patient and should be looking for the following key signs. A cardinal sign to look for is localized bony tenderness, i.e., pain upon palpating the fracture site. This sign is best elicited by gently feeling along the bone and watching the patient for discomfort associated with pressing a discrete area over a bone. Deformity of the limb may not be present if the fracture is undisplaced, therefore localized bony tenderness is the key sign.

Once the probability of a fracture being present has been assessed, the next step is to assess the amount of pain that the injury is causing the patient and the patient's understanding of the possible injury. Patient compliance with treatment will only be fully forthcoming if the patient understands fully the nature of the injury.

The neurovascular state of the limb should be assessed distal to the injury by feeling for a pulse, the location of which should be marked on the skin. Serious damage can occur if a blood vessel or nerve is involved in the fracture. *Dykes*, recommends nurses remember the 5 'p's of pain, pulses, paraesthesia, pallor and paralysis in assessing injured limbs. They should all be checked for distal to the fracture to ensure there are no signs of neurovascular damage. Any wound present should be examined with the possibility of an open fracture borne in mind.

Patient assessment should not be confined to the one limb where there may be an obvious fracture. If there has been sufficient force to break one bone, there may be other less obvious injuries as well, including fractures of other limbs. *Taylor et al.* showed, in a survey of 250 consecutive patients with fractured shafts of femur, that 85 had other serious injuries. Of this sample, 37 were motorcyclists and 92 were pedestrians; well over half of these patients had other significant injuries, yet in the 81 patients whose fractured shaft of femur stemmed from falls, only 7 had significant other injuries.

The type of accident, therefore has a major role in determining the risk of further injuries. Vital signs should be recorded to give a baseline from which any deviation indicative of hypovolaemic shock may be detected. The blood loss from fractures alone may cause this condition, in addition to which there is the possible loss of blood from soft tissue injury. As a rule of thumb, an open fracture has twice the blood loss of a closed one.

The psychological and social status of the patient should not be overlooked. This is of great importance in dealing with the elderly because very often it is these factors rather than physical problems that determine management. Similar considerations apply if the patient has a dislocated joint. Lack of normal joint movement, pain and deformity are the key signs that the nurse will find present upon assessment.

INTERVENTION

Provided that there is no other life-threatening problem immediately identified, the first goal of intervention should be pain relief. Immobilization of the fracture will make a contribution towards this goal. Home-made or ambulance splints should be removed to allow adequate assessment of the limb (using Entonox as required) and should be replaced with one of two kinds of splint.

If there is a femoral shaft fracture, traction will be required. The traditional method was the use of the Thomas splint with skin traction to overcome the very strong pull of the thigh muscles and to immobilize the fracture. A more modern approach involves the use of the telescopic Traesplint system developed in the USA.

For fractures of the other long bones, traction is not required in A & E. The best method of immobilization for these fractures involves the use of a vacuum splint. This is a bag full of polystyrene beads that can be placed around the limb; when evacuated by use of the wall suction, it collapses under atmospheric pressure, forming a rigid splint and moulding to the shape of the limb. Such a system is far superior to old-fashioned methods involving bandaging the injured limb to a rigid splint. In the new system, the limb is not under pressure, the splint *is* radiotranslucent and the limb is fully visible all the time to allow continual observation of its vascular status. Furthermore, in application, the new vacuum splint is far less painful for rhepatient.

The next step in relieving pain is to try to minimize swelling by elevation. Hand and wrist fractures should be in a sling;

fractures of the lower limb should be elevated by elevating the foot of the trolley. Rings and other constricting jewellery should be removed as soon as possible before swelling becomes a problem.

Movement of the injured limb should be minimized. The situation should not be allowed where successive doctors all want to look at the fracture, resulting in the splint being removed and reapplied several times. Entonox can be freely used for pain relief and in head injury cases this may still be used as the powerful opioids may be withheld for fear of depressing the level of consciousness.

Fear and anxiety will only increase the pain felt by the patient and tend to make for less cooperation. Clear explanation of what is happening and why, together with attention being paid to matters such as informing next of kin, will make a substantial contribution to pain control and the patient's well-being. The pain of a dislocation may be partly relieved by supporting the limb, thereby removing any weight that the joint has to take. Psychological support and Entonox will also be useful for pain relief.

If the injury involves a wound, steps should be taken to wash out any gross contamination with a litre of normal saline immediately. A dressing should be applied, consisting of saline soaks and gauze pads soaked in iodine solution (e.g., Betadine). It may be assumed that the patient will be going to theatre soon; therefore, hospital protocols should be followed as for any patient going to theatre. Formal toilet and debridement in theatre is essential to prevent infection by washing out all traces of contamination and excising all dead or dubious tissue from the wound.

If a fracture is displaced or a joint dislocated, manipulation is required to restore the normal anatomical position of the bones involved. This is frequently undertaken in the A & E department. As nursing assistance will be required, the nurse needs to know something of the procedures which may be carried out.

Gross fracture dislocations of the ankle (the foot rotated at 90 relative to the tibia) require immediate reduction under Entonox by disimpacting the fracture and rotating the foot back to the normal position. If reduction is not immediate, serious neurovascular damage will result. This is a first priority *before* X-ray. Severe injuries of the lower part of the leg in particular may require amputation and, as *Clarke* and *Molion* have shown, primary amputation results in discharge home in half the time compared to patients where amputation is delayed. Criteria for primary amputation are discussed by these authors and include complete disruption of the posterior tibial nerve, severe crush injury and serious associated multiple injuries.

The most commonly manipulated fracture in A & E is the *Colles fracture* using the *Bier's block technique*. A double cuff tourniquet is placed around the top of the arm which is then elevated to allow venous drainage before the cuff is pumped up to above arterial pressure as recorded by the attached pressure gauge. Local anaesthetic is then infiltrated into the arm via a butterfly, effectively anaesthetizing the whole forearm.

The danger is that the anaesthetic drug may leak past the cuff if it deflates. If this occurs before the drug has been bound and rendered inert by plasma proteins, a serious and possibly fetal reaction may occur. For this reason lignocaine and Marcaine are no longer used, the safer prilocaine being preferred. Even with this safer drug, however, the cuff must remain inflated for at least 20 minutes. It is essential that a nurse stay with the patient throughout the manipulation and check X-ray stage, observing the cuff pressure gauge to ensure there is no leak, and observing the patient, who will be probably very grateful for somebody to talk to.

Another common manipulation carried out in A & E is for dislocated shoulders. This technique involves the administration of intravenous diazepam (muscle relaxant) and an opioid analgesic e.g., pethidine before manipulation. The patient is, therefore, not anaesthetized, but will be very drowsy. There is a signficant hazard of respiratory depression, so close nursing observation is required in the post-manipulation period.

After the fracture has been successfully manipulated, if necessary and immobilized in plaster of Paris, the nurse must consider the problems associated with discharge. These include transportation to home, a follow-up appointment usually the following day to check the plaster, whether the patient fully understands how to use crutches and/or what precautions need to be taken with the plaster, and finally, whether the patient can cope. In dealing with the elderly, especially those who live alone, it is often the case that the fall that brought about the current injury was the final episode in a steadily deteriorating situation.

The A & E nurse must, therefore, carefully assess the patient's ability to cope at home and if there is any doubt, discuss the matter further with the medical staff, remembering the nurse's role as patient advocate, in order to mobilize fully community support or explore the possibility of admission to a care of the elderly ward. The final thought before discharging the patient should behave they got any analgesia. A timely reminder to the medical staff can save a lot of unnecessary pain with a quick prescription.

If the patient is being admitted because of the fracture, preparation for theatre in accordance with hospital protocols is required. In addition, an intravenous infusion is mandatory for fractures of the femoral shaft to prevent hypovolaemic shock. Fractures of the neck of femur, however, bleed very little and do not require an IVI to prevent hypovolaemia, although one may be erected to ensure adequate hydration of the patient in the pre-operative phase.

Elderly patients with fractures of the femur have a very high risk of developing pressure sores. It seems that the causes are largely to be found outside trauma wards in the form of hard A & E, theatre or X-ray trolleys, where elderly patients lie immobile for hours on end. Turning such a patient in A & E is impractical.

However, Spenco mattresses are available in sizes which fit trolleys and at least one such mattress should be available in A & E. Every effort should be made to transfer the patient to a ward bed where pressure area care may be instituted as rapidly as possible. Note that sheepskins will be of little use in A & E for such patients as they only prevent friction.

EVALUATION

The effectiveness of pain-relieving intervention should be continually checked, together with the neurovascular status of the limb. Although a limb has been elevated to reduce swelling, it should not be assumed that it will stay that way. Slings can slip and pillows can mysteriously vanish from under legs. Similarly, splinting should be checked at periodic intervals to ensure that it is still functioning effectively.

In evaluating the effectiveness of instruction given to the patient about either plaster of Paris or the use of crutches, it is important that the patient be asked to demonstrate that they have learnt what has been taught. Therefore, the patient should be asked to repeat the plaster instructions to ensure they know what to look for and the patient should be observed walking with crutches. It is not what has been taught that is important, but what has been learnt, and the only way to evaluate patient instruction is to assess what has been learnt.

If the patient is experiencing a minimum amount of pain and anxiety, if their injured limb is safely immobilized, and if its neurovascular status is secure, then the nursing intervention can be evaluated as successful.

SOME COMMON FRACTURES

FRACTURES OF THE UPPER LIMB

(a) Arm Bone (Humerus)

Humerus can be broken near the shoulder joint, middle part or near the elbow.

Fracture Upper End of Humerus

The fracture is slightly difficult to manage, as upper arm has got strong muscles and these muscles produce pull and overlapping of ends that get broken.

If the fracture is close to shoulder, Place a pad in the axilia. Lightly tie the arm to the chest. Bend the elbow, and, with the hand on the op posite shoulder, apply a collar and cuffsling.

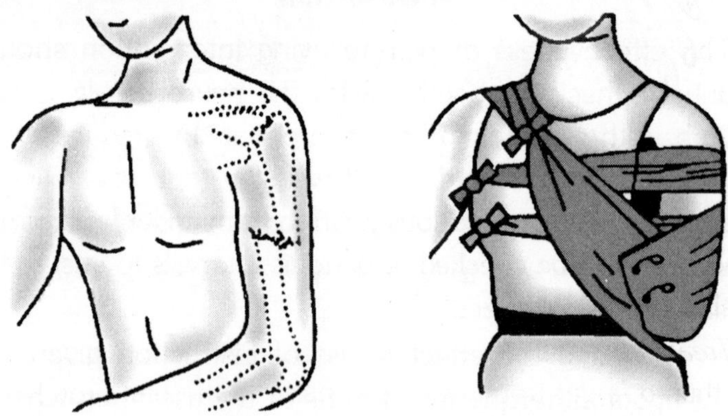

Fig. 22.4: *Fracture of upper arm.*

Fracture Middle of Humerus

There is likelihood of shortening due to muscle pull. If the fracture is in the Mid Shaft. Place a pad between arm and chest. Tie the upper arm firmly to the chest, one bandage above and the other below the site of fracture. Support the forearm in Collar bone the sling.

Fracture of Humerus Near Elbow Joint

If the elbow can be bent, tie the arm to the chest and support the forearm in a triangular sling. If the elbow cannot be bent, get the casually to lie down, and tie the arm to the trunk in extended position.

(b) Fracture of Forearm

There are two bones, i.e., radius and ulna. Forearm fractures are the only fractures where external splintage is definitely required. *Colles's fracture*, near to the wrist, is very common. It is caused by a fall on the outstretched hand. There will be swelling and deformity at the wrist.

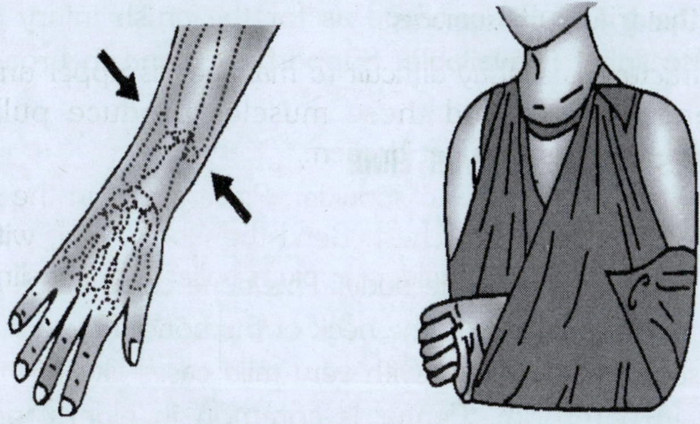

Fig. 22.5: *Fracture of forearm.*

It is best to use a splint for first aid in forearm fractures. A folded newspaper or magazine will serve well, if it extends from the elbow to the fingers.

Treatment—Place the forearm across the chest at right angle with thumb finger uppermost and palm of the hand towards the body. Roll the folded newaspaper or magazine around the forearm. Apply one bandage above the fracture and a second, as a figure of eight, around the wrist and hand. Support the arm in a sling with fingers, slightly higher than the elbow. Watch the fingers for signs of interference with the blood circulation, in which case, loosen the bandage slightly.

Fracture of the Hand and the Fingers

These fracture are mostly due to direct injury. There may also be severe bleeding into the palm if palmar arch (artial blood supply) is broken.

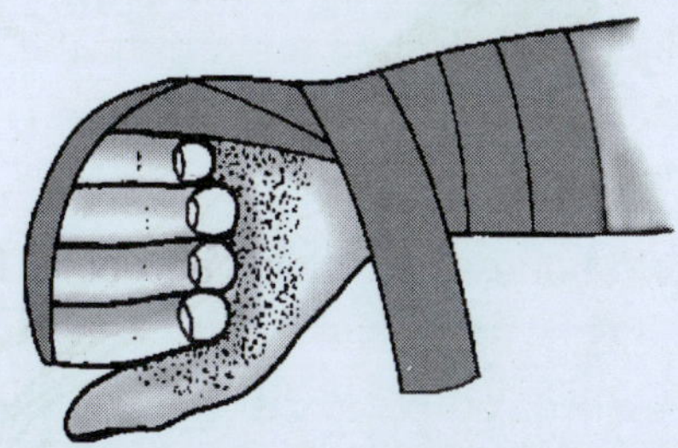

Fig. 22.6: *Fracture of hand and fingers.*

Tie the triangular bandage as for the crush injury of the hand. Use splint if available. Support the hand in broad arm sling.

FRACTURES OF THE LOWER LIMB

Femur

It is longest bone of the body. This bone could break at any place along its length or at the neck of the bone. Fracture of the neck is seen in old people with very mild cases like tripping or slipping in bathroom. Femur is common in elderly people. Fracture of the femur are always serious due to bleeding into the surrounding tissues.

The *signs and symptoms* of this fracture are pain, swelling and shock. Shortening of limb. The foot on the injured side, lies turned to the outside.

Treatment—Treat for shock. Pad between the legs and brings the good leg along side the injured one. Tie together the knees, ankles, hips, above and below the fracture. If there is a long and difficult journey to the hospital, two well paded splints should be applied. One, between the legs, the other, on the outside extending from axilia to the foot. Secure the splints with bandages around the chest, pelvis, knees, above and below the fracture, lower legs, a figure of eight around the ankles and knee.

Fracture of Knee Cap (Patella)

Fracture of the patella may occur due to direct force, but is more often, due to muscular action.

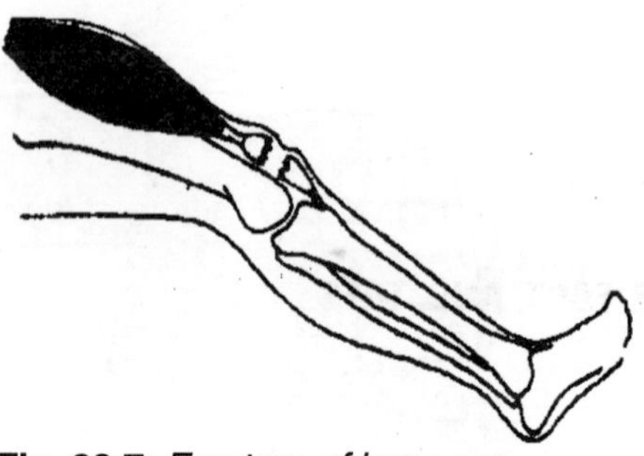

Fig. 22.7: *Fracture of knee cap.*

Signs and symptoms—The limb is helpless. There is much swelling. The gap may be felt between the two bits of bone.

Treatment—Support the casualty in a sitting position. Raise the injured leg gently and place the uninjured leg under for support. Tie the ankles together, and raise the legs on a box. The legs may be tied together by means of a narrow bandage above the knee in a figure of eight bandage. If a splint is available, apply it to the base of the limb, it should reach from the buttock to beyond the heel, pad under the ankle, and secure the splint to the limb by bandages round the thigh, ankle and figure of eight, above and below the knee.

FRACTURE OF LOWER LEG

The tibia only, or both and fibula may be broken. All the signs of fracture are seen in these cases. If the tibia only is much swelling around, the ankle fracture of ankle bones also, should be suspected.

Treatment—Treat as for femur fracture, but without the long splint. One or both of the bones may be broken. When both the bones broken then pain, swelling, shock, etc., occurs, but when fibula only is broken no deformity is visible because it is splinted by the tibia. Fracture of bones of ankle should be suspected in swelling around the ankle.

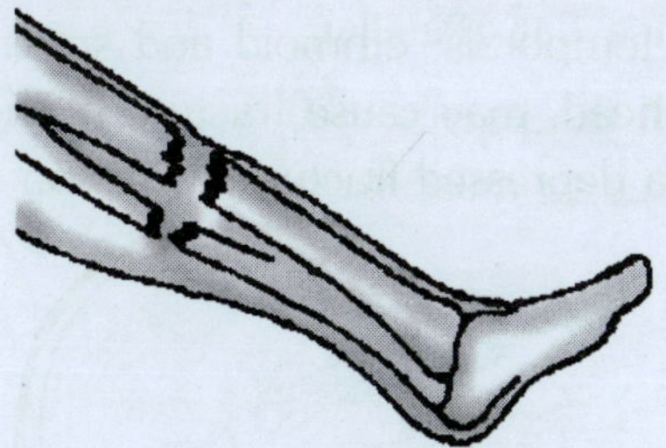

Fig. 22.8: *Fracture of leg.*

FRACTURE FOOT AND TOES

This fracture is caused by direct force, like a crush injuries due to heavy items falling on the foot or wheel passing over the foot. There could be wound and severe bleeding.

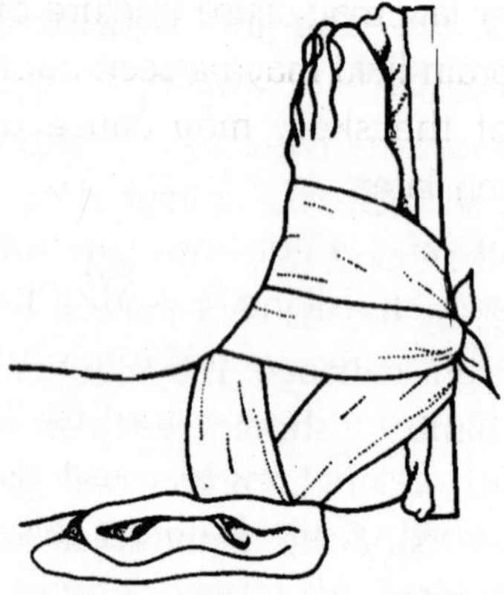

Fig. 22.9: *Fracture of foot and toes.*

Treatment: Remove footwear and treat wounds. Raise and support the foot. Apply a padded splint to the sole of the foot. Secure the splint with a figure of eight bandage. Start with the centre of broad bandage on the splints, cross the ends over the instep and carry them to the back of the ankle and again cross once more, to bring them to the front of the ankle. Cross once more to bring the ends to the foot, cross and tie it off over the centre of the splint. Transport the casualty by stretcher with the foot raised.

FRACTURE OF SKULL BONES

Skull consists of 8 bones namely frontal, two parietal, occipital, two temporals, ethmoid and sphenoid. A direct blow or fall on the head, may cause fracture of the upper part of the skull, is often a depressed fracture. A fall on the feet or buttocks

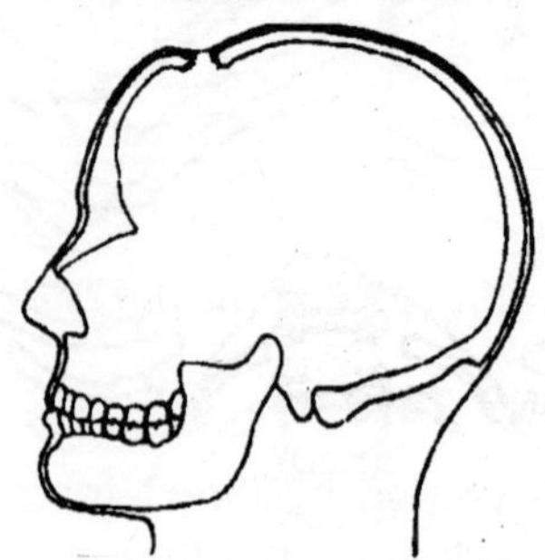

Fig. 22.10: *Fracture of skull bone.*

or a blow to the lower jaw may cause fracture of the base of the skull when blood or brain fluid may be seen coming from the ear or nose. Fracture of the skull, may cause unconsciousness immediately or coming later.

Treatment—If breathing is not noisy, lay the casualty on his back with head and shoulder slightly raised. If breathing is noisy, place the casualty into the recovery position with head to one side. If there is bleeding from the ear, turn the head so that, the bleeding side is down. Do not try to rouse the casualty. Keep him quiet and undisturbed. Keep the head still during transport, using sand bags or pads. Treat for shock and refer immediately.

FRACTURE OF RIB

Ribs may be broken by direct force, or indirectly by a crush injury. There is danger that the broken ribs may be driven inwardly causing injury to the lungs.

Signs and Symptoms—Pain that is made worse by coughing or deep breathing. The casualty taken short, shallow breaths, so that, the ribs do not move and increase the pain. If the lung is injured, blood may be coughed up. If there is an open wound in the chest, air is sucked in and blows out as the casualty breaths. This is a serious complication.

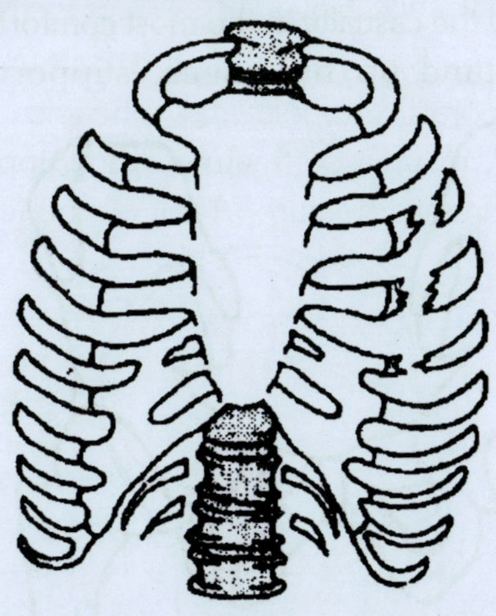

Fig. 22.11: *Fracture of ribs.*

Treatment—(a) If the fracture is *uncomplicated*—Apply two broad bandages to the area of pain. The upper bandage should overlap the lower one by half its width. Tie them lightly first after the casualty has breathed out, with knotsnear the front on the uninjured side. Support the arm to the injured side in a sling. (b) If the fracture is *complicated* fracture of the ribs—If there is a sucking wound, cover it with a dry dressing pad bandage firmly. In other cases, do not apply bandages. Support the casualty with head and shoulders raised and turned towards the injured side, transport carefully in the position on a stretcher. A sling may be applied to the arm on the injured side.

FRACTURE OF PELVIS (HIP BONE)

Fracture of the pelvis, usually, occurs due to direct force such as in the crush injuries, road accidents (specially of two wheelers). Especially, the urinary bladder or urethra passage are the main organs of pelvic cavity, they may be injured causing urinary complication.

Signs and Symptoms—Pain in the hips when they are pressed together. The casualty is unable to stand, nor to move the legs without pain. There may be an urge to pass urine, but he is unable to do so or finds it difficult. There may be internal bleeding.

Treatment—Lay the casualty in the most comfortable position. If he wants to stand up his knees, support them with

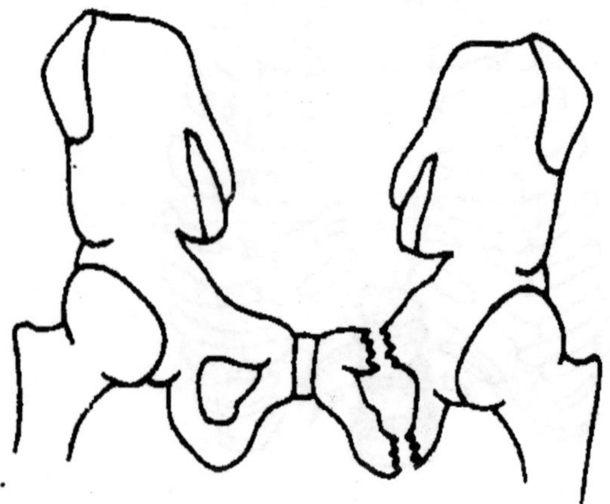

Fig. 22.12: *Fracture of pelvis.*

folded clothing or pillow. Ask him to avoid passing urine. If a hospital is near, transport him on a stretcher without bandaging. If the journey is long and on rough roads, apply pads between the knees and ankles, then tie two overlapping broad bandages or a towel around the pelvis. Bandages should be tied on the uninjured side. Tie the knees together, with a broad bandage. Tie a figure of eight bandage around the ankles and feet.

FRACTURE OF SPINE

Spine or vertebral column is formed of a series of bones called vertebrae. In youth the vertebrae are 33 in numbers,

7 cervical (in neck)

12 thorax (in thorax)

5 lumber (in loins regions)

5 sacral (in the pelvis)

4 coccygeal (in the pelvis)

Sacral and coccygeal vertebrae are firmly united and are fixed while others are separate and movable. Spine has to bear the weight of the head and trunck.

Spinal fracture due to indirect force include:

Neck fracture in whiplash injuries, thrown forward suddenly in a moving vehicle. Pull on vertebrae while lifting heavy weights.

Spinal fracture due to direct force include:

Fall of heavy weight on the back, falling from height on the back, earthquakes, landslides, stampedes in fairs etc.

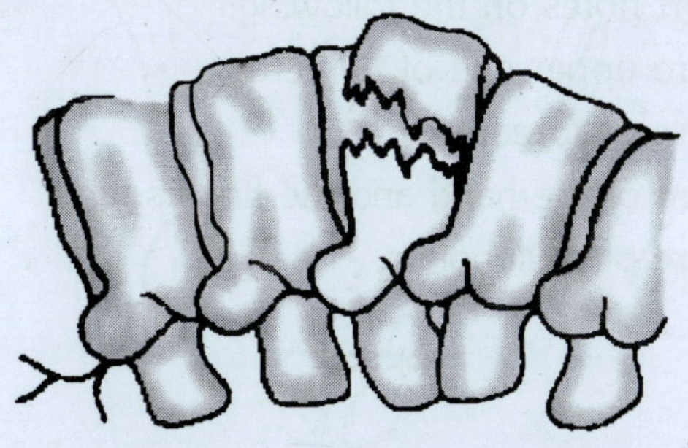

Fig. 22.13: *Fracture of spine.*

The casualty complains of pain at the side. The spinal cord may be damaged causing paralysis and loss of sensation below the side of the fracture. By good first aid treatment, paralysis may be prevented.

Treatment—Warn the casualty not to move. Treat for shock. Get a long enough board on which the casualty can lie. Collect padding material, bandages and blanket or rug. Cover the board with a folded blanket and paice small pillows or pads to fit the neck and middle of the back. Atleast four helpers are needed to get the casualty lying on the board. First place padding between legs. Tie together the ankles and feet with figure of eight bandage, and to his knees together.

When all are ready, the helper must carry together and be very careful not to bend or twist the spine as they either roll the casualty or lift him to get him on the prepared board. One should hold the head firmly and keep the neck straight. Another hold the legs near the ankles, while other keep the shoulder and hips steady and in line. Tie the casualty to the board to prevent movement during transport. If there is a neck injury, do not use a pillow under the neck, but place bags of sand or firm pads on each side of the bed to keep from moving. Take the casualty to hospital or health centre, as soon as possible.

STUDY-QUESTIONS

1. What do you mean by healing of fracture?
2. Write short notes on the following:
   (a) Fracture upper end of humerus;
   (b) Fracture of forearm;
   (c) Fracture of the hand and the fingers; and
   (d) Fracture of skull bones.

***

23 CHAPTER

BANDAGE AND DRESSING

BANDAGES

Bandage is used to protect or support the hurt part of the body. It is long piece of thin cloth which is wound around an injured part of the body. It should not be applied so tight as to cause injury to the part or to reduce the circulation of the blood. Bandages are used to maintain direct pressure over a dressing to control bleeding, to support for a limb or joint and restrict movement. It should be applied firm enough to keep dressing and splints in position. A bluish tinge and loss of sensation of the finger or nails may be the danger sign to indicate the bandages are too tight.

TYPES OF BANDAGES

Standard bandages are made from gauze, muslin, flannel, rubber or adhesive, crinoline. For first aid, bandages can be improvised by tie, stocking, scarf, handkerchief or sareefalls. There are many types of bandages in use these days, first aider requires to learn about *triangular* and *roller* bandages because they are easily available and do not require many precautions and skills.

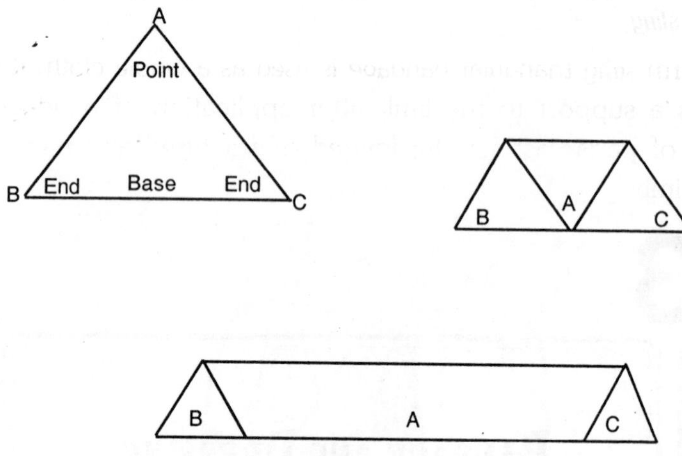

Fig. 23.1: *Triangular bandage.*

(1) Triangular Bandage
(2) Roller Bandage

1. Triangular Bandage

It may be used in nursing and for slings to support an arr after injury. It is made up of cutting diagonally a square piece c calico 100 cms. (40 inchs) in length, so that two bandages ar formed.

It has three borders—the longest is base, and the other tw sides. There are three corners; the one opposite the base i called the point and the other two are called ends. There are tw types of triangular bandages—Reef Knot and Slings.

(i) Reef Knot

For tying the triangular bandage a reef knot must always be used. Take the ends of the bandage one in each hand, cross the end in the right hand under and then over the end in the left hand thus making a turn. Then cross the end now in the right hand, thus making a second turn.

(ii) Slings

Slings are mainly used for upper limb to support an injured part and are used to prevent pull by upper limb of injuries to chest, shoulder and the neck. There are three types of slings:

(a) Arm sling

In arm sling triangular bandage is used as a whole cloth. It is used as a support to the limb after application of bandage, plaster of paris cast for the injured or fractured any part of upper limb.

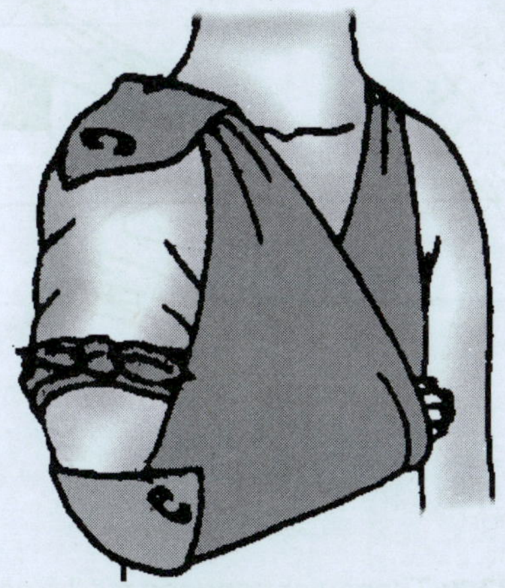

Fig. 23.2: *Arm sling.*

(b) Cuff and collar slings

This bandage is applied at the wrist and tied at the neck. This sling is used to support the injuries or fractures of wrist.

(c) Triangular slings

It is the modification of arm sling. It is used for supporting arm in cases of fractured collar bone.

USE OF TRIANGULAR BANDAGES FOR OTHER BODY PARTS

(i) Scalp—Fold in a hem along the base of triangular bandage. Then place it on the forehead joint above the level of eyebrows. Take the two ends backwards after placing the body of the bandage over the head, the point hanging near the nape of the neck. Cross the two ends, take them forward

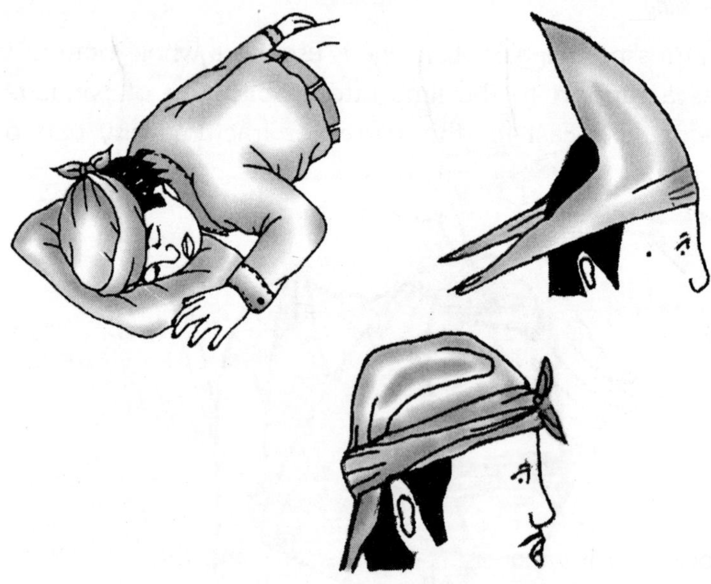

Fig. 23.3: *Triangular bandage for the scalp.*

round the ears to meet on forehead. Tie both these ends on the forehead making a reef knot. Pull the point firmly downwards and pin it to the bandage tucking the point inwards.

(ii) **Eye**—Place the center of the bandage over the injured part (eye/ear) and wind the bandage around the part. Tie in a place away from wound.

(iii) **Hand**—Place the open bandage in such a way that the injury is uppermost. Place the fingers towards the point and the wrist above the base. Now turn the point over so that it reaches the wrist. Make a narrow inward hem, pass the ends around the wrist, cross over. Tie it up over the point. Turn the point over the knot and pin it.

(iv) **Wrist**—Place the centre of a narrow bandage across the palm of a hand. Collect the ends and carry them to the back of the hand leaving out the thumb. Cross the ends on the

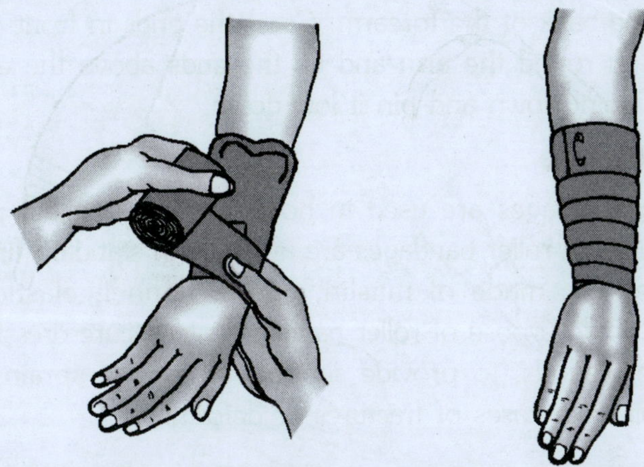

Fig. 23.4: *Wrist bandage.*

back of the hand and carry them around the wrist at the lower end of the forearm. Tie on the middle of the back of the limb.

(v) **Shoulder**—Place the center of the open bandage on the shoulder with the point over the side of the neck. Take the ends around the middle of the arm and tie the knot on the outer side. Now take another triangular bandage and apply arm sling to the injured limb. Turn down the point of the bandage over the sling knot and pin it.

(vi) **Elbow**—Bend the elbow to a right angle if it is safe to do so. Fold a suitable hem of the base of a triangular bandage and apply it as follows:

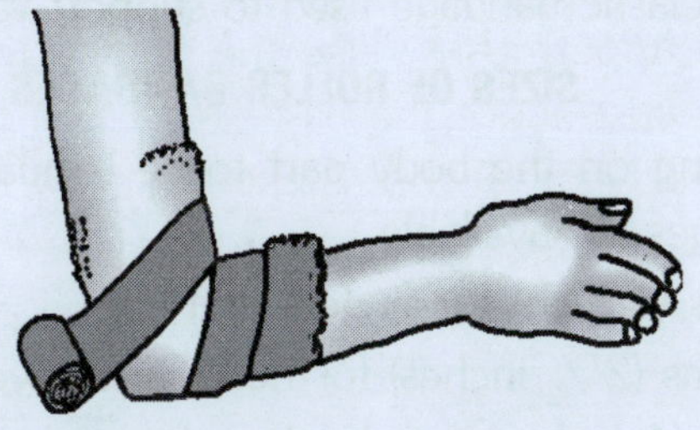

Fig. 23.5: *Elbow bandage.*

Lay the point on the back of the arm, in the middle of the base on the back of the forearm. Cross the ends in front of the elbow, then round the arm and tie the ends above the elbow. Turn the point down and pin it low down.

2. Roller Bandage

Roller bandages are used in hospitals and first aid posts. Various sizes of roller bandages are available in standard first aid box. They are made of muslin, gauze, flannel, elastic and adhesive. The purpose of roller bandage is to secure dressing to cover the wounds, to provide support in case of sprains, to secure splints in cases of fractures or deformity.

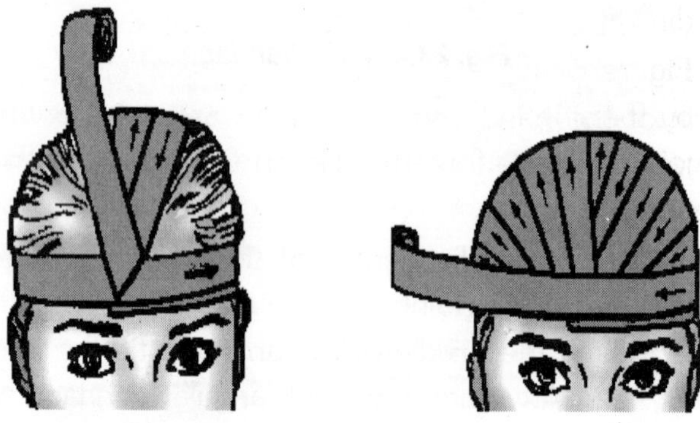

Fig. 23.6: *Roller bandage.*

The material used for making roller bandages is cotton-loosely woven cotton bandage is used for dressing and to secure splints and for support. Flannel to providce warmth to the part. Crepe bandage or elastic bandage used to support varisoce veins.

SIZES OF ROLLER BANDAGES

Depending on the body part to be bandaged various sized roller bandages are available.

1. 2.5 cms (1 inch) for fingers and toes.
2. 6.25 cms ($2^1/_2$ inches) for head, arm, eye and ear.
3. 10 cms (4 inches) for shoulder, leg and thigh.
4. 15 cms (6 inches) for chest, abdomen and groin.

BASIC BANDAGE PATTERNS

The roller bandage is—applied by using singly or in combination the five basic bandage patterns. They are circular, spiral, spiral reverse, figure of eight and recurrent.

1. **Recurrent Bandage**—The recurrent bandage pattern is used to retain a dressing on the head, on a stump or on the end of a finger. It is made by fixing the bandage with two circular turns. The roll of bandage is then turned to cover the middle of the area. Next turns alternate on each side of the midline, passing back to front and front to back. Each turn overlaps one half the previous turn. When the entire area is covered, the bandage is ended with a circular turn directly over the first circular turn.
2. **Figure of Eight Bandage**—This bandage pattern is begun by forming two loops or turns, one above and one below a joint. Succeeding turns alternate above, where they descend, and below from where they ascend until the joint is covered. This pattern is modified to form the spica bandage, where one circumference is much bigger than the other.

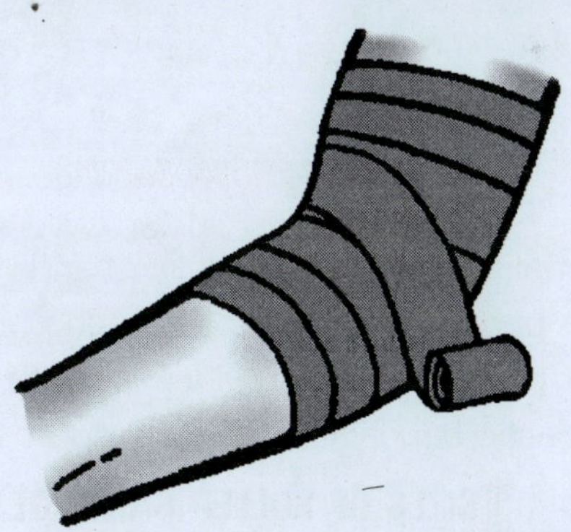

Fig. 23.7: *Figure of eight bandage.*

3. **Circular Bandage**—In application of the circular bandage pattern, each succeeding turn overlaps the entire width of the previous turn. This patten is used to secure the bandage at the start of tying a bandage.

4. **Simple Spiral Bandage**—The spiral bandage pattern is used to cover an area of uniform circumference. Each turn overlaps one-half or two-thirds of the previous turn. It is used for lower 1/3rd of forearm or leg.
5. **Spiral Reverse**—The spiral reverse bandage pattern is used on a cone shaped part such as the forearm or leg. After the bandage is secured by two circular turns, reverses (turning the bandage top to bottom) are made after each turn. Reverse pattern prevents gaps and ensures a smooth bandage.

STUDY–QUESTIONS

1. Describe the various types of bandage.
2. Elaborate the use of triangular bandages to bandaging other body parts.

24

CHAPTER

EFFECTS OF HEAT

HEAT EXHAUSTION

This condition often occurs when people exercise (work or play) in a hot, humid place and body fluids are lost through sweating, causing the body to overheat. The person's temperature may be elevated, but not above 104°F.

HEAT STROKE

This type of medical condition is life-threatening. The person's cooling system, which is controlled by the brain, stops working and the internal body temperature rises to the point where brain damage or damage to other internal organs may result (temperature may reach 105°F).

CAUSES OF HEAT EXHAUSTION AND HEAT STROKE

HEAT EXHAUSTION

Heat exhaustion is typically caused when people who are not well adjusted to heat exercise in a hot, humid environment.

- At high temperatures, the body cools itself largely through evaporation of sweat.

- When it is very humid, this mechanism does not work properly.
- The body loses a combination of fluids and salts (electrolytes).
- When this is accompanied by an inadequate replacement of fluids, disturbances in the circulation may result that are similar to a mild form of shock.

HEAT STROKE

Heat stroke may often develop rapidly.

- Medical conditions or medications that impair the body's ability to sweat may predispose people to this problem.
- Heat stroke happens in the following ways:
    - The classic form occurs in people whose cooling mechanisms are impaired.
    - The exertional form occurs in previously healthy people who are undergoing strenuous activity in a hot environment.
    - Infants and the elderly are more likely to have this problem, as are those who are taking antihistamines and certain types of medication for high blood pressure or depression.

HEAT EXHAUSTION AND HEAT STROKE SYMPTOMS

HEAT EXHAUSTION

- Often pale with cool, moist skin
- Sweating profusely
- Muscle cramps or pains
- Feels faint or dizzy
- May complain of headache, weakness, thirst, and nausea
- Core (rectal) temperature elevated—usually more than 100°F— and the pulse rate increased

HEAT STROKE

- Unconscious or has a markedly abnormal mental status (dizziness, confusion, hallucinations, or coma)

- Flushed, hot, and dry skin (although it may be moist initially from previous sweating or from attempts to cool the person with water)
- May have slightly elevated blood pressure at first that falls later
- May be hyperventilating
- Rectal (core) temperature of 105°F or more

WHEN TO SEEK MEDICAL CARE

As with all other medical problems, a doctor should be called if you are not sure what is wrong, if you do not know what to do for the problem, or if the person is not responding to what you are doing for them.

- Call a doctor for heat exhaustion if the person is unable to keep fluids down or if their mental status begins to deteriorate. Symptoms of shortness of breath, chest pain, or abdominal pain may indicate that the heat exhaustion is accompanied by more serious medical problems.
- Suspected heat stroke is a true, life-threatening medical emergency. Call for an ambulance and request information as to what to do until the ambulance arrives.

A person with suspected heat stroke should always go to the hospital or call for an ambulance at once.

For heat exhaustion, a person should go to the hospital if any of the following are present:

- Loss of consciousness, confusion, or delirium.
- Chest or abdominal pain.
- Inability to drink fluids.
- Continuous vomiting.
- Temperature more than 104°F.
- Temperature that is rising despite attempts to cool the person.
- Any person with other serious ongoing medical problems.

For a heat exposure emergency, the treating doctor needs some important information:

- Past medical history
- Medicines the patient is currently taking (prescription and over-the-counter)
- Symptoms the patient is experiencing

Blood tests to check for organ damage may be indicated, however, no specific radiologic (imaging) tests are necessary.

SELF-CARE AT HOME

Home care is appropriate for mild forms of heat exhaustion. Heat stroke is a medical emergency, and an ambulance should be called immediately.

- For mild cases of heat exhaustion
- Rest in a cool, shaded area.
- Give cool fluids such as water or sports drinks (that will replace the salt that has been lost). Salty snacks are appropriate as tolerated.
- Loosen or remove clothing.
- Apply cool water to skin.
- Do not use an alcohol rub.
- Do not give any beverages containing alcohol or caffeine.

Heat stroke (do not attempt to treat a case of heat stroke at home, but you can help while waiting for medical assistance to arrive.)

- Move the person to a cooler environment, or place him or her in a cool bath of water (as long as he or she is conscious and can be attended continuously).
- Alternatively, moisten the skin with lukewarm water and use a fan to blow cool air across the skin.
- Give cool beverages by mouth only if the person has a normal mental state and can tolerate it.

MEDICAL TREATMENT

The treatment is directed at cooling the patient in a controlled fashion while making sure that the patient stays hydrated and that their blood flow is normal.

- Treatment of heat exhaustion.
- Because heat exhaustion generally develops gradually, a person will often be dehydrated. Usually they may be given something to drink, and a cool sport beverage (with 6% or less glucose) should be used. IV fluid may be used if the person does not tolerate oral replacement (if he or she cannot keep anything down).
- The patient should stay in a cool environment and avoid strenuous activity for several days.
- Treatment of heat stroke.
- Treatment is aimed at reducing the patient's core temperature to normal as quickly as possible.
- The doctor may use immersion, evaporative, or invasive cooling techniques.
- In the evaporative technique, cold or ice packs may be placed in the armpits or groin. The skin is kept moist with cool fluid, and fans are directed to blow across the body.
- An IV will be started and fluids are given rapidly.
- The patient's urine output will be monitored.
- Treatment will continue until the patient's body core temperature is 101.3-102.2°F (38.5-39°C) and then stopped to keep from making the patient too cold.
- The patient most likely be admitted to the hospital for further blood tests and observation.

SUNBURN

A sunburn is a burn to living tissue such as skin produced by overexposure to ultraviolet (UV) radiation, commonly from the sun's rays. Exposure of the skin to lesser amounts of UV will often produce a suntan. Usual mild symptoms in humans and animals are red or reddish skin that is hot to the touch, general fatigue, and mild dizziness. Sunburn can be life-threatening and is a leading cause of skin cancer. Sunburn can easily be prevented through the use of sunscreen, clothing and hats, and by limiting solar exposure, especially during the middle of the day. The only cure for sunburn is slow healing, although skin creams can help.

CAUSE

The condition occurs when incident UV radiation exceeds the existing protective capacity of melanin in the skin. Concentrations of this pigment vary greatly among individuals, but in general, darker-skinned people have more melanin than those with lighter skin. Correspondingly, the incidence of sunburn among dark-skinned individuals is lower.

The sun is not the only origin — a similar burn can be produced by overexposure to other sources of UV such as from tanning lamps, or occupationally, such as from welding arcs.

SYMPTOMS

Typically there is initial redness (erythema), followed by varying degrees of pain, both proportional in severity to the duration and intensity of exposure.

Other symptoms are edema, itching, red and/or peeling skin, rash, nausea and fever. Also, a small amount of heat is given off from the burn, giving a warm feeling to the affected area. Sunburns may be first- or second-degree burns.

VARIATIONS

Minor sunburns typically cause nothing more than slight redness and tenderness to the affected areas. In more serious cases blistering can occur. Extreme sunburns can be painful to the point of debilitation and may require hospital care.

DURATION

Sunburn can occur in less than 15 minutes. Nevertheless, the inflicted harm is often not immediately obvious. It is thought that you need to be in the sun for at least 6 minutes to be affected by UV rays.

After the exposure, skin may turn red in as little as 30 minutes but most often takes 2 to 6 hours. Pain is usually most extreme 6 to 48 hours after exposure. The burn continues to develop for 24 to 72 hours occasionally followed by peeling skin in 3 to 8 days. Some peeling and itching may continue for several weeks.

STUDY–QUESTIONS

Write short notes on the following:

(a) Heat exhaustion.

(b) Heat stroke.

(c) Sunburn.

25 CHAPTER

EFFECTS OF COLD

CHILBLAINS

Chilblains, also called perniosis or blain, when occurring on the feet, is a medical condition that is often confused with frostbite and trench foot. Chilblains are acral ulcers that occur when a predisposed individual is exposed to cold and humidity. Causes are idiopathic or manifestations of serious medical conditions that need to be investigated. Chilblains can be prevented by keeping the feet and hands warm in cold weather. Smoking cessation is advised. A consultation with a dermatologist is mandatory.

SYMPTOMS AND DURATION

- Ulceration of the digits and toes
- Itchy skin inflammation
- Skin redness
- Toe skin inflammation
- Finger skin inflammation
- Earlobe inflammation

With treatment, chilblains usually heal within 3 weeks.

MEDICAL CARE

Once chilblain have occurred - avoid direct heat to the affected area, but keep the feet warm by the use of woolen socks and footwear. Do not rub or scratch chilblains. If you think the skin is broken, use an antiseptic dressing to prevent the chilblain becoming infected. Corns and callus are common in the pressure areas where chilblains can occur, so reduction of these will give some pain relief.

PREVENTING CHILBLAIN

Your doctor and a Podiatrist can help you in chilblains prevention. Some methods of preventing chilblain are:

1. Keeping your feet warm is an important way to prevent chilblains - wear several layers of clothing, which trap body heat more efficiently than one bulky layer.
2. Padding and pressure relief may give some relief for the chilblain symptoms.
3. Make sure your shoes are comfortable and don't squeeze your toes.
4. Do not let the feet become exposed to any direct source of heat, especially if the foot is very cold - this is a common factor causing chilblain.
5. Regularly pamper and condition the skin of your feet with home pedicures.
6. Wear warm clothes.
7. Thermal or insulating insoles can help keep the foot warm to prevent chilblain.
8. Exercise regularly to improve peripheral circulation.

TREATMENT

The list of treatments mentioned in various sources for Chilblain includes the following list. Always seek professional medical advice about any treatment or change in treatment plans.

- Keep area warm
- Avoid scratching
- Anti-itch creams, such as Calamine lotion
- Zambuk ointment
- Nifedipine may be used in more severe or recurrent cases. Its vasodilation helps reduce pain, facilitate healing and prevent recurrences.
- Self-medication can be provided by urinating on affected area and leaving to absorb for approximately 30 seconds. This should be repeated regularly during cold months.

The best treatment is to avoid having the chilblain problem in the first place by - wearing proper protection against the cold. Even though you may be used to working in the cold you should not overlook the effects of prolonged exposure, while in some circumstances which make you feel hot, e.g. skiing it is easy to underestimate the effects of cold on exposed areas.

The extremities and nose should be properly protected for proper cure of chilblain. If you do notice a white spot of damaged skin try to get into the warm and to warm up the area affected by rubbing it. Antibiotic creams may be useful if the skin ulcerates.

NATURAL HOME REMEDIES

There are a number of natural or home remedies that are recommended for the treatment of chilblains. Some suggestions for treating chilblain at home are follows here -

1. Egg and Honey : Honey will cicatrize open chilblain.Take a tablespoon of honey, a little glycerin, and one egg white. Then add to this a little flour to make a paste. Apply all over the chilblain. Leave it on for 6-8 hours and then wash off gently.
2. Lanolin (Heparin ointment) or similar rubbed into the feet will help retain body heat.
3. Wash ulcerated chilblains with tincture of myrrh diluted with warm water.

4. Use soothing lotions such as witch hazel and calamine.
5. Anoint cracked chilblain with Sultana pomatum, and cover with a soft, fine cloth. Cracked chilblains are difficult to cure in winter.
6. Gentle exercise will improve circulation to your feet.

PROFESSIONAL TREATMENT

Severe, ulcerating or recurring chilblain need professional attention. A qualified podiatrist can treat your chilblain and offer advice on prevention. If you have a pre-existing condition such as diabetes, see your doctor if your chilblain ulcerate.

FROSTBITE

Frostbite (*congelatio* in medical terminology) is the medical condition whereby damage is caused to skin and other tissues due to extreme cold. At or below 0°C (32°F), blood vessels close to the skin start to narrow (constrict). This helps to preserve core body temperature. In extreme cold or when the body is exposed to cold for long periods, this protective strategy can reduce blood flow in some areas of the body to dangerously low levels. The combination of cold temperature and poor blood flow can cause severe tissue injury by freezing the tissue.

Frostbite is most likely to happen in body parts farthest from the heart, and those with a lot of surface area exposed to cold. The initial stages of frostbite are sometimes called "frostnip". Risk factors for frostbite include using beta-blockers and having conditions such as diabetes and peripheral neuropathy.

SYMPTOMS

Generally, frostbite is accompanied by discoloration of the skin, along with burning and/or tingling sensations, partial or complete numbness, and possibly intense pain. If the nerves and blood vessels have been severely damaged, gangrene may follow, and amputation may eventually be required. If left untreated, frostbitten skin gradually darkens after a few hours. Skin destroyed by frostbite is completely black, and looks loose and flayed, as if burnt.

TREATMENT

Treatment of frostbite is not initiated until it is likely that the affected areas can remain thawed, as thawing followed by re-freezing can lead to more extensive and severe damage to the frostbitten tissue. In severe cases a body part that has frozen can cause the heart to stop when it thaws as the cold blood starts to circulate and shocks the heart as it flows through it, therefore it's important to warm someone who has had severe frostbite very carefully.

If medical attention is available, the victim is moved to a warm but never hot, safe area. The frostbitten areas are dressed, but not rubbed or massaged as ice crystals that have formed in the body act as tiny knives and ruin body tissue when rubbed. Also, beating or slapping the affected area is also very harmful, although it was once done to increase blood flow to the area.

If medical attention is not immediately available, the affected areas are placed in warm, but not hot, water, until tissues are soft and sensation has returned. The water temperature must be 107.6°F (42°C), and any major fluctuation from this can cause serious harm. At 113°F (45°C) the water will scald the frostbitten tissue, and below 107.6 has also proven to cause harm. Afterward, when the tissues have reached 98.6°F (37°C), the tissues are wrapped in clean, sterile dressings, and moved normally. It is crucial to keep the frostbitten skin from refreezing, as this is very harmful.

PREVENTION

Factors that contribute to frostbite include extreme cold, wet clothes, wind chill and poor circulation. This can be caused by tight clothing or boots, cramped positions, fatigue, certain medications, smoking, alcohol use or diseases that affect the blood vessels, such as diabetes.

Before anticipated prolonged exposure to cold, one should not drink alcohol or smoke, and get adequate food and rest.

Multiple layers of clothing, especially wind and water-proof synthetic fabrics, are the best protection against frostbite. Gloves and a hat that covers the ears are especially important. One should not wear fabrics like cotton, which retain moisture. If caught in a severe snowstorm, one should find shelter early or increase physical activity to maintain body warmth.

HYPOTHERMIA

Even when the weather is warm, do not forget that in many areas the water can be very, very cold. A sudden unexpected wake or other "unbalancing event" can land you in the frigid water. Although the possibility of drowning from falling into the water is a real threat, so too is hypothermia.

Hypothermia is a condition that exists when the body's temperature drops below ninety-five degrees. This can be caused by exposure to water or air. The loss of body heat results in loss of dexterity, loss of consciousness, and eventually loss of life. A few minutes in cold water makes it very difficult to swim, even to keep yourself afloat. In addition, a sudden, unexpected entry into cold water may cause a reflexive "gasp" allowing water to enter the lungs. Drowning can be almost instantaneous.

Your body can cool down 25 times faster in cold water than in air. If you examine the chart below you will see that survival time can be as short as 15 minutes. Water temperature, body size, amount of body fat, and movement in the water all play a part in cold water survival. Small people cool faster than large people and children cool faster than adults.

PFDs can help you stay alive longer in cold water. You can float without using energy and they cover part of your body thereby providing some protection from the cold water. When boating in cold water you should consider using a flotation coat or deck-suit style PFD. They cover more of your body and provide even more protection.

Hypothermia is progressive—the body passes through several stages before an individual lapses into an unconscious state. The extent of a person's hypothermia can be determined from the following:

1. Mild Hypothermia—the person feels cold, has violent shivering and slurred speech.
2. Medium Hypothermia—the person has a certain loss of muscle control, drowsiness, incoherence, stupor and exhaustion.
3. Severe Hypothermia—the person collapses and is unconscious and shows signs of respiratory distress and/or cardiac arrest probably leading to death.

Conservation of heat is the foremost objective for a person in the water. To accomplish this, limit body movement. Don't swim unless you can reach a nearby boat or floating object. Swimming lowers your body temperature and even good swimmers can drown in cold water.

If you can pull yourself partially out of the water - do so. The more of your body that is out of the water (on top of an overturned boat or anything that floats), the less heat you will lose. Especially keep your head out of the water if at all possible - this will lessen heat loss and increase survival time.

Wearing a PFD in the water is a key to survival. A PFD allows you float with a minimum of energy expended and allows you to assume the heat escape lessening position - H. E. L. P.

This position, commonly referred to as the fetal position, permits you to float effortlessly and protect those areas most susceptible to heat loss including the armpits, sides of the chest, groin, and the back of the knees. If you find yourself in the water with others, you should huddle as a group to help lessen heat loss.

Treatment of hypothermia can be accomplished by gradually raising the body temperature back to normal. Re-establishing body temperature can be as simple as sharing a sleeping bag or blanket with another individual, or applying warm moist towels to the individual's neck, sides of chest and groin. Remove wet clothes as they inhibit heat retention. A warm bath could be used for mild to medium hypothermia, gradually increasing the temperature. Keep arms and legs out of the water and do not attempt to raise the body temperature too quickly.

Do not massage the victim's arms and legs. Massage will cause the circulatory system to take cold blood from the surface into the body's core, resulting in further temperature drop. Do not give alcohol, which causes loss of body heat, or coffee and tea which are stimulants (and cause vasodilation) and may have the same effect as massage.

STUDY–QUESTIONS

Write short notes on the following:

(a) Hypothermia.

(b) Frostbite.

(c) Chilblain.

***

26

CHAPTER

Handling and Transportation of Casualty

INTRODUCTION

The aim of first aid treatment is transporting of injured people to the nearest medical hospital/clinic. Before transporting, the first aider has to ensure that casualty's respiration is normal, heart is beating, bleeding is arrested and injured limbs are well supported. A first aider acting alone or with unskilled help, may easily cause more damage trying to move the casualty than by dealing with him at the site of accident. Hence, first aider must remember that casualties should be handled minimum. All body parts must be examined only once and in one go.

As the first aider rescues the causalities from fire, collapsing building or poisonous environment, he examines the casualties and then makes necessary arrangements to transport them to the nearest medical aid/hospital/clinic.

REMOVAL OF CAUSALITIES

Casualties may be removed to shelter or to medical aid (if near by) following methods:

(i) Support of single helper.

(ii) Handseats and the kitchen chair carry.

(iii) Blanket Lift.

(iv) Stretcher.

(v) Wheeled transport (ambulance, car, bus).

(vi) Air and sea travel.

METHODS OF CARRYING OF CASUALTY

There are various methods of carrying of casualties. Depending on availability of helpers, methods are adopted.

A. Cradle—This method is used when the casualty is light weight or he is a child. In this method, the injured person should be carried from below the shoulder and knee with the hands.

B. Human Crutch—This method is used when injured person is able to walk with assistance. In this case, the casualty by putting your arm around his waist grasping the clothing at his hip and placing his arm round your neck, holding his hand with your free hand.

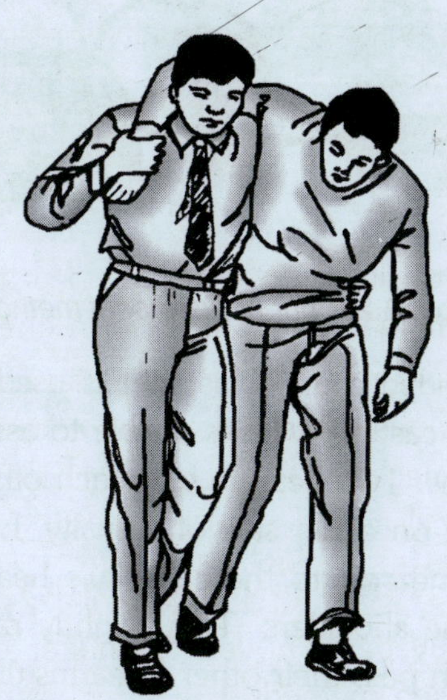

Fig. 26.1: *Human crutch*

C. Pick a Back—This method is used when the casualty is small, light and able to hold arm.

Methods adopted when two or more bearers are available:

A. **The four handed seat**—This seat is used when the casualty is able to assist the bearer by using one or both arms. Two bearers face each other behind the casualty and clasp their left wrists with their right hands and each other's right wrist with their left hands. The casualty is instructed to place one arm round the neck of each bearer, so that he may raise himself to sit on their hands and steady himself during transport. The bearers rise together and step off. The bearer on the right hand side of the casualty with the right foot and the left hand bearer with the left foot.

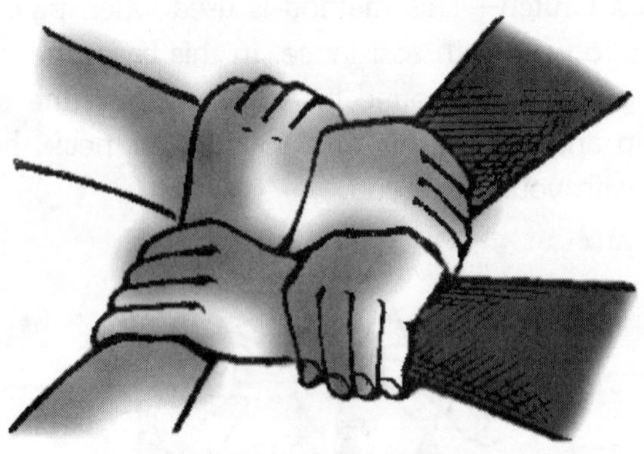

Fig. 26.2: *Four handed seat method.*

B. **The two handed seat**—This seat is used for the purpose of carrying a casualty who is unable to assist the bearers by using his arms. Two bearers face each other and stoop (not to kneel) one on either side of casualty. Each bearer passes his forearm nearest to the casualty's head under his back just below the shoulders. They slightly raise the casualty's back and then pass their other forearms under the middle of his thighs and clasp their hands, the bearer on the left of the casualty with his palm upwards and holding a folded kerchief to prevent hurting by the fingernails, the bearer on the right of the casualty with his palm downwards making a hook grip. In all cases of carrying by hand seats the bearers have to walk with the cross over steps and not by paces.

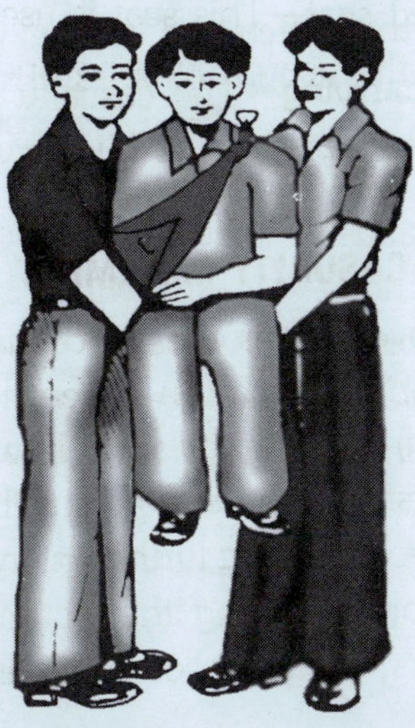

Fig. 26.3: *Two handed seat method.*

C. Fore and aft method—This method is used to place one unconscious casualty on to a stretcher or a carry chair. One bearer stands between the legs of the casualty, facing the feet, bends down and grasps the casualty under his knees. The other bearer takes a position behind the casualty and

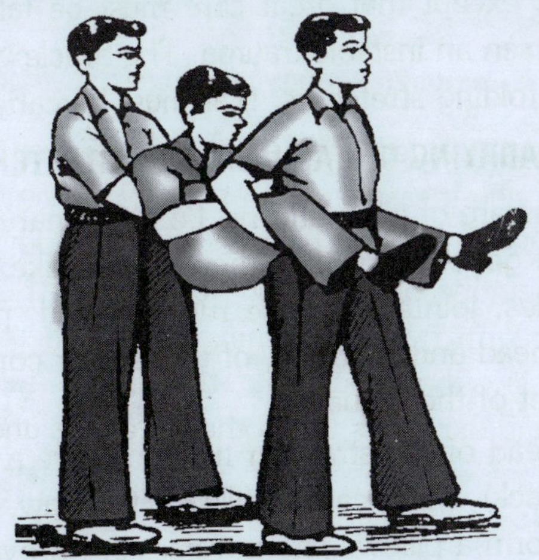

Fig. 26.4: *Fore and aft method.*

after raising his trunk passes his hands under casualty's armpits and grasps his own wrist on the casualty's chest. The casualty is then lifted and bearers walk in step.

D. **Kitchen chair carrying**—The casualty is made to sit on a chair and bearers walk in step by carrying the patient in a chair.

CASUALTY MOVEMENT

The casualty movement is the procedures used to move a casualty from the initial location (street, home, workplace, wilderness, battlefield) to the ambulance. In wilderness or combat conditions, it may first be necessary to stabilize the patient prior to moving them to avoid causing further injury. In such situations, evacuation may involve carrying the victim some distance on improvised stretchers, a travois or other improvised carrying gear.

Once the patient is ready to be moved, the first step is the casualty lifting, to put him/her on a stretcher. The final step is the patient transfer from the stretcher to the hospital bed. The present article is only about the handling of the stretcher once the casualty is on it. The use of wheeled stretchers, usually used in most developed emergency services, does not need much explanation, except that great care must be taken in order to avoid to worsen an instable trauma. The article will focus on the handling of folding stretchers, that must be caried.

CARRYING OF CASUALTIES ON STRETCHERS

Stretchers are of two patterns, i.e., 'Ordinary and Telescopic Handled'. In general principle they are all alike, and consist of poles, handles, jointed traverse runners, bed, pillow sack and slings. The head and foot end, of a stretcher correspond to the head and feet of the casualty.

At the head of the stretcher there may be a canvas overlay (the pillow sack) which can be filled with straw, hay, cotton or clothing to form a pillow. The traverses are provided with joints for opening or closing the stretcher. The telescopic handled pattern is similar but its length can be reduced to 6 feet by sliding the handles underneath the poles. When closed the poles of a stretcher lie close together, the traverse bar being bent-inwards, the canvas bed neatly folded on top of the poles and held in position by the slings, which are laid along with canvas and secured by strap which is placed transversely at the end of each sling and pass through the large loop of the other and round the poles and bed.

STRETCHER

Stretchers are used to carry seriously ill or injured casualties to an ambulance or to a shelter. For stretcher exercise, i.e., loading of casualty, to stretcher, then to ambulance and again unloading requires four bearers to carry out all procedures correctly and without causing any further discomfort to the casualty.

TYPES OF STRETCHERS

(i) **Improvised stretchers**—This is used in case of emergency when proper stretcher is not available. In this method, the button of the shirt of the injured person are opened and the open flaps of the shirt are folded and are caught by the helpers. The legs and head is held by other helpers and the person is made to lie on stretcher.

(ii) **Utila folding stretcher**—This is light weight stretcher. It consists of telescopic lifting handles and pull bars, guard rails, straps for safety and wheel brakes. In this trolley height, tilt knee and backrest can be adjusted to suit the casualty's condition.

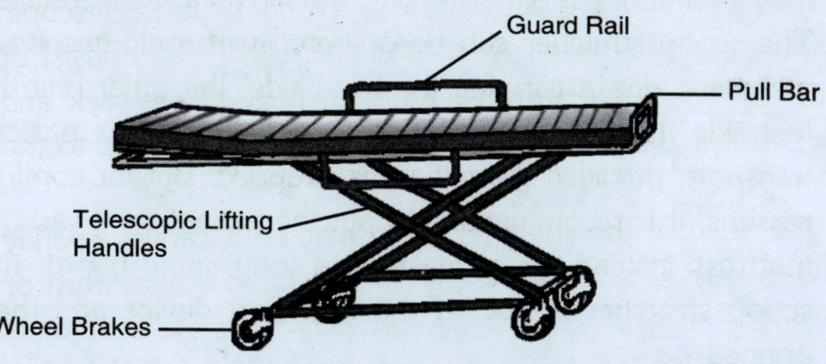

Fig. 26.5: *Utila folding stretcher.*

(iii) **Standard furlley stretcher**—Furely stretcher is the standard first aid equipment. It consists of poles, handles, traverse and canvas bed. The traverses are so jointed, that the stretcher can be opened and closed. When closed, the poles lie close together with the canvas bed folded at the top.

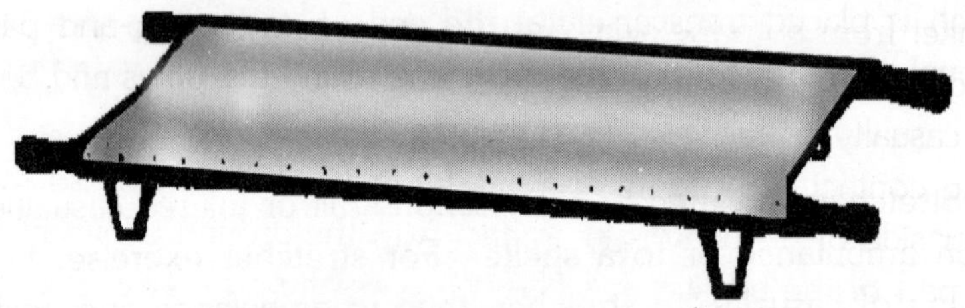

Fig. 26.6: *Standard furlley stretcher*

(iv) **Pole and canvas stretcher**—It consist of a canvas or plastic sheet with handles and side sleeves and a pair of carrying poles. Spreading bars are inserted over the ends of the poles to keep them apart and to make the stretcher firm and rigid. This stretchers is most commonly used for lifting a casualty from one to another stretcher to a trolley.

(v) **Scoop stretcher**—The scoop stretcher (or clamshell, Robertson Orthopedic Stretcher, or just scoop) is a device used specifically for casualty lifting. It is a tubular structure that can be split vertically into two parts; blades are fixed to the tubes. The two halves are put on each side of the casualty, and then clipped together; the blades go under the casualty and replace the hands of the first responders (as they are thinner, this less likely to worsen an instable trauma). The scoop stretcher can be operated with only two team members: one is carrying the head side, the other one the feet side. The scoop stretcher can be used for patient transport, provided the patient is strapped. But for comfort reasons, it is recommended to put the patient on a vacuum mattress instead, or at least on a long spine board: the scoop stretcher is put on the transport device and then opened.

LOADING STRETCHER

To transfer a casualty from the accident site to the stretcher is called *loading stretcher*.

1. Blanket Lift

If the injured person is lying on some blanket, then fold the blanket from both the sides. Instruct the two bearers to keep the head and ankles firm. Two other bearers then very gently turn the casualty on his side. Now, move the rolled part of blanket to be in contact with the casualty and gently roll him over, so that other side of his body is in contact with the ground. Now unroll the part of the blanket and place the casualty on his back in the centre of the blanket. The blanket is rolled tightly upto the sides of the casualty. Now four bearers, two on either side lift the casualty all together. If poles of good length (mosquito net set poles) and rigidity are available, roll the blanket over the poles, until the poles are pressed to the side of casualty. This makes lifting and carrying of casualty much easier.

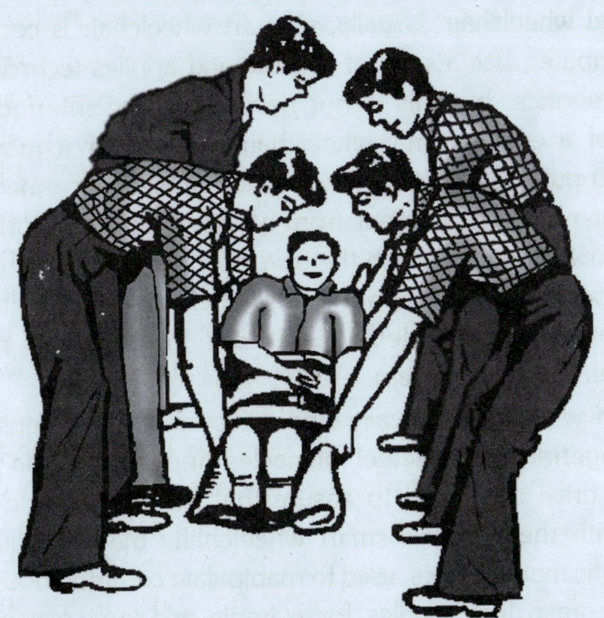

Fig. 26.7: *Blanket Lift*.

2. Manual Lift

If the casualty has a fractured spine, do not move him unless absolutely necessary. Sometimes you may have to lift the casualty on to a stretcher. When scoop stretcher cannot be used because of soft ground, ambulance cannot reach the site of the accident, and if danger dictates emergency movement, manual lift becomes necessary.

One person should kneel at the casualty's head and support his head and neck in the normal neutral position. Remove hard objects from his pockets. Put sufficient soft padding between his legs. Tie a figure of eight bandage around his knees. Place his arms across his chest.

SMART WHEELCHAIR

A smart wheelchair is any motorized platform with a chair designed to assist a user with a physical disability, where an artificial control system augments or replaces user control. Its purpose is to reduce or eliminate the user's task of driving a motorized wheelchair. Usually, a smart wheelchair is controlled by a computer, has a suite of sensors and applies techniques in mobile robotics, but this is not necessary. The interface may consist of a conventional wheelchair joystick, or it may be a "sipp and puff" device or a touch-sensitive display connected to a computer. This is different from a conventional motorized or electric wheelchair, in which the user exerts manual control over motor speed and direction via a joystick or other switch- or potentiometer-based device, without intervention by the wheelchair's control system.

Smart wheelchairs usually employ sonar, infrared sensors or laser rangefinders to detect obstacles and modify the user's intended drive command to ensure that the platform does not collide with them. Some smart wheelchairs may be equipped with robotic manipulators, used to manipulate common household objects or grasp door handles, for example, and some may employ computer vision techniques to visually detect obstacles or landmarks to assist in navigation.

Smart wheelchairs are designed for a variety of user types. Some platforms are designed for users with cognitive impairments, such as dementia, where these typically apply collision-avoidance techniques to ensure that users do not accidentally select a drive command that results in a collision. Other platforms focus on users living with severe motor disabilities, such as cerebral pulsae, or with paraplegia, and the role of the smart wheelchair is to interpret small muscular activations as high-level commands and execute them. Such platforms typically employ techniques from artificial intelligence, such as path-planning, artificial reasoning, and behavior-based control.

CARRYING A STRETCHER

After placing the casualty on the stretcher, the bearers should take up their positions at each end of the stretcher. Atleast two bearers are required to carry a stretcher and the person incharge of the casualty should be at the casualty's head. If bystanders are available, they should be used to help carrying the stretcher to spread the load. There should be atleast one trained bearer at each end of the stretcher. Unless a casualty is suffering from shock, the head should be kept higher than the feet. Hence, as a general rule, the casualty should be carried feet first. There are several exceptions.

1. When going upstairs or hills if the lower limbs are not injured.
2. When going downstairs or hills the casualty's lower limbs are injured or the casualty is suffering from hypothermia.
3. When carrying a casualty to the side or foot of a bed.
4. When loading casualty into an ambulance.

The stretcher is lowered with its head one pace from the door of the ambulance. The casually will be loaded head first. The bearers now stand to the stretcher and on the command 'load' the bearers turn inwards, stoop, grasp the poles of the stretcher, hands wide apart, palms uppermost, they rise slowly, lifting the stretcher, holding it at level at the full extent of the arms. They then take a side pace to the ambulance raising the stretcher evenly to the level of the berth to be loaded. The front bearers place the runners in the grooves and then assist the rear bearers to slide the stretcher into its place and secure it. If slings are used they should be kept with the stretcher.

Many ambulances are provided with upper and lower berths. In such cases the sequence of loading is upper right, upper left, lower right and lower left.

Unloading the Stretcher

The injured person is unloaded from the stretcher after being brought to the hospital or house. The methods applied for the unloading are same as loading patient on the stretcher described earlier. If the injured person is lying in bedsheet or blanket, then he is picked up by the four corners with the help of four persons and is made to lie on the bed, then the sheet is drawn out. If the person is not lying on the blanket, then the helpers sit around the person in all sides, then they rest their hands below the head, waist, chest, hips and legs of the injured person and lift him up from the stretcher.

STUDY–QUESTIONS

1. Discuss the various methods of carrying of casualty.
2. Explain the various types of methods adopted when two or more bearers are available.
3. Write short note on manual lift.

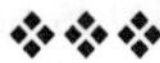

SECTION-IV

Emergency Management

Chapter: 27	Emergency Services	305–320
Chapter: 28	Ambulance	321–331
Chapter: 29	Major Disaster Management	332–346
Chapter: 30	Children in Accident and Emergency	347–358
Chapter: 31	Elderly People in Accident and Emergency	359–369
Chapter: 32	Eye Complaints and Emergencies	370–383
Chapter: 33	ENT and Dental Emergencies	384–395
Chapter: 34	Women's Health Problems in A & E	396–404
Chapter: 35	Medical Emergencies	405–484
Chapter: 36	Common Medical Problems	485–524

27 CHAPTER

EMERGENCY SERVICES

EMERGENCY

An emergency is a situation which poses an immediate risk to health, life, property or environment. Most emergencies require urgent intervention to prevent a worsening of the situation, although in some situations, mitigation may not be possible and agencies may only be able to offer palliative care for the aftermath.

Whilst some emergencies are self evident (such as a natural disaster which threatens many lives), many smaller incidents require the subjective opinion of an observer (or affected party) in order to decide whether it qualifies as an emergency.

The precise definition of an emergency, the agencies involved and the procedures used, vary by jurisdiction, and this is usually set by the government, whose agencies (emergency services) are responsible for emergency planning and management.

Whilst most emergency services agree on protecting human health, life and property, the environmental impacts are not considered sufficiently important by some agencies. This also extends to areas such as animal welfare, where some emergency organisations cover this element through the 'property' definition, where animals which are owned by a person are threatened (although this does not cover wild animals). This means that some agencies will not mount an 'emergency' response where it endangers wild animals or environment, although others will respond to such incidents (such as oil spills at sea which pose a threat to marine life). The attitude of the agencies involved is likely to reflect the predominant opinion of the government of the area.

TYPES OF EMERGENCY

DANGERS TO LIFE

Many emergencies cause an immediate danger to the life of people involved. This can range from emergencies affecting a single person, such as the entire range of medical emergencies which include heart attacks, strokes and trauma, to incidents affecting large numbers of people such as natural disasters including hurricanes, floods or mudslides.

Most agencies consider these to be the highest priority of emergency, which follows the general school of thought that nothing is more important than human life.

DANGERS TO HEALTH

Some emergencies are not immediately threatening to life, but might have serious implications for the continued health and well-being of a person or persons (although a health emergency can subsequently escalate to be threatening to life).

The causes of a 'health' emergency are often very similar to the causes of an emergency threatening to life, which includes medical emergencies and natural disasters, although the range of incidents which can be categorised here is far greater than those which cause a danger to life (such as broken limbs, which do not usually cause death, but immediate intervention is required if the person is to recover properly)

DANGERS TO PROPERTY

Other emergencies do not threaten any people, but do threaten peoples' property. An example of this would be a fire in a warehouse which has been evacuated. The situation is treated as an emergency as the fire may spread to other buildings, or may cause sufficient damage to make the business unable to continue (affecting livelihood of the employees).

Many agencies categorise property emergency as the lowest priority, and may not take as many risks in dealing with it. For instance, firefighters are unlikely to enter a burning building which they know to be empty, as the risk is unjustified, whereas they are more likely to enter a building where people are reported as trapped.

DANGERS TO THE ENVIRONMENT

Some emergencies do not immediately endanger life, health or property, but do affect the natural environment and creatures living within it. Not all agencies consider this to be a genuine emergency, but it can have far reaching effects on animals and the long term condition of the land. Examples would include forest fires and marine oil spills.

SYSTEMS OF CLASSIFYING EMERGENCIES

Agencies across the world have different systems for classifying incidents, but all of them serve to help them allocate finite resource, by prioritising between different emergencies.

The first stage in any classification is likely to be defining whether the incident qualifies as an emergency, and consequently if it warrants an emergency response. Some agencies may still respond to non-emergency calls, depending on their remit and availability of resource. An example of this would be a fire department responding to help retrieve a cat from a tree, where no life, health or property is immediately at risk.

Following this, many agencies assign a sub-classification to the emergency, prioritising incidents which have the most potential for risk to life, health or property (in that order). For instance, many ambulance services use a system called the Advanced Medical Priority Dispatch System (AMPDS) or a similar solution. The AMPDS categorises all calls to the ambulance service using it as either 'A' category (immediately life threatening), 'B' Category (immediately health threatening) or 'C' category (non-emergency call which still requires a response). Some services will now also have a fourth category, where they believe that no response is required after clinical questions are asked.

Another system for prioritizing medical calls is known as Emergency Medical Dispatch (EMD). Jurisdictions that use EMD typically assign a code of "alpha" (low priority), "bravo" (medium priority), "charlie" (requiring advanced life support), delta (high priority, requiring advanced life support) or "echo" (maximum possible priority, e.g., witnessed cardiac arrests) to each inbound request for service; these codes are then used to determine the appropriate level of response.

Other systems (especially as regards major incidents) use objective measures to direct resource. Two such systems are CHALET and ETHANE, which are both mnemonics to help emergency services staff classify incidents, and direct resource. Each of these acronyms helps ascertain the number of casualties (usually including the number of dead and number of non-injured people involved), how the incident has occurred, and what emergency services are required.

AGENCIES INVOLVED IN DEALING WITH EMERGENCIES

Most developed countries have a number of emergency services operating within them, whose purpose is to provide assistance in dealing with any emergency which may occur. They are often government operated, paid for from tax revenue as a public service, but in some cases, they may be private companies, responding to emergencies in return for payment, or they may be voluntary organisations, providing the assistance from funds raised from donations. Most developed countries operate three core emergency services which are:

- **Police** – who deal with security of person and property, which can cover all three categories of emergency. They may also deal with punishment of those who cause an emergency through their actions.
- **Fire service** – who deal with potentially harmful fires, but also often rescue operations such as dealing with road traffic

collisions. Their actions help to prevent loss of life, damage to health and damage to or loss of property.

- **Emergency medical service** (Ambulance service) – These services attempt to reduce loss of life or damage to health. This service is likely to be decisive in attempts to prevent loss of life and damage to health. In some countries or regions, two or more of these services may be provided by the same agency (e.g., the fire service providing emergency medical cover), and under different conditions (e.g. publicly funded fire service and police, but a private ambulance service). There may also be a number of secondary emergency services, which may be a part of one of the core agencies, or may be separate entities who assist the main agencies. This can include services providing specialist rescue (such as mountain rescue or mine rescue, bomb disposal or search and rescue.

EMERGENCY ACTION PRINCIPLES (EAP)

Emergency action principles are the key 'rules' which guide the actions of rescuers and potential rescuers. Because of the inherent nature of emergencies, no two are likely to be the same, so emergency action principles help to guide rescuers at incidents, by sticking to some basic tenets.

The adherence to (and contents of) the principles by would be rescuers varies widely based on the training the people involved in emergency have received, the support available from emergency services (and the time it will take to arrive) and the emergency itself. The key principle taught in almost all systems is that the rescuer, be they a lay person or a professional, should assess the situation for danger. The reason that an assessment for danger is given such high priority is that it is core to emergency management that rescuers do not become secondary victims of any incident, as this creates a further emergency that must be dealt with.

A typical assessment for danger would involve observation of the surroundings, starting with the cause of the accident (e.g.

a falling object) and expanding outwards to include any situational hazards (e.g. fast moving traffic) and history or secondary information given by witnesses, bystanders or the emergency services (e.g. an attacker still waiting nearby).

Once a primary danger assessment has been complete, this should not end the system of checking for danger, but should inform all other parts of the process. If at any time the risk from any hazard poses a significant danger (as a factor of likelihood and seriousness) to the rescuer, they should consider whether they should approach the scene (or leave the scene if appropriate).

EMERGENCY MANAGEMENT

There are many protocols which the emergency services use in dealing with an emergency, which usually start with planning before an emergency occurs. One commonly used system for demonstrating the phases is shown here on the right.

The planning phase starts at preparedness, where the agencies decide on how they will respond to a given incident or set of circumstances. This should ideally include lines of command and control, and division of activities between agencies. This avoids potentially negative situations such as three separate agencies all starting an official rest centre for victims of a disaster.

Following an emergency occurring, the agencies then move to a response phase, where they execute their plans, and may end up improvising some areas of their response (due to gaps in the planning phase, which are inevitable due to the individual nature of most incidents).

Agencies may then be involved in recovery following the incident, where they assist in the clear up from the incident, or help the people involved overcome their mental trauma.

The final phase in the circle is mitigation which involves taking steps to ensure that no re-occurrence is possible, or putting additional plans in place to ensure less damage is done. This should feed back in to the preparedness stage, with updated plans in place to deal with future emergencies, thus completing the circle.

STATE OF EMERGENCY

In the event of a major incident, such as civil unrest or a major disaster, many governments maintain the right to declare a state of emergency, which gives them extensive powers over the daily lives of their citizens, and may include temporary curtailment on certain civil rights, including the right to trial (for instance to discourage looting of an evacuated area, a shoot on sight policy may be in force)

PERSONAL EMERGENCIES

Some people undergo incidents which cause them to believe they are in an emergency situation. However, it does not pose a risk to their life, physical health or property. In some instances, people may feel that they are entitled to or deserve an emergency response from agencies they come in to contact with, which is a view that may or may not be shared by the agency.

Some of these cases may be genuine emergencies if they threaten the mental health and well-being of the person involved, but many agencies do not recognise this as valid. This is more likely to be dealt with by social services or a physician than by the traditional emergency service agencies.

EMERGENCY DEPARTMENT

The emergency department (ED), sometimes termed the emergency room (ER), emergency ward (EW), accident & emergency (A&E) department or casualty department is a hospital or primary care department that provides initial treatment to patients with a broad spectrum of illnesses and injuries, some of which may be life-threatening and requiring immediate attention. Emergency departments developed during the 20th century in response to an increased need for rapid assessment and management of critical illnesses. In some countries, emergency departments have become important entry points for those without other means of access to medical care.

Upon arrival in the ED, people typically undergo a brief triage, or sorting, interview to help determine the nature and severity of their illness. Individuals with serious illnesses are then seen by a physician more rapidly than those with less severe symptoms or injuries. After initial assessment and treatment, patients are either admitted to the hospital, stabilized and transferred to another hospital for various reasons, or discharged. The staff in emergency departments not only includes doctors and nurses with specialized training in emergency medicine but in house emergency medical technicians,respiratory therapists, radiology technicians, Physician Assistants (PAs)/Healthcare Assistants (HCAs), volunteers, and other support staff who all work as a team to treat emergency patients and provide support to anxious family members. The emergency departments of most hospitals operate around the clock, although staffing levels are usually much lower at night. Since a diagnosis must be made by an attending physician, the patient is initially assigned a *chief complaint* rather than a diagnosis. This is usually a symptom: headache, nausea, loss of consciousness. The chief complaint remains a primary fact until the attending physician makes a diagnosis.

CRITICAL CONDITIONS HANDLED

CARDIAC ARREST

Cardiac arrest may occur in the ED/A&E or a patient may be transported by ambulance to the emergency department already in this state. Treatment is basic and advanced life support as taught in the Advanced Life Support and Advanced Cardiac Life Support courses. This is an immediately life-threatening condition which requires immediate action in salvageable cases.

HEART ATTACK

Patients arriving to the emergency department with a myocardial infarction (heart attack) are likely to be triaged to the resuscitation area. They will receive oxygen and monitoring and have an early ECG; aspirin will be given if not contraindicated or not already administered by the ambulance team; morphine or diamorphine will be given for pain; sublingual (under the tongue) or buccal (between cheek and upper gum) glyceryl trinitrate (nitroglycerin) (GTN or NTG) will be given.

An ECG that reveals ST segment elevation or new left bundle branch block suggests complete blockage of one of the main coronary arteries. These patients require immediate reperfusion (re-opening) of the occluded vessel. This can be achieved in two ways: thrombolysis (clot-busting medication) or percutaneous transluminal coronary angioplasty (PTCA). Both of these are effective in reducing significantly the mortality of myocardial infarction. Many centers are now moving to the use of PTCA as it is somewhat more effective than thrombolysis if it can be administered early. This may involve transfer to a nearby facility with facilities for angioplasty.

TRAUMA

Major trauma, the term for patients with multiple injuries, often from a road traffic accident or a fall, is treated by a trauma team who have been trained using the principles taught in the internationally recognized Advanced Trauma Life Support (ATLS) course of the American College of Surgeons. Some other international training bodies have started to run similar courses based on the same principles.

The services that are provided in an emergency department can range from simple x-rays and the setting of broken bones to those of a full-scale trauma center. Emergency medical technicians often work as support staff in emergency departments under the supervision of nurses and doctors. A patients chances of survival are greatly improved if emergency care begins within one hour of an accident (such as a car accident) or onset of acute illness (such as a heart attack). This critical time frame is commonly known as the "golden hour."

Some emergency departments in smaller hospitals are located near a helipad which is used by helicopters to transport a patient to a trauma center. This inter-hospital transfer is often done when a patient requires advanced medical care unavailable at the local facility. In such cases the emergency department can only stabilize the patient for transport.

Some patients arrive at an emergency department for a complaint of mental illness. In many jurisdictions (including many U.S. states), patients who appear to be mentally ill and to present a danger to themselves or others may be brought against their will to an emergency department by law enforcement officers for psychiatric examination. From the emergency department, patients thought to be mentally ill may be transferred to a psychiatric unit (in many cases involuntarily).

ASTHMA AND COPD

Acute exacerbations of chronic respiratory diseases, mainly asthma and chronic obstructive pulmonary disease (COPD) are assessed as emergencies and treated with oxygen therapy, bronchodilators, steroids or theophylline, have an urgent chest X-ray and arterial blood gases and are referred for intensive care if necessary. Non invasive ventilation in the ED has reduced the requirement for intubation in many cases of severe exacerbations of COPD.

SPECIAL FACILITIES, TRAINING, AND EQUIPMENT

An ED requires different equipment and different approaches than most other hospital divisions. Patients frequently arrive with unstable conditions, and so must be treated quickly. They may be unconscious, and information such as their medical history, allergies, and blood type may be unavailable. ED staff are trained to work quickly and effectively even with minimal information.

ED staff must also interact efficiently with pre-hospital care providers such as EMTs, paramedics, and others who are occasionally based in an ED. The pre-hospital providers may use equipment unfamiliar to the average physician, but ED physicians must be expert in using (and safely removing) specialized equipment, since devices such as Military Anti-Shock Trousers ("MAST") and traction splints require special procedures. Among other reasons, given that they must be able to handle specialized equipment, physicians can now specialize in emergency medicine, and EDs employ many such specialists.

ED staff have much in common with ambulance and fire crews, combat medics, search and rescue teams, and disaster response teams. Often, joint training and practice drills are organized to improve the coordination of this complex response system. Busy EDs exchange a great deal of equipment with ambulance crews, and both must provide for replacing, returning, or reimbursing for costly items.

Cardiac arrest and major trauma are relatively common in EDs, so defibrillators, automatic ventilation and CPR machines, and bleeding control dressings are used heavily. Survival in such cases is greatly enhanced by shortening the wait for key interventions, and in recent years some of this specialized equipment has spread to pre-hospital settings. The best-known example is defibrillators, which spread first to ambulances, then in an automatic version to police cars, and most recently to public spaces such as airports, office buildings, hotels, and even shopping malls.

Because time is such an essential factor in emergency treatment, EDs typically have their own diagnostic equipment to avoid waiting for equipment installed elsewhere in the hospital. Nearly all have an X-ray room, and many now have full radiology facilities including CT scanners and ultrasonography equipment. Laboratory services may be handled on a priority basis by the hospital lab, or the ED may have its own "STAT Lab" for basic labs (blood counts, blood typing, toxicology screens, etc) that must be returned very rapidly.

EMERGENCY MEDICAL SERVICES PROVIDERS

Depending on your country, area within in country, or clinical need, EMS may be provided by one (or several) organisations, with different reasons for operating the service. Some countries closely regulate the industry (and may require anyone operating the EMS to be qualified to a set level), whereas others allow quite wide differences between types of operator.

- *Government EMS*—Operating separately from (although alongside) the fire and police service of the area, these ambulances are funded by local or national government. In some countries, these only tend to be found in big cities, whereas in countries such as the United Kingdom, almost all emergency ambulances are part of the NHS.
- *Fire or Police Linked Service*—In many countries (USA, France, Germany, Japan), many ambulances are operated by the local fire or police service. This is particularly common in rural areas, where maintaining a separate service is not necessarily cost effective. This can lead, in some instances, to an illness or injury being attended by a vehicle other than an ambulance, such as Fire truck.
- *Voluntary EMS*—Some charities or non-profit companies operate ambulances, both the an emergency and patient transport function. This may be along similar lines to volunteer Fire companies and either community or privately owned. They may be linked to a voluntary fire service, with volunteers providing both services. There are also charities who focus on providing ambulances for the community, or for cover at private events (sports etc.). The Red Cross provides this service in many countries across the world on a volunteer basis (and in others as a Private Ambulance Service), as do some other smaller organisations such as St John Ambulance. In some countries, these volunteer ambulances may be seen providing support to the full time ambulance crews during times of emergency.
- *Private Ambulance Service*—Normal commercial companies with paid employees, but often on contract to the local or national government. Many private companies provide only the patient transport elements of ambulance care (i.e. non urgent), but in some places, they are also contracted to provide emergency care, or to form a 'second tier' response, where they only respond to emergencies when all of the full-time emergency ambulance crews are busy or

to respond to non-emergency home calls, such as "pick up and put back" calls, which are made when a person falls without injury, but needs help getting up. Dependant on their contract they might also provide "first aid only" services, such as providing bandages (but not a trip to the hospital emergency room) to a child who skinned his/her knees at a playground. They may also be contracted by private clients to provide standby EMS for large events such as sports, conventions, or parades.

- *Combined Emergency Service*—These are full service emergency service agencies, which may be found in places such as airports or large colleges and universities. Their key feature is that all personnel are trained not only in ambulance (EMT) care, but as a firefighter and a peace officer (police function). They may also be found in some smaller towns and cities which do not have the resource or requirement for separate services. This multifunctionality allows to make the most of limited resource or budget, but having a single team respond to any emergency.
- *Hospital Based Service*—Some hospitals may provide their own ambulance service as a service to the community, or where ambulance care is unreliable or chargeable. Their use would be dependent on using the services of the providing hospital.

LEVELS OF CARE

A PHTLS exercise of the Israeli EMS involving Paramedics and Emergency medical technicians, and first responders utilising ALS equipment like EKGs as well as a backboard. Dependent on the country and area in which the service operates, and what type of provider it is, there may be any one of several levels of EMS crew. They can broadly be divided in to Basic Life Support (BLS) qualifications (responders, ambulance technicians) which usually involves non-invasive procedures and Advanced Life Support (ALS) qualifications (higher level technicians and paramedics) which includes more invasive procedures (such as intubation and infusion). Some of the most common qualification terms are:

- **First Responder**—A person who arrives first at the scene of an incident, and whose job is to provide early critical care such as CPR or using an AED. First responders may be dispatched by the ambulance service, may be passers-by, or may be dispatched to the scene from other agencies, such as the police or fire departments.
- **Ambulance Driver**—Some services employ staff with no medical qualification (or just a first aid certificate) whose job is to simply drive the patients from place to place
- **Ambulance Care Assistant**—Have varying levels of training across the world, but these staff are usually only required to perform patient transport duties (which can include stretcher or wheelchair cases), rather than acute care. Dependant on provider, they may be trained in first aid or extended stills such as use of an AED, oxygen therapy and other live saving or palliative skills. In some services, they may provide emergency cover when other units are not available, or when accompanied by a fully qualified technician or paramedic.
- **Emergency medical technician**—It is also known as Ambulance Technician.Technicians are usually able to perform a wide range of emergency care skills, such as defibrillation, spinal care, and oxygen therapy. Some countries split this term in to several levels (such as in the US, where there is EMT-I and EMT-II). This title is not protected in all countries, such as in Great Britain, where anyone can legally call themselves an EMT, even without any training.
- **Paramedic**—This is a high level of medical training and usually involves key skills not permissible for technicians, including cannulation (and with it the ability to use a range of drugs such as morphine), intubation and other skills such

as performing a cricothyrotomy[16]. In many countries, this is a protected title, and use of it without the relevant qualification may result in criminal prosecution.

- **Emergency Care Practitioner**—This is a position sometimes called a 'super paramedic' and is designed to bridge the link between ambulance care and the care of a general practitioner. ECPs are university graduates in Emergency Medical Care or qualified paramedics who have undergone further training, and are authorized to perform specialized emergency techniques using expert emergency drugs. Additionally some may prescribe medicines (from a limited list) for longer term care, such as antibiotics. With respect to a Primary Health Care setting, they are also educated in a range of Diagnostic techniques.
- **Registered Nurse (RN)**—Some services use nurses for ambulance work, and as with doctors, this is mostly as air-medical rescuers or critical care transport providers, often in conjunction with a technician or paramedic. They may bring extra skills to the care of the patient, especially those who may be critically ill or injured in locations that do not enjoy close proximity to a high level of definitive care such as trauma, cardiac, or stroke centers.
- **Doctor**—Some ambulance services - most notably air ambulances will employ physicians to attend on the ambulances, bringing a full range of additional skills such as use of prescription medicines

Depending on the service provider, but most commonly in the Fire and Police linked or combined services, the EMS crew members may also be certified or trained in skills such as water rescue or motor vehicle extrication using the jaws of life in medically directed rescue. Some EMS providers offer different kinds of rescue service including rope rescue, cave rescue, water rescue, extrication, search and rescue and more. Some EMS organisations may have a whole variety of vehicles including boats, response cars and ambulances to deal with the demands of their particular service. In some places, law requires that all rescue team members be medically certified and in others the main rescue service (such as a Fire Department) do not have medical staff and leave all rescue up to an EMS department.

STUDY–QUESTION

Write a detailed note on emergency service.

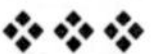

28 CHAPTER

AMBULANCE

AMBULANCE

The term ambulance derived from the Latin word ambulare, meaning to walk or move about which is a reference to early medical care where patients were moved by lifting or wheeling. The word ambulance is most commonly associated with the land-based, emergency motor vehicles that administer emergency care to those with acute illnesses or injuries, hereafter known as emergency ambulances. These are usually fitted with flashing warning lights and sirens to facilitate their movement through traffic. It is these emergency ambulances that are most likely to display the Star of Life, shown on the right, which represents the six stages of prehospital medical care.

There are other types of ambulance, with the most common being the patient transport ambulance. These vehicles are not usually (although there are exceptions) equipped with life-support equipment, and are usually crewed by staff with fewer qualifications than the crew of emergency ambulances. The purpose of emergecy ambulances is simply to transport patients to, from or between places of treatment. In most countries, these are not equipped with flashing lights or sirens.

Other vehicles used as ambulances include trucks, vans, station wagons, buses, helicopters, fixed-wing aircraft, boats, and even hospital ships.

DIFFERENT TYPES OF AMBULANCES

Ambulances can be grouped into types depending on whether or not they transport patients, and under what conditions:

(1) Functional Type

Emergency aAmbulance—The most common type of ambulance, which provide care to patients with an acute illness or injury. These can be road going vans, helicopters, fixed-wing aircraft (known as air ambulances) or even converted vehicles such as golf carts.

Patient Transport Ambulance—A vehicle which has the job of transporting patients to, from or between places of medical treatment, such as hospital or dialysis center, for non-urgent care. These can be vans, buses or other vehicles.

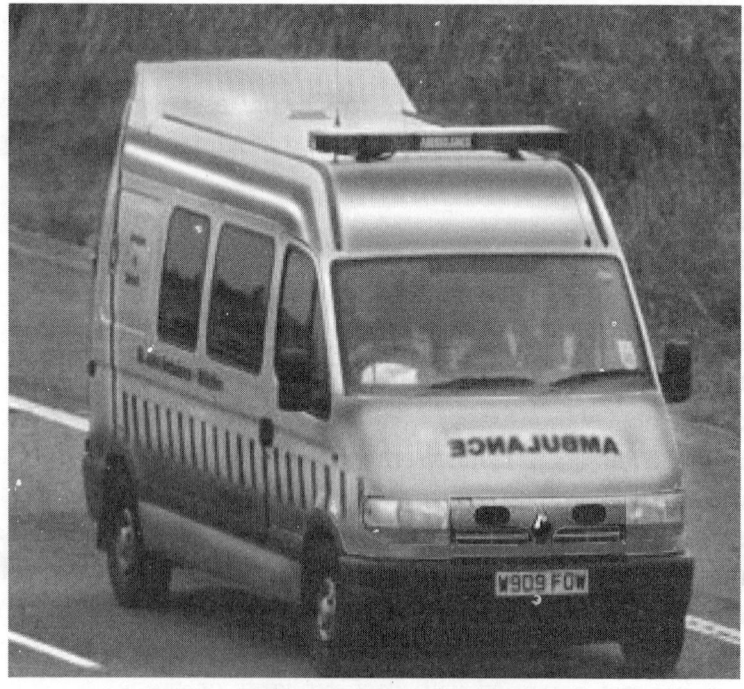

Fig. 28.1: *Ambulance.*

Response Unit Ambulence—Also known as a fly-car, which is a vehicle which is used to reach an acutely ill patient quickly, and provide on scene care, but lacks the capacity to transport the patient from the scene. Response units may be backed up by an emergency ambulance which can transport the patient, or may deal with the problem on scene, with no requirement for a transport ambulance. These can be a wide variety of vehicles, from standard cars, to modified vans, motorcycles, pedal cycles, quad bikes or horses. These units can function as a vehicle for officers or supervisors (similar to a fire chief's vehicle, but for ambulance services).

Charity Ambulance—A special type of patient transport ambulance is provided by a charity for the purpose of taking sick children or adults on trips or vacations away from hospitals, hospices or care homes where they are in long term care.

(2) Vehicle Types

Ambulances can be based on many types of vehicle, although emergency and disaster conditions may lead to other vehicles serving as makeshift ambulances:

Van—A typical ambulance is of a van construction, based on a standard chassis, usually with a maximum road weight loaded of between 3.5 and 7.5 tonnes. In North America, the large box type vehicles are referred to as "mods" (modular) and the smaller van type vehicle is often called a "high-top".

Car/SUV—can br used either as a fly-car for rapid response or for patients who can sit, these are standard car models adapted to the requirements of the service using them. Some cars are capable of taking a stretcher with a recumbent patient, but this often requires the removal of the front passenger seat, or the use of a particularly long car. This was often the case with early ambulances, which were converted (or even serving) hearses, as these were some of the few vehicles able to accept a human body in a supine position).

Motorcycle—In developed areas, these are used for rapid response in an emergency as they can travel through heavy traffic much faster than a car or van, although in the developing world, trailer or sidecar adaptations make these patient transporting units.

Bicycle—these are used for response, but usually in pedestrian only areas where large vehicles find access difficult. Like the motorcycle, a bicycle may be connected to a trailer for patient transport, most often in the developing world.

All Terrain Vehicle—Such as a 'quad bike', these are used for response off road,especially at events. ATVs can be modified to carry a stretcher, and are used for tasks such as mountain rescue in inaccessible areas.

Golf cart—Used for rapid response at events. Function similar to ATVs, with less rough terrain capability, but with less noise.

Helicopter—Usually used for emergency care, either in places inaccessible by road, or in areas where speed is of the essence, as they are able to travel significantly faster than a road ambulance.

Fixed-wing Aircraft—These can be used for either acute emergency care in remote areas (such as in Australia, with their 'Flying Doctors') or for patient transport over long distances (usually a re-patriation following an illness or injury in a foreign country.

Boat —Boats can be used to serve as ambulances, especially in island areas. Some lifeboats or lifeguard vessels may fit the description of an ambulance as they are used to transport a casualty.

Ship—Ships can be used as hospital ships, mostly operated by national military services, although some ships are operated by charities. This can meet the definition of ambulances as they provide transport to the sick and wounded (along with treatment). These are often send to disaster or war zones to provide care for the casualties of these events.

MODERN VEHICLES

Israeli EMS's contemporary civilian armored Mobile Intensive Care Unit. It is used for response to ongoing terrorist incidents, it is based off a super-duty Ford E-450 chassis. Modern ambulances are now often custom built, and as well as the specialist medical equipment now built in to the ambulances, industry wide improvements in vehicle design have had an impact, including improvements in audible and visual warning equipment to help protect crews in vulnerable situations (such as at a Road Traffic Collision), and general improvements such as ABS, which are particularly valuable for ambulances, due to the speeds reached and the weight carried. There have also been improvements to help safeguard the health and welfare of ambulance crews, such as the addition of patient tail lifts, ramps and winches, to cut down on the amount of manual handling a crew must perform.

Ambulance design is still evolving, largely due to the growing skills and role of Paramedics and other ambulance crew, which require specialist equipment. Other factors driving improvement include the need to help protect ambulance crews from common accidents, such as traffic collisions and rarer, but potentially catastrophic incidents such as terrorist activities.

DESIGN AND CONSTRUCTION OF AMBULANCE

Ambulance interiors are often cramped, as seen in this Brazilian ambulanceSuccessful ambulance design must take in to account the local conditions and available infrastructure. Maintained roads are necessary for the familiar road going ambulances to arrive on scene and then transport the patient to a hospital, though in rugged areas four-wheel drive or all-terrain vehicles can make up for a paucity of good roads. Appropriate fuel must be readily available and service facilities are necessary to maintain the vehicle.

Methods of summoning (e.g. telephone) and dispatching ambulances usually rely on electronic equipment, which itself often relies on an intact power grid. Similarly, modern ambulances are equipped with two-way radios or cellular telephones to enable them to contact hospitals, either to notify the appropriate hospital of the ambulance's pending arrival, or, in cases where physicians do not form part of the ambulance's crew, to confer with a physician for medical oversight.

Ambulances often have two manufacturers. The first is frequently a manufacturer of light trucks (or previously, cars) such as Mercedes-Benz or Ford. The second manufacturer purchases the vehicle (which is sometimes purchased incomplete, having no body or interior behind the driver's seat) and turns it into an ambulance by adding bodywork, emergency vehicle equipment, and interior fittings. This is done by one of two methods - either coachbuilding, where the modifications are started from scratch and built on to the vehicle, or using a modular system, where a pre-built 'box' is put on to the empty chassis of the ambulance, and then finished off.

Modern ambulances are typically powered by internal combustion engines, which can be powered by any conventional fuel, including diesel, gasoline or liquefied petroleum gas, depending on the preference of the operator and the availability of different options. Colder regions often use gasoline powered engines, as diesels can be difficult to start when they are cold. Warmer regions may favor diesel engines, as they are thought to be more efficient and more durable. Diesel power is sometimes chosen due to safety concerns, after a series of fires involving gasoline powered ambulances during the 1980s. These fires were ultimately attributed in part to gasoline's higher volatility in comparison to diesel fuel. The type of engine may be determined by the manufacturer: Ford will only sell vehicles for ambulance conversion if they are diesel powered.

SAFETY

Like all vehicles, ambulances may be involved in collisions. Ambulances, like other emergency vehicles, are required to operate in all weather conditions, including those during which civilian drivers often elect to stay off of the road. Also, the ambulance crew's responsibilities to their patient often preclude their use of safety devices such as seat belts. Research has shown that ambulances are more likely to be involved in motor vehicle collisions resulting in injury or death than either fire trucks or police cars. Unrestrained occupants, particularly those riding in the patient-care compartment, are particularly vulnerable. When compared to civilian vehicles of similar size, one study found that on a per-accident basis, ambulance collisions tend to involve more people, and result in more injuries. An eleven-year retrospective study concluded in 2001 found that although most fatal ambulance crashes occurred during emergency runs, they typically occurred on improved, straight, dry roads, during clear weather. Safety is thus of special concern in ambulance design.

EQUIPMENT

In addition to the equipment directly used for the treatment of patients, ambulances may be fitted with a range of additional equipment which is used in order to facilitate patient care. This could include:

Two Way Radio—One of the most important pieces of equipment in modern emergency medical services as it allows for the issuing of jobs to the ambulance, and can allow the crew to pass information back to control or to the hospital (for example a priority ASHICE message to alert the hospital of the impending arrival of a critical patient.) More recently many services world wide have moved from traditional UHF/VHF sets, which can be monitored externally, to more secure systems, such as those working on a GSM system, such as TETRA

Mobile Data Terminal—Some ambulances are fitted with Mobile Data Terminals (or MDTs), which are connected wirelessly to a central computer, usually at the control center. These terminals can function instead of or alongside the two way radio and can be used to pass details of jobs to the crew, and can log the time the crew was mobile to a patient, arrived, and left scene, or fulfill any other computer based function.

Evidence Gathering CCTV—Some ambulances are now being fitted with video cameras used to record activity either inside or outside the vehicle. They may also be fitted with sound recording facilities. This can be used as a form of protection from violence against ambulance crews, or in some cases (dependent on local laws) to prove or disprove cases where a member of crew stands accused of malpractice.

Tail Lift or Ramp—Ambulances can be fitted with a tail lift or ramp in order to facilitate loading a patient without having to undertake any lifting. This is especially important where the patient might be obese. There may also be equipment linked to this such as winches which are designed to pull heavy patients in to the vehicle.

Trauma Lighting—In addition to normal working lighting, ambulances can be fitted with special lighting (often blue or red) which is used when the patient becomes photosensitive.

Air Conditioning—Ambulances are often fitted with a separate air conditioning system to serve the working area from that which serves the cab. This helps to maintain an appropriate temperature for any patients being treated, but may also feature additional features such as filtering against airborne pathogens.

INTERMEDIATE TECHNOLOGY

In parts of the world which lack a high level of infrastructure, ambulances are designed to meet local conditions, being built using intermediate technology. Ambulances can also be trailers, which are pulled by bicycles, motorcycles, tractors, or animals. Animal-powered ambulances can particularly useful in regions that are subject to flooding. Three-wheeled motorcycles are also used, though they are subject to some of the same limitations as more traditional over-the-road ambulances. The level of care provided by these ambulances varies between merely providing transport to a medical clinic to providing on-scene and continuing care during transport.

The design of intermediate technology ambulances must take into account not only the operation and maintenance of the ambulance, but its construction as well. The robustness of the design becomes more important, as does the nature of the skills required to properly operate the vehicle. Cost-effectiveness can be a high priority.

APPEARANCE AND MARKINGS

Emergency ambulances are highly likely to be involved in hazardous situations, including incidents such as a road traffic collision, as these emergencies create people who are likely to be in need of treatment. They are required to gain access to patients as quickly as possible, and in many countries, are given dispensation from obeying certain traffic laws (for instance, they may be able to treat a red traffic light or stop sign as a yield ('give way') sign, or be permitted to break the speed limit. For these reasons, emergency ambulances are often fitted with visual and/or audible warnings to alert road users. Visual warnings on an ambulance can be of two types - either passive or active.

(i) Passive Visual Warnings

An ambulance in the UK fully marked with passive visual warnings (retro-reflective battenburg pattern)The passive visual warnings are usually part of the design of the vehicle, and involve the use of high contrast patterns. Older ambulances (and those in developing countries) are more likely to have their pattern painted on, whereas modern ambulances generally carry retro-reflective designs which reflect light from car headlights or torches. Popular patterns include 'checker board' (alternate coloured squares, sometimes called 'Battenburg', named after a type of cake), chevrons (arrowheads - often pointed towards the front of the vehicle if on the side, or pointing vertically upwards on the rear) or stripes along the side (these were the first type or retro-reflective device introduced, as the original reflective material, invented by 3M, only came in tape form). In addition to retro-reflective markings, some services now have the vehicles painted in a bright (sometimes fluorescent) yellow or orange for maximum visual impact.

(ii) Active Visual Warnings

The active visual warnings are usually in the form of flashing coloured lights (sometimes known as 'beacons' or 'lightbars'). These flash in order to attract the attention of other road users as the ambulance approaches, or to provide warning to motorists approaching a stopped ambulance in a dangerous position on the road. Common colours for ambulance warning beacons are blue and red, and this varies by country (and sometimes by operator).

There are several different technologies in use to achieve the flashing effect. The original method of producing flashing was to place a spinning mirror which moves around a light bulb, called a 'rotating beacon'. More modern methods include the use of strobe lights, which are usually brighter, and can be programed to produce specific patterns (such as a left -> right pattern when parked on the left hand side of the road, indicating to other road users that they should move out away from the vehicle). There is currently the more widespread use of LED flashing lights as they are low profile and low energy. More information on Emergency vehicle equipment.

In order to increase safety, it is best practice to have 360° coverage with the active warnings, improving the chance of the vehicle being seen from all sides.

AUDIBLE WARNINGS

In addition to visual warnings, ambulances can be fitted with audible warnings, sometimes known as sirens, which can alert people and vehicles to the presence of an ambulance before they can be seen. The first audible warnings were mechanical bells, mounted to either the front or roof of the ambulance. Most modern ambulances are now fitted with electronic sirens, which can produce a range of different noises. Ambulance services may specifically train their drivers to use different siren tones in different situations. For instance, on a clear road, approaching a junction, the 'wail' setting may be used, which gives a long up and down variation, with a unbroken tone, whereas, in heavy slow traffic, a 'yelp' setting may be preferred, which is like a wail, but speeded up.

Modern siren technology also includes 'dual tone' sirens, which can emit two different siren tones simultaneously and is beneficial for maneuvering through heavy traffic or approaching intersections.

The speakers for modern sirens can be integral to the lightbar, hidden in or flush to the grill. Ambulances cam additionally be fitted with airhorn audible warnings.

A more recent development is the use of the RDS system of car radios, whereby the ambulance can be fitted with a short range FM transmitter, set to RDS code 31, which interrupts the radio of all cars within range, in the manner of a traffic broadcast, but in such a way that the user of the receiving radio is unable to opt out of the message (as with traffic broadcasts). This feature is built in to every RDS radio for use in national emergency broadcast systems, but short range units on emergency vehicles can prove an effective means of alerting traffic to their presence. It is, however, unlikely that this system could replace traditional audible warnings, as it is, by design, unable to alert pedestrians, or those not using a compatible radio.

STUDY-QUESTION

Write a short note on ambulence.

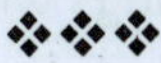

29 CHAPTER MAJOR DISASTER MANAGEMENT

INTRODUCTION

A disaster is the impact of a natural or man-made hazard that negatively affects society or environment.Disasters are characterised by their suddenness and unexpectedness, with the result that hospital plans need to be simple, flexible and integrated with the plans of all the other emergency services. They are always subject to improvement and should be continually reviewed in the light of lessons learnt the hard way as incidents occur.

The basic principle that should run through a good plan is that people perform best, especially under stressful conditions, when they are doing the things with which they are most familiar. Thus, plans should avoid major changes in work practices and departmental layout, aiming to have the department functioning like an ordinary, although very busy, day as far as possible.

A second important principle is that of flexibility and simplicity. A rigid plan that will cope with all eventualities is not possible as it is not possible to foresee all such eventualities. After all, if disasters could be predicted they could be largely avoided. Simplicity has the virtue of allowing flexibility while the simpler a plan is, the easier it is for staff to follow. The more there is in a plan that can go wrong, the more will go wrong.

Within the department, the person who should be in charge is the senior Sister/Charge Nurse on duty, in other words, the person who would normally be in charge. The place for senior management is doing what they normally do – organising the rest of the hospital, providing extra staff where needed and supplying the A & E unit with back-up facilities such as extra equipment, trolleys and pairs of hands.

Once the alert has been received, there is a need to evacuate A & E immediately of all patients, either by sending them to wards or moving them to a holding area (e.g., out-patients clinic), in order to free staff and facilities for casualty reception. A designated disaster ward that will receive all admitted casualties is essential, not only for immediately logistic reasons, but also for long-term psychological reasons in the days and weeks after the disaster when its victims can give each other vital mutual support.

Many of the patients that attend will be very distressed and tearful, but may be suffering little serious injury. In bombings patients will complain of headaches and deafness. Perforated eardrums may be common due to the blast effect.

Provision should be made for relatives of those involved to be accommodated away from the department as the large numbers that may be involved will be disruptive. Similarly, the media should be catered for elsewhere, and ideally the department should be closed by the police to all but staff and disaster casualties. Routine casualties should be informed of the situation and told that they will have to wait a long time before being seen dire to the disaster (assuming their clinical condition will permit such a delay) and advised to go to another hospital or their GP. The notion of attempting to operate a non-disaster A & E unit in tandem with a department on major disaster plan is clearly a non-starter and will only result in sub-standard care for everybody.

Action cards for staff which describe their various functions are an excellent idea, for it is likely to be quite chaotic preparing to receive casualties if different groups of staff are all trying to read through the same lengthy copy of the plan in an attempt to find 'their bit'.

Staff should realise that they may get no official notification of an incident occurring; the fires at Manchester Airport and Bradford City FC in 1985 were examples of this, while communication may remain non-existent with the field for hours on end, as happened in the Hungerford Massacre in 1987. More recently A & E staff at Charing Gross Hospital were reported to be 'stunned' to find a fleet of ambulances arriving with casualties from the Israeli Embassy bombing with no prior warning from the London Ambulance Service (Nursing Standard News).

Casualties may just start pouring through the doors, underlining the need for a speedy response and immediate triage. This means sorting the casualties into categories so that those who need the care first get it first, and are not delayed by either less urgent cases, or more problematically, those who will die whatever care they are given. This needs considerable expertise and the senior nursing and medical staff on duty will need to be involved in this function.

The A & E unit also has a responsibility to send a team to the site of the incident. This has been carefully discussed by *Salt* (1989) and he has stressed that the team should be equipped with weather-proof clothing that for safety reasons is brightly coloured, including fluorescent tabards marked 'Nurse' and 'Doctor'. There should also be helmets with lights and Wellington boots in a full range of sizes. Equipment should be carried in backpacks rather than in one big trunk that may be impossible to carry near to the site of the disaster, although a back-up trunk containing reserve equipment is worth while.

The functions of the mobile team are two-fold: first to provide life-saving measures where appropriate and pain relief for patients whose evacuation is not immediately possible. Triage on site is usually carried out by senior ambulance personnel in practice. The team need equipment to secure and maintain an airway and breathing (including chest drainage), IVIs, wound dressings, space blankets and analgesia. The only surgical pack that is worth including is an amputation set and saw, together with the means to give quick acting IV anaesthesia.

On-site triage is needed to ensure that the most appropriate casualties reach hospital first. Theoretically this may mean that patients with probably non-survivable injuries such as 80% burns or bilateral high traumatic amputation of legs should be put to one side, in order that other patients go to hospital first, and treated symptomatically with analgesia only. In practice in a civilian situation, this would be very difficult to do, but if the scale of the disaster were big enough, it would have to be done.

A second function on site is that of splitting up the case load so that the ambulances distribute the casualties among the various departments in the area. This may not be possible in a rural area where there may not be more than one department within 30 miles, but in urban areas this is possible and greatly to be desired. In the Harrods bombing, St. Stephen's Hospital received 39 casualties and the Westminster Hospital 37, a good example of sharing the workload.

The incidents that occurred in the 1980s produced two types of injury that many staff have little experience of coping with: major burns and high energy missile wounds. Apart from the need to improve knowledge among both medical and nursing staff about the care of such patients, the need for a national team of staff skilled in these areas of care is now apparent. The whole question of a national disaster plan is now firmly on the agenda, and it is to be hoped that A & E staff, both medical and nursing, will campaign for an integrated national action plan to cope with the disasters that lie ahead.

Psychological first aid is important as well as the obvious physical care needed by survivors. It is crucial they start the process of coming to terms with the horrific events they have survived by being able to talk about their experiences. A & E staff should recognise this need in the survivors and they should not try to switch the subject. *Haslum* (1989) has stressed that much needs to be learnt about the psychological needs of survivors and the *Bradford Fire* of 1985 seems to have marked the beginning of serious attempts to explore this area. Nobody could have remained unmoved at the spontaneous way the people of Liverpool transformed the Kop at Anfield into a memorial to the dead of Hillsborough just as the much smaller community of Aberfan still bears the scar of the terrible disaster that destroyed a school full of children, so, too, the much larger city of Liverpool will remember Hillsborough for many decades to come.

TYPES OF DISASTER

Wisner *et al* reflect a common opinion when they argue that all disasters can be seen as being man-made, their reasoning being that human actions before the strike of the hazard can prevent it developing into a disaster. All disasters are hence the result of human failure to introduce appropriate disaster management measures. Hazards are routinely divided into natural or human-made, although complex disasters, where there is no single root cause, are more common in developing countries. A specific disaster may spawn a secondary disaster that increases the impact. A classic example is an earthquake that causes a tsunami, resulting in coastal flooding.

(i) Natural Disasters

A natural disaster is the consequence of when a potential natural hazard becomes a physical event (e.g. volcanic eruption, earthquake, landslide, tsunami) and this interacts with human activities. Human vulnerability, caused by the lack of planning, lack of appropriate emergency management or the event being unexpected, leads to financial, structural, and human losses. The resulting loss depends on the capacity of the population to support or resist the disaster, their resilience. This understanding is concentrated in the formulation: "disasters occur when hazards meet vulnerability". A natural hazard will hence never result in a natural disaster in areas without vulnerability, e.g. strong earthquakes in uninhabited areas. The term natural has consequently been disputed because the events simply are not hazards or disasters without human involvement. The degree of potential loss can also depend on the nature of the hazard itself, ranging from a single lightning strike, which threatens a very small area, to impact events, which have the potential to end civilization.

(ii) Man-made Hazards

Disasters having an element of human intent, negligence, error or the ones involving the failure of a system are called man-made disasters. Man-made hazards are in turn categorised as technological or sociological. Technological hazards are results of failure of technology, such as engineering failures, transport accidents or environmental disasters. Sociological hazards have a strong human motive, such as crime, stampedes, riots and war.

EFFECTS OF DISASTER

Man-made disasters present a serious threat to the health and welfare of all people throughout the world. Due to disaster loss of life, environmental destruction, property damages, physical injuries, psychological trauma effects the health and welfare of all people. Therefore, there is a desperate need for community preparedness, particularly the healthcare system, especially hospitals, which should be prepared and equipped to mobilise all their facilities for maximum usage in whatever circumstance.

Nowadays, thermonuclear warfare is considered to be ultimate type of disaster but the local community striken by storm, fire, earthquake, or explosion may well face almost as high casualty rates as would be the nation in case of nuclear war. During disaster, the number of people will be its victim and whether they die or are crippled, will depend to a great extent on how well the community and its homes are prepared to meet such emergencies.

What happens to the average community or family in a disaster area? First of all, the electric power supply is impaired. Without electricity, there are no lights, radio and television station will no longer function. The telephone lines may well be out of operation making it difficult to summon help from the fire or police departments or to contact the family physician or local hospital. Even if they can be contacted, the condition of the roads and streets may make it impossible for them to reach you. If the grocery store faces the disaster, their contents may be so damaged to be unsafe to use. The water of many communities is pumped from a well, reservoir or lake by electric pumps. If the pumping station is damaged, the water supply will quickly be exhausted or the disaster may damage water mains so badly that contamination makes the water no longer safe.

Disease thrives under disaster condition. Prevention of disease, involves sanitation, isolation and immunisation. Sanitation involves the proper disposal of waste, especially, human waste and the control of whatever may carry disease. Disease carries include, rodents, house flies, mosquitoes and other insects.

THE PHASES OF DISASTER – HOW PEOPLE REACT

The phases of disaster are the time periods of series of events which vary according to the type of disaster. However, most include the following:

1. *Inventory phase* — During this phase, one tries to find out what has actually happened to him. Victims may exhibit fear, anger, sorrow, depression, anxiety, apprehension and other emotions.
2. *Remedy phase* — During this phase morale of survivors/ victims usually picks up as the work together with rescue personnel to get the community back on its feet. A spirit of co-operation often prevails. This phase is the longest post disaster period when reconstruction takes place.
3. *Restoration phase* — In this phase, the individuals regain the stability that they enjoyed prior to the disaster. The time required for a community to reach a state of eqilibrium

depends on the nature and intensity of disaster and the disaster relief available,

4. *Warning phase* — Some disasters give warning of their approach. In this, certain precautionary measures are undertaken to handle the disaster situation efficiently and selectively.
5. *Rescue phase* — During this post disaster period, the victims help each other to cope and begin to help with the rescue provide comfort to others and to re-establish shelter and other needs.
6. *Impact phase* — When disaster strikes, people may at first, be stunned. Then they begin to realise the magnitude of the effects of disaster such as injury, death, destruction etc.
7. *Threat phase* — This is a critical decision making period when one's activity is directed towards the survival action.

CARE OF DISASTER VICTIMS

The goal of care in any disaster situation is to provide the greatest chance of survival to the largest number of the disaster victims through a system of attending the most sick and seriously injured victims first, then the ones who are less serious and could wait for sometime to get medical attention. This system of prioritising victims is termed as *Triage.*

DISASTER TRIAGE

To determine the priorities of care, victims are classified into several groups. Some of classifications are as under:

1. *Classification according to priority of care*

(i) *Priority one—Emergency*: Persons who need immediate attention to save their lives.

(ii) *Priority two—Urgent:* Persons who need attention within a few hours; if they do not receive attention may be serious consequences.

(iii) *Priority three—Nonurgent:* Persons who can tolerate a delay in receiving attention. Victims in this group can be attended in order of arrival and will need assurance that they have not been forgotten about.

(iv) *Priority four—Nonacute :* Persons who do not require the services from rescuing/emergency department but can be examined by the medical staff as a regular or routine cases.

2. *Classification according to treatment need*

(i) *Minimal treatment*: Persons who may assist others after treatment is given.

(ii) *Immediate treatment:* Persons who will benefit most by treatment.

(iii) *Delayed treatment*: Persons who will not die if treatment is delayed.

(iv) *Expectant treatment:* Critically injured persons who will receive treatment if time permits.

DISASTER MANAGEMENT

The probability of avoiding a disaster is greatly improved when those potentially affected by them implement mitigative action and develop emergency preparedness plans. The science of disaster management deals with this issue. Although the term disaster is subjective, it is often used in the developed world to refer to situations where local emergency management resources are inadequate to counteract the negative effects of the event (Quarantelli 1998). Business continuity planning focus on the particular application of disaster management in the commercial domain.

COMMUNITY EMERGENCIES

(i) Fire Explosions

The fire explosions either due to electrical leakage or blasts can cause considerable damage to the buildings and surroundings where the people are dwelling. During the disaster, the first aider should attend to the minor burns, put off the main electrical line of fire is caused due to electricity, evacuate the victims from the house/building as early as possible. In case of major burns, treat for shock, if any, first, and send or accompany the victims to the nearby hospital for further treatment. In case of the explosion is of greater nature call for help from fire-fighting service who can help you in evacuating the victim from the place of fire-explosion.

(ii) Floods

Flood always has a warning signal. In case of floods, the dwellers should be evacuated to a safer place and the first aider, as fast as possible should try to minimise the damage going to happen to life and property. Adults, and aged must be helped to get into a safe place. In case the person drowned are treated with the first-aid measures taken routinely for drowning and asphyxia. If the victim require hospital management they should be sent to nearby health centres/hospitals for further treatment. Meanwhile help is taken from the concerned authorities, police and sometimes even divers to save the people who have drowned.

(iii) Earthquakes

In a major earthquake the victims number may go substantially high and which may include the conditions such as head injuries, fractures, unconsciousness, minor injuries and even deaths. A first-aider who witnesses the earthquake should be alert specially is isolating the victims and attending to the serious victims first according to priority. A helping squad from the nearby hospital should be summoned in case of medical team arrive late. The victim who need hospital management should be sent/or accompanied to the hospital.

The victims are given first-aid treatment according to the type of episode occurred, e.g., head injuries, unconsciousness etc. The first-aider should record all the observations on the patient and brief report may accompany to the patient to the hospital.

(iv) Famine

The first-aider in case of famine should contact the voluntary or government agencies to get assistance which may be in the field of either food or shelter or both. The first-aider can also help in arranging immediate requirement such as drinking water, milk, bread or other staple food from the nearby places or through some voluntary agencies.

(v) Rehabilitation

Rehabilitation of vulnerable weak classes in the above disasters require top priority beyond the condition become worse. The first-aider should have ready in hand informations regarding to different rehabilitation centres for different categories for disasters.

EMERGENCY SERVICES

(i) Police

The first-aider should contact the local police force for any kind of help and suggestion, either in controlling the mob, direct to individual to proper area, or in providing the basic needs of the victims. The police force itself is trained and equipped with personnel to meet any challenge at this time of crisis. Therefore, the police assistance is of great help to a first-aider.

(ii) Ambulance Service

Ambulances are nowadays fitted with radio communications to hospitals. The ambulance should have the necessary "Logo" and Bell system to have easy access to the hospital on the way. The nearest route may be used to reach the hospital. The victim and one of his relative may be permitted in the ambulance. The ambulance should have all facilities to meet any eventuality, during the transport of the patient. This includes Stretchers, Oxygen administration apparatus, B.P. apparatus, I.V. infusion stand, Emergency drugs, Airway, Pillows, Towels, Stethoscope. The first-aider should accompany the victim to the hospital preferably with a trained nurse who can handle the equipment and monitor the patient effectively.

(iii) Firemen

Primary role of the fireman is the extinguishing and prevention of fire. The tasks basically performed by the firemen are: Extinguishing and preventing fire, Rescue and First aid.

(iv) Armed Forces

The roles of the armed forces are assist police and firemen in their functions as needed and Organise and establish the pattern of communication, rescue, first aid, transportation of victims and direct relief operation.

(v) Doctors

The primary role of doctors is to save lives and to prevent further trauma and injury. The task responsibilities of doctors are first aid, surgical support, evaculation decision and providing basic life support measures to the victim in critical condition, i.e., basic airway maintenance and control of serious bleeding.

(vi) Nurses

Nurses play an important role in disaster operation by providing assessment of victims, giving basic life support measures to the victims in critical condition, i.e., basic airway maintenance and control of serious bleeding regulating flow of victims for first aid.

(vii) Red Cross Personnel

The role of the Red Cross personnel is to render assistance in disaster care by ambulance services, setting up first aid team, providing food, drink and temporary shelters for victims and rescuers, supplying drugs and equipment, helping in rehabilitation, supply of clothes, blankets etc.

(viii) Public Work Personnel

Public work personnel may perform any action which would lessen the chance of a secondary disaster. The tasks are — removing road blocks to clear traffic for relief vehicles, ambulances, prevention of any untoward effects, i.e., breakdown of power lines, water lines and gas lines, assistance to firemen in obtaining adequate water for fire fighting, removing victims from under debris.

INTERNATIONAL AGENCIES

1. Food and Agricultural Organisation

The Food and Agricultural Organisation (FAO) was found in 1945 with headquarters in Rome. The main aims of FAO are to help nations to raise living standard, to increase the efficiency in farming, forestry and fishers and to better the conditions of rural people.

2. World Health Organisation

World Health Organisation (WHO) is a specialised non-political health agency of the United Nations with headquarters in Geneva was established in 1946. The objective of the WHO is "The Attainment by all people of the highest level of health." WHO assists in many projects related to health and assists in developing education both medical and nursing. It also assists Epidemiological survey on Communicable diseases.

The WHO has also paid attention, in the programme of work to Non-communicable disease problems such as cancer, cardio-vascular diseases, genetic disorders, mental disorders, drug addiction and dental diseases. Promotion of environmental health has always been important an activity of the World Health Organization.

3. United Nations International Children's Emergency Fund

UNICEF (United Nations Children's Emergency Fund) is one of the specialised agencies of the United Nations. It was established in 1946. UNICEF works in close relationship with WHO and looksafter the welfare of Children both in preventive and curative aspects of disease.

BIOLOGICAL WARFARE

Much experimentation has been carried out into possible means of disabling enemy populations using bacterial or viral organisms or their toxins. Various insect vectors, such as mosquitos and flies, have also been studied in this context.

The choice of agent would depend upon the circumstances of war. Agents with a high mortality, such as anthrax, might be used to inflict heavy casualties, but suspicion of biological warfare, outlawed by the Geneva Convention, would soon be aroused. A more subtle approach, which might never be discovered, would involve the use of more 'usual' organisms, such as virulent influenza viruses or dysentery.

Biological agents, however, also present a risk to the aggressor in close geographical proximity. Natural or acquired immunity in the target population, and anticipation of attack, would render it much less effective. Suitable organisms would need to be able to survive storage in a virulent state and be very potent to be effective after dilution in the air or in water supplies. Some of the agents which might be considered for use in biological warfare are anthrax, botulism, cholera, various forms of dysentery, plague, typhoid, typhus, smallpox, influenza, encephalitis and other virulent viruses. Personal protection depends upon a high level of suspicion, scrupulous hygiene and protection by suitable clothing. The armed forces possess special suits and respirators (NBC suits) for this purpose. Civilian populations, however, are very much at risk from inhalation of organisms in the air.

Pest control methods must be strictly enforced. Most of the agents likely to be used will rapidly lose their virulence.Persistently virulent organisms would threaten the invading forces. Decontamination by thorough washing in hot soapy water and burning of clothing is feasible. Buildings should be washed down with bleach and all water boiled. Treatment of any established infection will be the normal medical management of the disease, including isolation procedures, immunisation and antibiotic treatment.

RADIATION CASUALTIES

After Chemobyl, no A & E unit can afford to pretend that it may never have to deal with radiation casualties. If nurses are to understand the principles of care, they first need to know a little about ionising radiation.

Atoms consist of a central nucleus composed of a cluster of positively charged particles (protons) and particles with no charge (neutrons), all held together by very strong forces. Surrounding the nucleus is a cloud of negatively charged particles called electrons that are almost one two-thousandth the mass of a proton and whose number equals that of the number of protons. The atom is, therefore, electrically neutral. Neutrons and protons are similar in mass, and the number of neutrons in the nucleus of a given element can vary.

STUDY-QUESTIONS

1. Explain the various types of community emergencies.
2. What do you mean by disaster?
3. Explain the different types of disaster.

CHAPTER 30

CHILDREN IN ACCIDENT AND EMERGENCY

INTRODUCTION

Children are a major group of patients in A & E with problems unique to themselves. Children should not be treated as small-scale adults. Their needs are totally different.

The staffing of such units is critical and a careful study should always be undertaken to identify those periods when children are most likely to present in order that registered children's nurses can be most effectively deployed. *Cliff* and *Li* looked at where accidents actually do happen, the most dangerous area is the living room, followed by the bedroom and finally the garden. The kitchen, stairs and bathroom were the least dangerous areas in their survey. Of the children involved, 72 per cent of their parents stated that they had no advice about home safety from a health professional.

THE WAY CHILDREN THINK AND HOW IT VARIES WITH AGE

The busy A & E department will see many children, both ill and injured, in the course of a day. It is important that the nursing staff are aware of some of the ways in which children differ from adults, starting with the way that children think.

A child's way of thinking and of perceiving the world is very different from that of an adult. It develops through stages, each of which is very different one from the others. In order that the nurse may communicate effectively with the young child, due recognition of the child's cognitive development has to be made. It is to the work of *Jean Piaget,* and his co-workers that nurses should look for guidance in describing the thought or cognitive processes of a child.

According to *Atkinson et al., Piaget's* ideas may be summarised by saying that children pass through the following stages:

1. *The sensory-motor stage, age 0-2*—At this age, the child is said to be egocentric, gradually learning that the world around is not just an extension of self. For the first 7 months of life, the child is without the concept of object permanence; therefore, if something cannot be seen it does not exist to the child. That something includes both mother and nurse! It is 18 months before the child's actions can be described as purposeful, i.e., the child can work out how to do something before doing it.
2. *Pre-conceptual thought, age 2-4*—Egocentricity is still very pronounced; the child believes that others, including the nurse, think and see the world in the same way that the child does. There is no idea of groups or classes, therefore, the child is unlikely to realise that the nurse who has just appeared is the same sort of person as the nurse who was looking after him or her but who has now gone to lunch. The child cannot deduce as adults can, with the result that if X and Y are alike in some respects, the child may claim that they are alike in all respects. Thus, if one medicine tastes nasty, the child may decide that all medicines taste nasty.
3. *Intuitive thought, age 4-7*—According to *Piaget*, it is at this age that the child begins to see things from other

people's point of view. But the child is still unable to reverse mental processes with the result that understanding quantity is beyond the child of this age. If liquid is poured from one container into another of different shape, the child will claim that there is more in the container with a higher liquid level and will not be able to see that the volume remains the same. Thus in giving medicine to a reluctant 5 year old, a more successful approach may be to pour the medicine onto a spoon from the measuring pot as the child may think of this as a smaller volume.

4. *Concrete operational thought, age 7-11*—The child develops thought that is defined as logical by adult standards. Reversibility and the ability to group and classify are now developed. However, the child cannot deal with abstract concepts, only with those that can be derived from first-hand reality. Thus when a 9-year old Tarzan falls out of a tree and fractures his arm. The instructions to the boy upon discharge should centre upon care of the POP which he can see and understand rather than the healing process of the broken bones which he cannot see and which involves abstract concepts that will not be understood.
5. *Formal operational thought, age 12-14*—It is only in this age range that the child learns to handle the abstract thought patterns and concepts that are taken for granted by adults.

In summarising the debate around *Piaget's* ideas, *Atkinson et al.* point out that recent work suggests factors such as intelligence and environment play a big part in determining the rate at which children progress. It also appears that *Piaget* may have seriously underestimated children's developmental rates. A & E nurses must however consider that children of different ages tend to think in different ways and utilise *Piaget's* ideas as a guide.

In describing the child's physical development, there are the well-researched milestones which can be summarised by charts such as the *Denver Developmental Screening Test.* The use of such detailed screening tests is the role of the health visitor rather than the A & E nurse. However, in assessing young children in A & E, especially in cases of suspected child abuse, it is essential to know what the child should be able to achieve, as underachievement indicates possible under-stimulation and neglect. Furthermore, in planning A & E facilities for young children, their developmental level is essential knowledge if sensible plans are to be made.

CHILD ABUSE

Abused children present to A & E every day of the week. Therefore, it is important for nurses to understand something of the background and the tell-tale signs that should make the nurse suspicious of child abuse—be it physical, mental or sexual. Child abuse is a large-scale problem and the situation is not helped by the subjective nature of the term and a lack of clarity of definition. *Wheeler* points out that different agencies make different definitions of child abuse and also reminds us that communication failures are a depressingly common theme that is throughout all the enquiries that have been held into child deaths from abuse.

Dingwall is critical of the way many professional workers identify non-accidental injury cases by stereotyping parents such as single mothers as likely abusers yet excluding others from any possibility of abusing their children by virtue of social class. In his research, *Dingwall* did find that nursing staff in A & E units were more alert to and more effective in detecting child abuse than doctors who he criticises for not looking beyond the physical evidence.

There is another dimension to this debate, however, for as *Niven*, points out there is a strong statistical association between sociodemographic factors such as financial deprivation, single mothers, young parental age, marital disruption and lack of social support with child abuse. However, the vast majority of children from such backgrounds, as *Niven* reminds us, are not abused, hence the importance of avoiding stereotyping.

In assessing any child in A & E for the risk of abuse the following factors should be noted as warning signs:

1. Whether delay in seeking treatment.
2. Whether there is an inadequate explanation of the injury.
3. Whether the explanation is inappropriate for the extent or type of injury.
4. Whether there are signs of previous injury, such as fading bruises.
5. Whether there is defensiveness and hostility, or alternatively apathy and disinterest towards the child by the parent.
6. Whether there is silence and withdrawal on the part of the child.
7. Whether there is evidence of failure to thrive; if the child has not reached appropriate milestones both for physical or mental development.
8. Whether there are frequent parental attendances at A & E (often for non-specific reasons) with the child.
9. Whether there are signs of physical neglect.

If any of the above factors are present, the child should be completely undressed to allow a thorough examination. The behaviour of the child and the parent or parents should be carefully watched as this may reveal clues to abuse that may not be noted if just the physical signs are searched for (*Helberg*), Mental cruelty, isolation and neglect of the child's developing mind does not leave physical evidence.

Sexual abuse may not either, although the genitalia and rectum should be included in the physical examination. The incidence of sexual abuse of children is difficult to estimate because the better known the person is to the child, the less likely the case is to be reported to the police.

At some stage in the proceedings, the child should be carefully questioned in private, out of earshot of the parents if this is possible. The stage of cognitive development of the child should be considered in phrasing questions. A doll may be helpful in the case of a young child who can demonstrate which parts of their body were interfered with more readily than they can describe with words where sexual abuse is suspected. The important role of A & E nurses in helping to select cases of child sex abuse cannot be underestimated.

If there is a possibility of child abuse, it is usual procedure to contact the paediatric services who will involve Social Services. Meticulous attention to detail is necessary in recording injuries and marks on the child together with the child's general appearance as the case may well end up in court.

Dimond lists the following key sections from the 1989 Children Act which are relevant:

Section 43. Child Assessment Order; this gives legal authority for a detailed assessment to be carried out.

Section 44: Emergency Protection Order; this allows a local authority to take a child into care for protection.

Section 46: Police Powers; this permits a constable to remove a child to a place of safety or prevent anyone removing a child from a hospital or other accommodation.

Cases of child abuse can be very distressing for the staff involved. Feelings of anger and outrage at the sight of a pathetic rag doll of a child covered in bruises and burns are understandable human emotions. The suspicion of sexual abuse may also fill the nurse with revulsion and anger. However, anger is not a constructive force that will help the child. The child is, after all, the victim of anger and may have mixed emotions of guilt and anger as a result of the abuse.

The nurse must be in control of him or herself if he or she is to be in control of the situation and to act for the child in the child's best interests. Remember we are not employed as judges; it is for others to pass judgement on the parents. It is worth noting the findings of *Ward et al.*, that the mothers of assaulted children are more likely than other women to become the victims of assault themselves.

SOME COMMON CHILDHOOD EMERGENCIES

1. Accidental Poisoning

Burton found that in a study of 319 children presenting at a major A & E department, the most common age was 2-3 years old. Tablets were the most common substance taken (31 per cent) followed by liquid medications (15 per cent), household cleaners and paint thinners (10 per cent each). He comments that taste and smell are no deterrent to young children and also that many parents stated they thought substances were safe because they were in high cupboards. This ignores the climbing ability of even young toddlers.

In the assessment of the child, nurses need to discover exactly what was taken, how much, when, and if there has been any vomiting since ingestion. Questioning should be tailored to the child's level of cognitive development and also to the parent or guardian's level of anxiety which can be very high and as a result interfere with their ability to think clearly.

There are few specific antidotes to ingested poisons; the approach is, therefore, to attempt to eliminate the substance before further absorption can occur. Gastric lavage is to be avoided if possible in children, and instead emesis is induced by giving 15 ml of syrup of ipecacuanha followed by about 200 ml of water which should be flavoured according to the child's taste with squash. If this does not work, the dose may be repeated. Vomiting is usual within 20-30 minutes and in the majority of cases admission is not needed. Gastric lavage is only considered if ipecacuanha has failed or if the child's level of consciousness makes vomiting hazardous. If this is the case for lavage to be safely performed, the airway needs securing by insulation.

If a corrosive substance e.g., bleach or a hydrocarbon-based chemical such as turpentine has been swallowed, emesis is to be avoided and drinks of milk given instead. One of the most common and serious poisonings is that due to iron capsules prescribed for the mother's anaemia; they present a very attractive sight to the young toddler. The result is necrosis of the gastrointestinal wall and poisoning by the iron as it is so rapidly absorbed. Desferriox-amine IV should always be available to deal with this serious emergency.

In dealing with the accidentally poisoned child, we should be acutely aware of the mother's distress and guilt feelings. Awareness about safety might be raised tactfully if it is appropriate, as in Burton's study almost 20 per cent of parents said they had never received any advice about the safe storage of drugs in the home.

2. Febrile Convulsion

Children react to illness very quickly, and an acute infection can produce a rapid climb in temperature to over 39°C. It is during this phase of rising temperature that a convulsion is most likely with children aged 6 months to 5 years. Such a convulsion can be a very alarming experience for the parents, who usually wrap their child up in a blanket, increasing the risk of further convulsions by raising the temperature even further, and then rush off to the nearest A & E department in a state of great anxiety.

Great reassurance is necessary, together with an accurate temperature reading (with the thermometer at least 5 minutes *in situ*, under the axilla). The use of the rectum is unsafe and unreliable and this traditional method should no longer be used with children. If the child is indeed pyrexial, then cooling should commence by removal of clothing, blankets etc. but extreme measures such as tepid sponging are not recommended (*Rogers*). The nurse should be explaining to the parents all the time what is being done and why. Medication to reduce the child's temperature such as Calpol should be commenced as soon as the child is able to cooperate.

Epilepsy still has a major stigma attached to it in the minds of many parents, and this thought will be paramount in their minds in many cases. It is best to avoid the word 'fit' and handle the parents with great tact. It has been found, however, that about 2.5% of children who have a febrile convulsion subsequently develop epilepsy.

3. Acute Respiratory Distress

Pathology—The most common causes of acute respiratory distress in children are:

(a) *Foreign body*—Commonly nuts or beans cause an inflammatory response in addition to obstruction; can be anywhere between the nasopharynx and bronchus.

(b) *Infectious disease causing obstruction of the airway*—A common problem is tonsillitis or a tonsillar abscess. Epiglottitis is a serious emergency as the swollen epiglottis can easily occlude the airway; the child is pyrexial, dysphagic, drooling, hypoventilating but not coughing. No attempt must be made to examine the epiglottis as this can cause spasm and respiratory arrest.

(c) *Croup*—A bacterial infection of the larynx, trachea and bronchi leading to inflammation of the lining of the trachea and larynx. The child is very distressed, exhibits respiratory stridor and has great difficulty breathing.

(d) *Asthma*—The bronchioles are in spasm leading to expiratory wheeze.

(e) *Bronchiolitis/pneumonia*—The young child can be acutely ill as a result of infection of the lower respiratory tract. Parents may not always contact their GP and can bring such an ill child to A & E at any time of the day or night.

4. Children with Burns

It is worth raising the subject here to remind nurses that children are different to adults. This is particularly relevant in view of the findings of Irwin et al., who surveyed 100 children with burns referred to a regional burns unit. Of these children, 53 were injured by hot liquids, the most common causes being flame burns (12 cases), domestic irons (8) and radiators (6). In

60 per cent of cases for example no estimate of burn area was made and in 51 per cent of cases, no estimate of burn depth.

A final reminder of how A & E units can let down children with burn injury comes from Cox, who developed a written information pack to be given to parents of children with burns upon leaving A & E. She found that, in a follow-up study of twenty-three children seen and discharged with burns, the A & E nursing staff only remembered to give the leaflet to five parents.

5. Sudden Infant Death Syndrome (SIDS)

Perhaps one of the most tragic scenes of all in A & E is played out several times as an ambulance rushes to hospital with the lifeless body of a young baby and a totally distraught mother who found her apparently healthy baby dead in the cot where she had laid him to rest not long before. The rate of SIDS has remained constant and, therefore, is now the commonest cause of post-perinatal mortality in infancy, accounting for 2000 deaths in 1991.

The age most at risk is 2-4 months and, according to some authorities, in this age range SIDS accounts for more deaths than all other diseases put together. The evidence is that most deaths occur in the early hours of the morning when infant and family are all asleep. There are several factors involved, there is a strong consensus that if babies are not placed face down to sleep, then the risk of SIDS will be substantially reduced.

Returning to A & E and the nurse confronted with this situation, it has to be said that usually there is nothing that can be done for the infant, who is usually beyond resuscitation. The nurse's attention has to focus on the parents. The nurse will readily appreciate the guilt feelings associated with this situation, especially if the baby has been left with a baby-sitter. It is imperative to try to dissipate this guilt by pointing out that there is no blame to attach and that there is nothing that could have been done. Accidental suffocation is a common idea that springs to the parents' mind in this situation. It is an idea that can be safely dispelled as this is not the cause of SIDS.

The grieving process begins in the resuscitation room and the parents should be encouraged to hold the baby. It is the first step in coming to terms with the reality of death, of accepting rather than denying death, of letting go.

It is essential to arrange support for the family; assistance should be given to contact other members of the family and friends. The health visitor, GP and Coroner's Office should be contacted. A post-mortem will be required. Support for the parents may be obtained from the Foundation for the Study of Infant Deaths. Their address is given at the end of the chapter. They are a world famous organisation offering counselling and support through a network of local self-help groups, among their many other activities.

It remains to say that, in addition to the grief of the family, there is also the grief of the staff. Such grief is to be expected as a normal human response to any death, particularly a child's death, and staff should therefore be encouraged to verbalise their feelings and emotions. Students in particular find this situation very difficult to handle. In this day and age, there is no place for tears in the sluice and a brusque 'Pull yourself together, girl' from Sister, but rather there should be discussion of the event and support for staff. The dangerous myth of being 'too soft for nursing' should be laid firmly to rest. It is the senior nurses' responsibility to see that such discussion takes place and that staff feelings are thoroughly explored.

NURSING INTERVENTIONS

The following key points are essential to remember in A & E because children are different in significant ways not least of which is the obvious fact that a child's airway is smaller than an adult's. Airway blockage is, therefore, easier in children whether the cause is a foreign body or oedema. The immature anatomy of an infant means that the normal process of clearing the airway by extending the neck has the opposite effect as this will compress the larynx; therefore, the jaw thrust manoeuvre should always be used (Soud). A much narrower endotracheal tube will be used with small children which means the risk of occlusion is always greater and, therefore, greater attention should be paid to suctioning the tube. If the child is conscious, he or she should be allowed to find the most comfortable position, which may be sitting upright on a parent's lap.

Children are much less likely than adults to tolerate an oxygen mask although the presence of a parent may help, especially if combined with the use of nasal cannula. In a child with serious respiratory distress, pulse oximetry and close observation of respiratory rate and effort, along with pulse, are essential throughout. The nurse should always remember the extreme anxiety of the parents involved as well as the fear of the child, in such a situation.

Children with acute asthmatic attacks may be seen frequently in A & E. Some 10 per cent of children are estimated to have asthma. The normal adult inhaler is not suitable for young children and the A & E nurse must be familiar with paediatric equipment such as the large volume spacers (Hurrell). Every effort should be made to encourage parents to try and allow their child to have as normal a lifestyle as possible (Wooler) and the A & E nurse should reinforce this message, although with sensitivity, and the parents may well be very anxious after their child has had an acute attack.

STUDY–QUESTIONS

1. Discuss the various stages of children in which they pass through.
2. Write a short notes on the following:
   (a) Accidental poisoning;
   (b) Acute respiratory distress;
   (c) Children with burns; and
   (d) Nursing interventions.

***

31 CHAPTER

ELDERLY PEOPLE IN ACCIDENT AND EMERGENCY

INTRODUCTION

Just as it is not proper to think of children as adults only smaller, in the same way. It is wrong to think of the elderly as the same as everyone else only older. The complete physiological, psychological and sociological changes associated with ageing mean that nurses must consider the elderly as having a unique field of problems that is deserving of special consideration.

As a person ages, he or she becomes more likely to be affected by various degenerative disease processes which will make that person more likely to attend A & E as an emergency e.g., after a stroke or myocardial infraction. However, ageing also makes a person much more likely to have accidents and falls and brings with it increasing social problems for many elderly people. The social circumstances of the elderly patient must receive careful consideration by the nurse before discharge from A & E, and there are times when the patient advocate role of the nurse must be strongly to the fore.

PHYSIOLOGICAL CHANGES IN ELDERLY PEOPLE

There will be a general deterioration of bodily function with age. This is only to be expected, but there are certain key areas which are worth focusing on in some detail, starting with the musculoskeletal system.

There is a loss of muscle bulk and osteoarthritis of various joints leading to pain and stiffness. Such changes seem to affect most old people. In addition there is also thinning of the bone, *osteoporosis*, which affects females more than males. Loss of bone mass increases fracture risk but the relationship between these two variables is complicated by other factors such as the effects of bone density decrease being more pronounced on cancellous rather than cortical bone . Other pathological processes affecting bone become more common in the elderly such as osteomalacia, *Paget's* disease and bony mestastases from malignancy.

It is inappropriate to think that the elderly do not experience pain as much as younger people because of degeneration of the nervous system. It has already been stated that pain is an individual experience and the nurse must assess pain for each individual. Many of today's elderly population grew up in hard times and were firmly taught that pain was something to bear and stoicism a virtue. An elderly person is, therefore, more likely to bear pain with less complaint than might be expected.

Temperature regulation which deteriorates with age in some people is the major problem area. Consequently, the elderly are prone to hypothermia. A range of social factors such as poverty and poor housing act with other physical factors such as lack of mobility and side effects of drugs to make hypothermia the problem it is today.

The elderly experience many problems with the special senses. Vision deteriorates with age due to changes in the cornea and lens shape that affect focusing, leading most commonly to long-sightedness. Diminishing pupillary size and opacification of the lens with old age reduces the amount of light entering the eye to such an extent that a person of 85 needs eight times as much light to see objects as brightly as a younger person.

Problems such as cataracts, chronic glaucoma and retinal detachment all threaten the sight of the elderly. If an elderly person is brought to A & E without a pair of spectacles, the nurse's assumption should not be that their sight is so good that they do not need spectacles, but rather that they may have left them behind somewhere in the process of being brought to hospital. The simple solution is to ask the patient or relative if the person normally wear glasses.

Hearing impairment increases sharply with age. Degenerative changes in the auditory nerve and cochlea cause a preferential loss of hearing for high frequency sounds, i.e., consonants, which are essential for understanding speech. Problems in sound conduction contribute further to deafness and many old people, therefore, rely on lip reading to understand what is being said. However, staff should be wary of the stereotypical assumption that all elderly people are deaf and should certainly refrain from shouting at a person who is hard of hearing. Slower, carefully enunciated speech, ensuring that the patient can see the speaker's lips, and a careful check on any hearing aid (is it switched on?) will be more productive.

The A & E nursc must care for the elderly person as an individual, not a collection of stereotypes. Respect and dignity must be afforded the patient, not childish sobriquets such as 'dearie'. The nurse who assumes that a woman patient will be incontinent, deaf, confused and probably will not feel much pain simply because she is 82 years old has no place in A & E or any other form of nursing.

THE PSYCHOLOGY OF AGEING

Confusion is often the first psychological problem to spring to mind in considering the psychological changes of ageing. It can either be a progressive chronic state, for example, dementia, or it can be an acute episode brought on by physical factors and known as acute brain failure. The nurse therefore, needs to know the patient's normal level of mental functioning before making a judgement about any confusional state. Cerebral hypoxia may induce an acute confusional state secondary to a chest infection or heart failure, while other metabolic disturbances e.g., electrolyte imbalance can have the same effect.

However, confusion in the elderly may not have a simple physical cause, but may be situational in nature, i.e., it may be the environment and situation that the patient is in that is causing the confusion. It is important to recognize this possibility as simple environmental manipulation by the nurse may control and diminish the patient's confusion.

Mitchell, looked at sensory deprivation in relation to nursing and described three situations which make the old particularly prone to suffer from this effect. *Mitchell's* three types of sensory/perceptual deprivation apply particularly to A & E.

She first talked of a 'therapeutically restricted environment' which corresponds to a typical A & E cubicle: bare walls, no indication of day or night or time of day—an environment totally lacking in stimuli. Nurses can try lying flat on one of their own trolleys in a cubicle to see how long it takes to get bored.) Mitchell then talks of a 'socially restricted environment' typical of many old people living alone and isolated and also typical of many A & E cubicles where the old person lies for hours, while busy A & E staff go about their work elsewhere. Finally, she describes 'sensory-perceptual deficits' associated with the deterioration of the special senses described already and which will be made worse if the patient's spectacles or hearing aid are not available.

If a patient who cannot hear or see properly is put in an environment with little or no sensory input, the patient will experience severe sensory/perceptual restriction. Experiments on sensory deprivation have produced mood changes, thought disorder and hallucinations in a matter of a few hours in young volunteers (*Atkinson et al.*). Therefore, nurses may considerably reduce confusion in elderly patients by providing them with an environment rich in stimuli and interaction with other people. A & E nurses should encourage friends/relatives to be with elderly patients at all times. Nurses should try to find time to talk to elderly patients, should arrange cubicles so that there are clues to time and date, should repeatedly tell patients where they are and why they are there (for short-term memory characteristically fails with age) and should make every effort to compensate for the elderly patient's failing eyesight and hearing. In short, nurses must provide an informative and stimulating sensory environment for elderly people in A & E.

Finally, nurses ought to consider the ageing patient as a whole and how he or she views the current situation they are in. Physical limitations on activity can produce frustration; for some people retirement brings hours of empty time and a feeling of worthlessness which results in a fall in self-esteem. Death becomes all too familiar as lifelong friends and relatives succumb to the inevitable passing of the years and this leads to isolation. Anxiety and depression are commonly encountered in old age. The presenting symptoms of depression in the elderly can be confused with early dementia; these include memory impairment, poor communication, apathy and muddled thought processes. This only underlines the importance of not stereotyping elderly patients.

SOCIOLOGICAL ASPECT OF AGEING

A & E departments generally encounter with elderly patients who cannot look after themselves but who are not suffering from an injury or medical condition that alone requires admission. As a result, A & E staff may question how caring and responsible the patient's family are being.

The traditional view of the extended, pre-industrial family caring for its elderly members in a way not seen today has little or no evidence to support it. However, there are three times as many frail elderly people cared for at home than in institutions and more women are now caring for elderly dependants than they are under 16 year olds. Many families actually perform heroics at great cost to themselves to care for elderly relatives and it is usually as a result of intolerable stresses and strains that they might leave an elderly relative in A & E with the statement that 'We just can't cope anymore'.

The evidence therefore suggests that the elderly person brought to A & E in a state of neglect will be unlikely to have a family to look after them, while if a family states that they cannot look after granny and she will have to stay in hospital, there are usually good reasons for the family to say so. It is certainly in the patient's best interest not to have conflict between family and hospital, which may easily arise if the A & E staff try to force the issue.

ELDERLY PEOPLE WHO FALL OVER

Having briefly considered some of the physiological, psychological and sociological problems that are relevant to the care of the elderly in A & E, this chapter concludes by looking at what is probably the most common reason for the elderly to attend A & E apart from illness, and that is a fall. Much of what is said, however, applies equally well to old people who attend A & E for other reasons.

Joint stiffness, muscle wasting and bone disease are mobility problems. All these are compounded by decay in neuromuscular coordination, cardiovascular function, environmental factors and drugs. Elderly people are therefore more likely to lose their balance than younger persons, and once they have done so, are less able to correct their posture, leading to a fall. Falls may be seen, therefore, in terms of intrinsic factors such as postural hypotension and extrinsic factors such as loose carpets or poorly fitting slippers. The frequency of falls in the elderly has been found to lie in the 28-35 per cent per annum range in most studies which have looked at the elderly living at home. The rate amongst those in institutions is probably much higher.

Terms used by the elderly tend to be very vague such as giddiness, blackout, and light-headedness, which makes retrospective medical diagnosis imprecise. The nurse in A & E is more concerned with the effects of the fall which can vary from the obvious immediate injury to a loss of confidence, which leads to the person becoming house-bound, chair and then bedbound, becoming increasingly more immobile and dependent.

Common injuries suffered by the elderly in falls include fractures to the upper end of the femur, wrist (Colles fracture) and upper humerus, dislocation of the shoulder, and lacerations of the shin, scalp and face. Great care has to be exercised with the case of the confused elderly person with a head injury. Is the confusion due to the head injury? The sudden move to hospital in the middle of the night after falling out of bed? Or was the person already confused?

A fracture of the upper end of the femur is a serious injury that most A & E departments see in an elderly person every day on average. The classic clinical sign is shortening and external rotation of the injured leg. Two recent large-scale studies both reported mortality rates of 12 per cent for such patients and a female to male ratio of over 6:1. The study by *Fox et al.* showed the mean hospital stay was 31 days but those patients with dementia averaged 56 days and those with pressure sores 53 days. The *Holt* study found the best predictor of discharge mobility and post-operative complications were age and mobility pre-injury. The most common complication was chest infection, although the incidence of pressure sores is not referred to.

Every effort should be made to ward such patients as quickly as possible to prevent problems such as pressure sore formation. In order to fix the fracture internally, surgery is performed as the alternative conservative treatment requires a lengthy period of traction and bed rest. The complications of immobility are such that the elderly person would be unlikely to survive the period of time involved. Fractures of the wrist are usually reduced and plastered in A & E under regional anaesthesia and followed up on an out-patient basis; similarly dislocations of the shoulder are relocated using IV sedation and analgesia. Fractures of the neck of humerus require pain relief and a sling, but can be managed with minimal interference on an out-patient basis. Lacerations in elderly people are better steristripped rather than sutured in many cases due to the fragile nature of the skin. This is especially true of flap lacerations over the shins where careful application of steristrips, a non-adherent dressing and an elasticated tubular bandage (never crepe as it always falls down) will produce the best results. On occasions, however, skin grafting is necessary.

ASSESSMENT

The psychological and social setting of the patient should be assessed. Vital information about the state of the person's home can be obtained from the ambulance crew who bring the person to hospital: is it clean, warm and looked after or dirty, cold and neglected? What is the situation with regard to neighbours and family? This and much more key social information is to be gained from the ambulance crew. In undressing the patient, further information may be gleaned about social background by looking at the state of the clothes, skin and general hygiene. According to *Bennett* and *Ebrahim*, the assessment of the patient's social networks in A & E is just as important as the physical state.

Talking to the patient will enable further information to be gleaned. A first assessment should be made of how oriented the patient is, and of any disabilities due to visual or hearing impairment. Short-term memory should be checked by asking the patient to remember some item and then repeating the question five minutes later. Some elderly people suffer from pathological short-term memory loss yet are able to keep a remarkably good facade of normally in conversation, so short-term memory should always be checked. Does the patient know where they are and why? This may seem an obvious question, but nurses will be surprised about how many elderly patients do not-small wonder they are then labelled confused!

The principle of multiple pathology should always be considered in assessing the patient for physical injuries. Just because there is an obvious fracture of the upper femur, nurses should not forget to look at the wrists and shoulders for possible fractures there also. A full set of vital signs is needed as there may be a whole range of cardiovascular, respiratory, urinary tract, gastrointestinal and endocrine pathologies present as well. Careful temperature recording is essential to eliminate the possibility of hypothermia. An ECG is fairly standard procedure to eliminate cardiac arrhythmias or a silent MI. Blood sugar should be tested by pin prick and a 'stix' method while urine should also be tested and an MSU obtained if possible.

INTERVENTION

Every effort must be made to keep the patient oriented in time and space using reality orientation techniques. Provision must be made for the poor memory if present by repeating vital information. Spectacles and hearing aid should be obtained if at all possible and great care exercised to secure effective communication. Consideration should be given to having a reality orientation board which includes a large clock, the date and a notice of where the patient is. The nurse should remember to use language that the patient will understand.

A & E trolleys are notoriously hard, and pressure sores can have their origins in a long wait in A & E. Pressure area care is therefore essential if patients are to be in A & E for over 2 hours. Turning is difficult but not impossible on narrow trolleys. If the patient has a fracture of the femur turning, will be impossible since the fracture will not be stabilized. The Spenco mattress offers a solution, as it is available in widths that fit trolleys. Sheepskins may be of value in relieving friction, but rubber rings should be discontinued as a pressure-relieving aid as they are of little value and are of positive harm.

The availability of a commode in the department will help many patients for whom perching on a bedpan is very difficult. Small points make a big difference in caring for the elderly. Have they a call button available? The urge to micturate can come suddenly in many elderly patients, leading to the humiliation of apparent incontinence, which could have been avoided.

Hypothermia needs to be treated with a space blanket which by virtue of its high reflectivity warms the patient by reflecting their own body heat. The blanket should cover the scalp, from which a very high proportion of heat loss occurs and it should be next to the body. ECG monitoring may be required.

Old people are more likely to accept their lot uncomplainingly; they should not be forgotten therefore in the hustle of a busy A & E department. The offer of a cup of tea while waiting (if they are not waiting for a general anaesthetic) and a few kind words can mean a great deal, and can also obtain for the nurse information that might not have been otherwise volunteered. Elderly people often see real problems as 'something that you just have to put up with', rather than an important symptom.

The problems associated with discharging patients have been discussed elsewhere; however, they are never more pressing than in the case of the elderly. A clear picture of the social background to which we are discharging our elderly patient is necessary before such a step is taken. Given the communication difficulties that arise from declining vision, hearing and short-term memory, it is obviously important to be sure that what has been taught has been learnt with regard to points such as plaster instructions, medication, and follow-up appointments. Simple instruction cards in bold type and medicine bottles that can be opened by the elderly, whose manual dexterity may have declined, are simple examples of planning for the special needs of the elderly.

If care is planned around Orem's self-care model, nurses are more likely to appreciate potential problems from the patient's point of view and, therefore, to make more realistic plans for the patient on discharge. At the end of the day, the nurse should not forget her or his role as patient advocate, and if you are unhappy about a medical decision that since the old lady did not break anything when she fell over she must go home, then you must say so. Busy but junior and inexperienced medical staff often overlook the social element of how the patient will cope at home. At the very least, you should ask the doctor to see if the patient can walk unaided, the basic requirement for going home. Many intended discharge decisions have been reversed by such a simple step. Most casualty officers are willing to listen to advice from nursing staff about the care of elderly people and their suitability for discharge or about how to get the community services involved, provided that the nursing staff go about it in a constructive way.

EVALUATION

Evaluation of nurses attempts to maintain an old person's orientation in time and space is achieved by talking to the patient, and always in language that they will understand. How effective instructions about care of an arm in plaster or about taking medication have been will be seen when the patient next returns, so to some extent we are shutting the stable door after the horse has bolted.

While the patient is in A & E, evaluation can be carried out by checking the condition of the patient at regular intervals to make sure that the trolley is not wet and that pressure points are being relieved.

STUDY–QUESTIONS

1. Discuss the physiological changes with age in brief.
2. Write a short note on sociology of ageing.

***

32

CHAPTER

EYE COMPLAINTS AND EMERGENCIES

INTRODUCTION

The human eye has been well-endowed by nature with defences such as the bony orbit and a very fast blink reflex. Despite these defences, however, eye injuries are common. In addition, the A & E nurse will see many patients who bring themselves to the department with a wide variety of eye complaints of a non-traumatic origin, although eye trauma remains the single most likely reason for attendance.

NON-PENETRATING EYE INJURY

The bony orbit that surrounds the eye may be fractured as a result of facial or head injury. The injury may be an isolated fracture which is called a 'blow out' fracture or it may be a component of either a facio-maxillary injury or a fractured base of the skull. In a blow out fracture, the cause is a blow to the front of the orbit; the force from the blow is conducted as shock waves by the orbital floor and causes a sudden rise in intra-orbital pressure, the result being that an isolated piece of bone is blown into the adjacent sinus. The problem that this injury causes is that tissue, including muscle, herniates through the hole and becomes trapped; the mobility of the eye is restricted and double vision or diplopia develops.

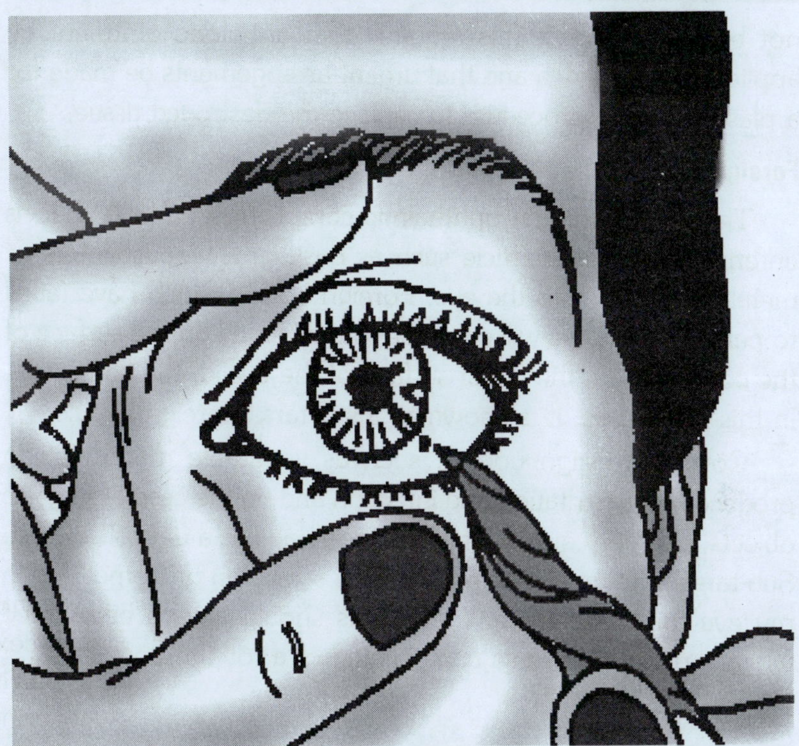

Fig. 32.1.

In the more serious cases, where the orbital fracture is part of other fractures, the eye can be impaired by damage to the optic nerve, or one of the other facial nerves. It leads to the development of a nerve palsy.

Soft tissue injury to the eyelids is a common situation; it usually causes bruising which resolves with the passage of time. Most lacerations are easily stitched or closed with tissue glue; however, *Wardrope* and *Smith,* recommend that lacerations which go through both surfaces of the lid or involved structures such as the lachrymal duct should be referred to a specialist. Due to the speed with which swelling of the lids can develop, it is essential to examine the damaged eye promptly, as soon afterwards examination may be rendered virtually impossible by the swollen and bruised lids. In burns cases, it may be impossible to close the lids due to the burn damage. As the cornea must not be left exposed, this requires that antibiotic ointment be applied to the cornea and that urgent arrangements be made for a plastic surgery procedure to replace the destroyed tissue.

Foreign Body

The most common ophthalmic complaint seen in A & E, is entering any small particle such as dust, grit, woodsplinters or metal fragments into the eye. Foreign bodies which have failed to penetrate the eye will either be found lodged on the surface of the cornea or on the under-surface of the eyelid, the conjuctiva. In this latter case, it is known as a sub-tarsal foreign body.

Corneal foreign bodies, such as vegetable material, can produce severe irritation and infection and, in the case of metallic objects, can very quickly stain the cornea with a deposit of rust. Sub-tarsal foreign bodies produce the sensation of 'something in my eye' and, therefore, the eyelids should always be everted when a patient presents complaining of a foreign body.

Corneal Abrasion

This is an extremely painful condition in which the epithelium of the cornea is removed from the damaged part. It is usually caused by a glancing blow to the eye from any number of objects such as a finger nail, towel or newspaper.

Chemical Injury

The extent of the injury is related to the nature and concentration of the agent involved. Alkalis are the most damaging (e.g., substances containing lime such as wet cement) as they can rapidly penetrate the cornea and produce severe damage to the iris, ciliary body and lens while also causing ischaemia. Acids of equivalent strength are less damaging than alkalis as they combine with tissue components to precipitate deposits of protein which form a barrier against further penetration. Nevertheless, whether the injury is caused by an acid or alkali chemical, the effects can be devastating.

Radiation Injury

Ultra-violet is the usual culprit, damage to the superficial layers of the epithelium of the cornea. Pain, photophobia and watering are the usual symptoms the patient presents with a few hours after exposure. Sun lamps and welding without proper goggles are the usual causes, the latter giving rise to the name of 'are eye' by which this condition is informally known.

Keratitis or inflammation of the cornea is the usual result of exposure to other forms of radiation. Cataract formation is a long-term complication of ionizing radiation exposure. This is well-documented in survivors of the Japanese atom bombs, the cataracts tending to develop some 5 years after the bombing.

Contusion and Concussion Injury

Contusion refers to injury from the direct impact of the force involved. Damage to the eyelids has already been mentioned; the cornea can also be affected by contusion. The result can vary from corneal oedema through to rupture of the whole globe, depending on the force involved.

Concussion refers to the conduction of shock waves from the point of impact to other parts of the eye. The blow out fracture has already been discussed as an example of this type of injury. Within the globe itself, various very severe injuries are possible, including detachment of the retina or the ciliary body, vitreous or retinal haemorrhages, and/or the development of a hyphaemia. A hyphaemia is bleeding into the anterior chamber and can have devastating effects on sight due to the development of secondary glaucoma and corneal staining. Cataract of the lens or the dislocation of the lens may result from a concussion injury; the iris sphincter may be ruptured in concussion, leading again to the long-term risk of glaucoma.

PENETRATING EYE INJURY

Penetrating eye injuries may be classified into two groups:

(i) Those in which the object responsible is withdrawn after penetration and;

(ii) Those in which the object is retained in the eye, forming an intraocular foreign body. Dust, insect, coal particles, loose eye lashes and iron particle get lodged in the eyes. They causes considerable pain, redness and itching in the eye. These foreign bodies mainly iron particles get lodged in the cornea causing serious trouble.

The prognosis for vision depends upon the size of the laceration in the cornea or sclera, and upon which part of the eye is involved. Penetration to the posterior chamber carries the worst prognosis.

In order that a foreign body may penetrate the eye, it must possess a large amount of energy. Typical objects are glass from a car windscreen, flying debris from industrial processes such as drilling, and material propelled by a blast after an explosion. The most common form of retained foreign body within the eye is metallic-iron and steel account for between 85 and 98% of intraocular foreign bodies caused by industrial accidents, a similar proportion to that found in war casualties.

A much feared complication of penetrating eye injury is sympathetic ophthaimitis, where after injury to one eye, the uninjured eye develops a severe inflammation some time after (from 3 weeks to 4 months has been reported). If untreated, this inflammation may lead to loss of useful vision in the uninjured eye. Prompt post-traumatic surgery and early enueleation of the injured eye, together with the use of steroid therapy, have greatly reduced the incidence of this complication which can lead to complete blindness.

In addition to the obviously disastrous effects that the foreign body may have on the delicate structures of the eye, there is a further risk of siderosis bulbi if the foreign body contains iron. This condition stems from the chemical reactions which occur within the eye due to the iron, its effects being seen some time after the injury. As the iron dissolves, it becomes incorporated into the cells of the eye, leading to chronic damage and eventually blindness. For this reason, it is mandatory that all ferrous intra-ocular foreign bodies be removed. An electromagnet is commonly used to do this.

INFLAMMATION OF THE EYE

Not only traum but there are also many varied eye conditions that bring patients to A & E other than trauma. There is not space to describe all of them, but it is worth noting some of the conditions that give rise to inflammation of the eye, for this is the most common eye problem after trauma.

ASSESSMENT

The first step is to obtain a history of the complaint from the patient. Important symptoms that may be mentioned and which should alert the nurse to give a patient high priority in the queue include: haloes around lights (classically indicative of an early attack of glaucoma), 'floaters' described by the patient as visible wisps or strands (indicating inflammation or debris from trauma), flashing lights (retinal damage) and, of course, sudden blindness. Other less helpful symptoms (less helpful because they are so non-specific) include photophobia, which may be associated with inflammation of the eye but can be associated with many other illnesses such as migraine and pain in the eye. Pain may be of ocular origin (e.g., inflammation of the cornea), but it may also be caused by many other conditions such as sinusitis, where the patient attributes the pain to the eyeball. Furthermore, the pain of acute glaucoma can be described by some patients as being in the forehead and nowhere near the eyes.

COMMON CAUSES OF INFLAMMATION OF THE EYE

The common causes of inflammation of the eyes are:

(i) Stye—Boil on lid margin.

(ii) Chalazion—Cyst within tarsal plate (eyelid).

(iii) Allergy—Reaction affecting both eyelid and conjunctiva.

(iv) Conjunctivitis—Redness of conjunctiva. There is discharge but no pain. Bacteria are the usual cause.

(v) Keratitis—Painful inflammation of cornea. Common causes are an extension of existing conjunctivitis. Corneal exposure, or the herpes simplex virus which leads to the formation of a dendritic ulcer.

(vi) Iritis—Acute inflammation of the iris.

(vii) Glaucoma—Raised intra-ocular pressure. Common cause is blockage of the aqueous circulation from the ciliary body via the pupils to the drainage angle in the anterior chamber. It can be either acute. Chronic or secondary tò some other condition such as iritis or hyphaernia. This is a potentially blinding condition.

It is also possible that the patient may present as an emergency complaining of sudden visual disturbances and loss of visual acuity which turn out to be associated with AIDS. According to *Plena* and *Schremp,* in the USA 75 per cent of AIDS patients develop ocular conditions and comment that the person may be totally unaware that they are HIV positive when they present. Typical pathological findings include cytomegalovirus (CMV) infections, Kaposi's sarcoma of the conjunctiva, retinal haemorrhages and vasculitis. There are many other systemic diseases which can affect vision of course, such as diabetes, but none perhaps so devastating as AIDS.

If the patient is presenting with a foreign body, it is essential to find out if it was a high energy or low energy accident due to the risk of penetration and if possible what the foreign body might be composed of. Similarly, if it is a chemical injury to the eye that the patient has sustained, then nurses need to know what chemical, how long ago and what first aid measures have been taken (hopefully copious irrigation with cold water).

After obtaining a history, the next step is to assess vision. Simple finger counting will assess whether there is any double vision present. The use of the standard Snellen Visual Acuity

Test is strongly recommended for all patients with eye complaints. The chart consists of lines of letters of differing sizes which the average eye should be able to read at varying distances, depending on the size of the letters.

The patient is asked to read the chart from a distance of 6 metres, one eye at a time, the other eye being occluded. The results of each eye are carefully recorded, noting the last line to be read correctly. If the patient wears spectacles, this test should be carried out both with and without the spectacles. Each line has a number which refers to the distance at which the average eye should be able to read that line. The result is, therefore, recorded as a fraction, the top number referring to the distance at which the patient stood from the chart, the bottom number being the line number that was correctly read (i.e., the distance at which an average eye would be able to read that line). Thus, vision recorded as 616 means that at a range of 6 metres the patient can read the same size letters that the average eye can read at 6 metres.

If the patient is not able to read or very young an E chart is used, consisting of rows of the capital letter E pointing in different directions. The patient is asked to indicate using three fingers the position of the E. After assessing visual acuity, the nurse should move on to the eye itself, working inwards in a regular sequence which the A & E nurse will find helpful to have as a standard pattern for assessing eyes. Both eyes should always be examined.

The eyelids should first be examined for evidence of disease or damage. This should include eversion to examine the under-surface of the lid (the conjunctiva). This is best done by asking the patient to look downwards, grasping the eyelashes, then gently pulling down, round and up while depressing the upper margin of the tarsal plate with a cotton applicator or similar implement. The under-surface of the eyelid should be readily visualized by this technique.

A bright pen torch is used for assessment of the eye itself. First the pupil responses and the shape of the pupil should be tested to cheek they are brisk to respond and equal and regular in size and shape. A pear-shaped pupil indicates significant eye trauma and disruption of internal ocular structures (*Hartland*). The cornea should be examined for evidence of a foreign body, a corneal wound or redness indicative of inflammation. Damage to the corneal epithelium is difficult to visualize under normal conditions, but the addition of a drop of sodium fluorescein will show the damaged area in bright green which is easily visible. Ocular position and movement should also be checked; a blow out fracture of the orbit is often associated with an apparently recessed eye, for example (Hartiand).

Finally, the person as a whole must be assessed. Eye injuries produce great fear of blindness in many patients. Patients are, therefore, likely to be very frightened and anxious. Thus an assessment of the psychological state of the patient is needed as nursing intervention is required in this area as much as for the actual eye injury.

Amongst those patients who do lose their sight, the greatest psychological trauma has been shown to occur at the actual time of sight loss rather than later, which underlines the importance of the A & E nurse approaching such patients holistically rather that just focusing on the immediate physical problem. According to *Vader,* amongst those who lose their sight as a result of trauma there is profound remorse and recrimination together with anger, denial and self-pity. *Plona* and *Schremp,* indicate that in AIDS patients, the fear of blindness acts to increase the already high suicide risk as there is no greater fear than the fear of blindness.

The medical assessment will include a test of the field of vision, a detailed examination using both an ophthalmoscope and a slit lamp. A slit lamp is a binocular microscope with a strong light source that provides a well-illuminated and highly magnified view of the area in question. X-rays will be required if there is a risk of penetrating injury or fractures.

INTERVENTION

The victim of an accident who has suffered serious eye injury will need considerable and immediate psychological support due to the fear of blindness which will probably be uppermost in his or her mind. It will be the lot of the nurse to deal with difficult questions such as 'Will my sight be alright?' and 'Am I going to be blind?' from a patient whose face will probably be swathed in bloody bandages.

If chemicals have been spilt into the eye, copious irrigation with water is the correct first aid procedure, and removal of contact lenses if worn. Irrigation will then be continued in A & E, with a sterile solution of water or saline. *Tannen* and *Marsden* recommend the use of an ordinary IV giving set, first accustoming the patient to the temperature of the solution by running it onto the check. The procedure is best carried out with the patient lying flat and the nurse standing at the patient's head. For effective irrigation to occur, the eyelids must be opened. This will require a great deal of tact and gentleness on the part of the nurse, for most people with an already irritable and possibly painful eye are understandably reluctant to have that eye held open while somebody pours fluid into it. Local anaesthetic such as amethocaine 1per cent applied in advance may facilitate this procedure. Nurses would do well to try to imagine themselves in the patient's position when deciding how to handle the victim of eye trauma. A kidney dish should be held against the face in order to catch the irrigation fluid and the fluid should not be allowed to soak into the patient's clothes. The nurse should work from the inner, nasal part of the eye outwards when irrigating and ensure that there is a constant flow of fluid over the eye, but that it is not under pressure – a gentle trickle provides sufficient force.

A subtarsal foreign body can be readily removed with the help of a cotton applicator or a glass rod after eversion of the eyelid. Gentleness and reassurance are required in carrying out the procedure as the patient may find it frightening. Corneal foreign bodies are removed frequently with nothing more than a sterile hypodermic needle; however, the cornea first needs anaesthetizing.

Nurses are frequently required to instil various drops and oinments into the patients' eyes. These include antibiotic ointment, mydriatics to dilate the pupil and local anaesthetic agents for pain relief. After treatment, consideration should be given to padding the eye. However, eye pads do cause great inconvenience due to the monocular vision they produce (e.g., for drivers) which has significant implications for the patient's self-care demand. They should be used, therefore, only after careful consideration of how the patient will manage with monocular vision.

The indication for padding an eye is if there is a defect in the corneal epithelium which will heal more quickly under a closed lid. Instillation of antibiotic ointment and padding may be carried out on a daily basis until healing is complete. The pad is best secured with tape (e.g., Micropore) and a short piece of elasticated tubular bandage. In serious conditions such as a hyphaemia or detached retina, rest is essential as further sudden movements can exacerbate the situation. It is as well, therefore, to have a general rule in A & E that movement should be minimised for patients suffering from any eye injury. Effective channels of communication must exist between A & E and the nearest ophthalmic unit to ensure prompt specialist treatment for serious eye conditions.

Finally, before discharging a patient home from A & E, nurses must be sure that the patient understands what is required in terms of self-care of their eyes and that they are aware of the correct way to apply the ointment or cream that has been prescribed.

EVALUATION

Continual assessment of the patient's psychological status is needed to assess how they are coping with the mental stress caused by the fear of blindness.

When the irrigation process if completed, the nurse should carefully check the eye to ensure that there is no obvious material present, including by everting the eyelid. The degree of understanding of the patient of self-care requirements should be ascertained before discharge, for it is not what is taught, but what is learnt that counts.

ABNORMALITIES AND MEDICAL EMERGENCY

- Cataract—In this abnormality, the lens becomes either partially or completely opaque. This opacity is either due to the degeneration of cells in the lens or their replacement with non transparent fibrous proteins. In this, there is a progressive painless loss of vision. In cataract one or both eyes may be affected. A cataract may develop over the years or more rapidly. It may be hard or soft. There are four varieties of cataract:
- Congenital—Those of familial origin or due to intra-uterine rubella in early pregnancy.
- Traumatic—The extent of the cataract depends on the amount of destruction of lens substance.
- Diabetic—This form is thought to be due to lack of nutrition. It occurs in patients with diabetes.
- Senile—This is the commonest type of cataract, which occurs most often between 50 and 60 years of age and is due to degenerative changes taking place in the lens.
- Glaucoma—It is an increase of intra-ocular tension when the pressure within the eye is raised above the normal value 15-20 mm. Hg.) It is a very serious condition and results in blindness. In this the aquous humor does not return into the blood stream through the *canal of Schlemm* as quickly as it is formed. The fluid accumulates and, by compressing the lens into the vitreous humor, puts pressure on the neurons of the retina. If the condition is prolonged it destroys the neurons and brings about blindness.

- Myopia—It is a disorder of vision due to the deformity of the eye ball. In this, the lens of the eye is too convex, and rays of light are focused at a point of the retina, instead of upon it. The result is that the individual can only see near objects, that is why the stage is said to be the *short sightedness.* Glasses with concave lenses of proper refractive power are used.
- Hypermetropia—It is commonly known as *long sightedness.* In this condition the eye ball is too short or the lens is in its most relaxed or non-accommodating state. The affected person feels difficulty in seeing objects near them because the rays of light fall on a point of focus behind the retina. Headache is frequently a troublesome symptom of this condition; the treatment is the correction of vision by the use of convex glasses.
- Astigmatism—In this abnormality the light rays are not brought to a point focus on the retina. The rays are focussed at two different points on the retina. The focus for horizontal rays differs from that of the vertical rays. Hence, an astigmatic subject looking at a piece of graph paper may focus on the vertical lines and may fail to focus the horizontal lines and vice versa. In this defect, the accommodation results in headache. This defect is due to the uneven curvature of the lens or irregular cornea. In astigmatism cylindrical lenses are used which produce refraction in one plane alone.
- Presbyopla— In old age, the lens of the eye loses its elasticity and ability to accommodate and the lens is not made efficiently convex. This decreased range of accommodation is *termed presbyopia.* Presbyopic vision occurs at any time after the age of 35. It is handled by the use of two pairs of glasses, or one pair with two different lenses, called *bifocals.*
- Trachoma—It is the greatest single cause of serious and progressive loss of sight in the world, often leading to total blindness. It is caused by a viral organism called *virus*

conjunctivitis. Trachoma is characterized by many granulations or fleshy projections on the eyelids. The disease produces an excessive growth of sub-conjunctival tissue and the invasion of blood vessels in front of cornea. The cornea may be ulcerated and vision is lost. The disease can also be spread by flies which settle on the eyes.

- Conjuctivitis—Inflammation of the conjuctiva may be acute or chronic and generally affects both eyes. Conjuctivitis can be caused by micro-organisms or by a number of irrtants including dust, smoke, wined, air pollution and excessive glare.
- Strabismus—An eve muscle disorder commonly known as "crossed eyes" or *squint.* The eyeballs do not move in unison and image does not fall upon corresponding points of the two retina. It may be caused by lack of coordination of the extrinsic eye muscles. As a result, two images are seen, a condition termed *diplopia.*

STUDY–QUESTIONS

1. Write short notes on the following:

   (a) Non-penetrating eye injury;

   (b) Contusion and concussion injury; and

   (c) Inflammation of the eye.

33

CHAPTER ENT AND DENTAL EMERGENCIES

ENT

ENT stands for ear, nose and throat.

THE EAR

The external part of the ear, the pinna, is composed of cartilage and is commonly involved in injury. It may be lacerated, in which case it may be sutured and treated as any other wound,

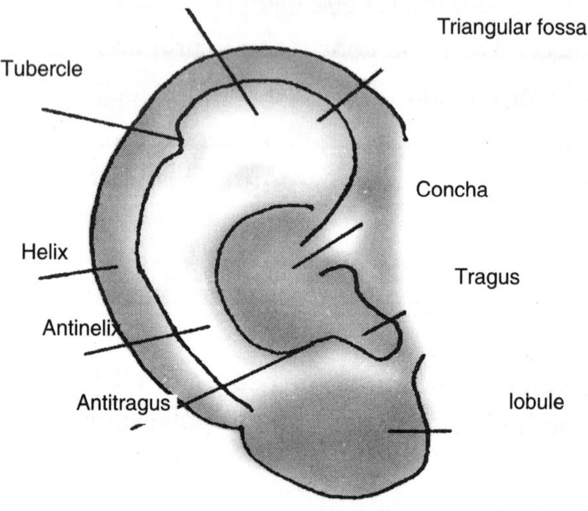

Fig. 33.1: *Right auricle lateral aspect.*

or it can suffer blunt trauma leading to the formation of a haematoma. If this is not properly treated, this will lead to deformity and the formation of a 'cauliflower ear'.

In severe injuries the whole of the pinna may be cut or torn off, e.g., in a knife fight. In such cases reattachment may be possible; therefore, the wound site should be covered with a saline soak and the missing part retained, preferably dry and in a refrigerator though not frozen.

FOREIGN BODIES IN THE EAR

Foreign bodies in the external auditory meatus are common problems with small children. They vary from beads to live insects in which latter case they should be drowned with olive oil before removal is attempted, as the insects are easier to remove dead than alive. The nursing staff need to great skill to gain the cooperation and confidence of the parents and the child. The best approach after explaining to the parents what is going to happen is to sit the child on the parent's lap, wrapped tightly in a blanket so as to keep little hands and arms safely out of the way, and then attempt once to remove the object. If the casualty officer cannot remove it immediately, it is best left and the case referred to an ENT specialist. Further attempts with a struggling child may well lead to the object being pushed further into the ear, risking perforation of the eardrum.

The eardrum is most frequently damaged as a result of a sudden pressure change, e.g., after an explosion or in landing or take-off when flying. A blow to the ear with the hand flat or slightly cupped can produce the same effect. Small perforations will usually heal themselves but large tears may require surgical repair. The usual result of a perforated eardrum is deafness on the affected side.

A common reaction is for people to hit themselves on the side of the head affected or to try to poke something down their ear. Both should be discouraged as they may lead to further damage to the delicate structures of the middle ear. In making disaster plans, it should be taken into account that if an explosion has occurred there may be large numbers of people with perforated eardrums and deafness as a result. It is important to attempt to convey the likely temporary nature of such deafness to people in order to allay anxiety.

DISEASES OF THE EAR

It is properly true to say that in an ideal world people with diseases of the ear would not often be seen in A & E as they should have seen their GP who would have arranged the appropriate ENT specialist referral, if needed.

A & E staff should not, however, be too dismissive of people with earache for two reasons. *First*, the ear may be very painful and the patients may be in considerable distress, especially if they cannot get an appointment to see their GP for two days, and *second*, ear pain may indicate a disease process which could have serious consequences for the patient if untreated.

The usual cause of a painful ear is infection: otitis externa, otitis media (which can be acute or chronic), or mastoiditis. Chronic disease of the middle ear (chronic suppurative otitis media) is sometimes proved to be very fatal and leads to complications such as meningitis, brain abscess, and erosion and destruction of bone.

Chronic otitis media requires a careful toilet of the ear, a swab should be taken for culture of fungi and bacteria, and topical antibiotics applied, typically gentamicin and neomycin with a steroid. The nurse should enquire tactfully about personal hygiene as health education could significantly reduce the incidence of future episodes. *Ludman* indicates that cleaning the ear with a dirty towel, particularly after swimming, is the best way to produce otitis media.

Infections of the pinna of the ear include herpes (which may be accompanied by involvement of the inner ear leading to deafness, giddiness and vomiting) and the inflamed crusts of a staphylococcal infection seen in children with impetigo. If herpes is suspected it is essential the patient is given a triage category which ensures he/she see a doctor. A swollen painful earlobe may be associated with a recently pierced car which has become infected. The earring should be removed and the person advised about hygiene.

One disease involving the ear that can lead patients to attend A & E in a very distressed emergency condition is vertigo. This condition gives rise to an illusion of movement, either that the person is moving, or that the environment is in motion. The cause is a conflict of information from the vestibular sources within the inner ear with information from other sensory systems, or alternatively, when the information supplied by the vestibular system about body movement cannot be coherently assessed by the central nervous system.

Vertigo always produces imbalance, although imbalance is not always caused by vertigo. The person suffering from an attack of vertigo will often fall to the ground and vomiting and nausea are common. The patient will present at A & E collapsed with vomiting. The patient should be laid flat on a trolley with cot sides in place and a vomit bowl available. Acute episodes of vertigo can be very frightening for the patient, therefore, considerable psychological support is necessary. An intramuscular injection of *prochlorperazine* (Stemetil) 12.5 mg is often prescribed to help relieve the symptoms.

A common cause of vertigo is *Meniere's disease*, affecting one ear only and most common in onset in people between 30 and 60 years of age. The result is a violent paroxysmal attack, rotary in nature, associated with tinnitus and deafness, which may be one of several attacks clustered together. Migraine is another common cause of vertigo, particularly in adolescent girls.

THE NOSE

Fracture of the nasal bones is the most common facial fracture and is usually due to blunt trauma, e.g., a fall on the face or assault. Deformity which may be obvious at first will quickly be obscured by soft tissue swelling. Reduction should occur before 3 weeks, as fractured nasal bones will set within 3 weeks, but after one week in order to allow the swelling to go down. The need is, therefore, to make an ENT appointment for 7 to 10 days' time in order that the ENT specialists can manage the problem thereafter.

Nose Bleeds

There are many reasons for nose bleeds, ranging from trauma or simply blowing the nose too hard in young people through to hypertension and degenerative arterial disease in the elderly. In young people bleeding is usually venous, while in the elderly an area of multiple arterial anastomosis is located on the septum Little's area, is usually the culprit giving rise to arterial bleeding.

Nose bleeds in elderly people are potentially very serious. They should be carefully assessed by the nurse in the same way that any other serious bleed would be assessed. Blood loss should be assessed by interviewing the patient to find out how long the bleed has been going on, by examining any evidence such as a towel used to try to stop the bleeding, and by asking if the patient has been swallowing any blood as well as spitting it out. Blood pressure and pulse must be measured as hypotension and hypovolaemic shock are possible; an alternative finding is that the patient is hypertensive, and the hypertension has given rise to the nose bleed.

If the patient is hypovolaemic, then the full resuscitation procedure should be activated and should take priority over controlling bleeding in the first stages. According to *Ludman* that 'An elderly patient who has lost a lot of blood is more likely to die during the next few hours from the effect of loss already sustained than from the results of continued bleeding.'

The effective method to arrest bleeding is to show the patient how to squeeze the *soft* lower part of the nose tightly. This will control bleeding by compression. Compression should be applied continuously for 20 to 30 minutes. The application of ice packs to the bridge of the nose may also be beneficial due to their vasoconstrictor effect. The patients should be made to sit upright if possible with their head tilted slightly forward and they should be supplied with a bowl and instructed to expectorate any blood that drips into their mouth. The patient should be instructed not to swallow the blood because it will lead to vomiting and also prevent measurement of the blood loss. If direct pressure is controlling bleeding, however, there should be little or no blood dripping down into the mouth.

If the patient is shocked from the bleed, his position should be modified to promote venous return and perfusion of the vital centres by elevating the legs and lying the patient as flat as possible. We see in nose bleeds a good example of Orem's self-care model of nursing at work, as under nursing guidance the patient meets his own self-care demand in stopping the bleeding.

A spray of cocaine solution (2.5-10 per cent), a head light and mirror, silver nitrate cauterization sticks, and a nasal packing set will be required by the medical staff to control the bleeding if direct pressure fails. The medical techniques used in A & E are either cauterization or nasal packing. The nursing staff must ensure that they know where this essential equipment is kept.

The sight of blood can have a very distressing effect on some people and, young or old, the patient suffering from a nose bleed may need considerable psychological support and encouragement from the nursing staff who should be aware that this is a potentially fatal condition. This is especially true of the situation where the patient is required to compress their own nose for 30 minutes. The temptation to let go soon becomes very great and all the good work done by 10 minutes of compression can be undone by 10 seconds' curiosity in wanting to see if the bleeding really has stopped.

THE THROAT

Foreign bodies lodging in the throat often creates serious problems. Small objects like peanuts, peas, fish bone or a safety pin can get struck in the throat and get lodged there. The foreign body may irritate the throat and produce a tighting of the vocal cord muscles. In such situation leads to causes noisy band difficult breathing. The need to deal urgently with neck injuries due to the twin threats posed by spinal injury and damage to the soft tissues of the throat which may lead to swelling and airway obstruction. A common problem encountered in A & E is that of adults who feel they have 'something stuck in their throat', usually a fish or chicken bone. Such objects are usually found at the level of the tonsils or in the upper part of the oesophagus.

In assessing the patient, the nurse should be alerted by the patient describing a sensation of sharp pain on swallowing, especially if it radiates to the ear, difficulty in swallowing saliva, and tenderness over the trachea. Any of these symptoms indicate a real risk of an object being lodged in the throat or upper oesophagus. Unfortunately many such objects are radiotranslucent, e.g., fish bones and many dental plates, but radiography is standard procedure still. If a perforation has occurred, even though the causative object may not show on X-ray, air in the soft tissues will allow the medical staff to make a diagnosis.

The picture is complicated by the fact that a sharp object that is swallowed may well scratch soft tissue, leaving behind a sensation of something sticking in the throat, even though the object has long gone on its way down the alimentary canal. Despite reassurance that there is not a problem and that nothing is stuck, the patient can still feel the sensation of something sticking there, and may not be convinced of the diagnosis. Considerable tact and diplomacy are required sometimes in this situation.

Perforation of the oesophagus or the development of an abscess in the upper respiratory tract due to impaction of a foreign body can have very serious consequences. It is advisable, therefore, to err on the side of caution and most A & E departments refer their patients on to ENT specialists if there is any chance of an impacted foreign body. If the patient is discharged, the nurse should reinforce patient instructions to return if symptoms do not improve or if any feeling of being unwell and feverish or if pain in the upper chest and neck region should develop. Mediastinitis developing from a perforation of the oesophagus will make the patient seriously ill, while if a pharyngeal abscess were to develop, there is a risk of occluding the airway.

HOARSENESS AND STRIDOR IN CHILDREN

Stridor in a child with a previously adequate airway is usually caused by infection, but inhaled foreign bodies, trauma from ingesting corrosive agents and allergic oedema are other possible causes.

Croup is caused by acute laryngitis and can be a very frightening experience for both parent and child, a fact that should be remembered by the nurse. Dyspnoea is usually associated with more serious infections of the respiratory tract from the epiglottis downwards, rarely but most seriously epiglottitis. The throat and larynx of such young children in respiratory distress should only be examined by medical staff with considerable experience due to the risk of provoking laryngeal spasm which will lead to a total airway obstruction and cardiac arrest. Tracheotomy in a situation such as this is extremely difficult and the only way of providing an airway may well be by inserting needles into the trachea.

FACIAL AND DENTAL EMERGENCIES

Facial Trauma

Trauma in the form of a direct blow to the face tends to produce one of several characteristic fracture patterns, which may also involve the base of the skull, leading to CSF leakage (rhinorrhoea from the nose and otorrhoea from the ear).

Blunt trauma to the side of the face is most likely to fracture the cheek or zygoma characteristically in three places, the zygomatic arch, the posterior half of the infra-orbital rim and the frontal zygomatic suture, giving rise to what is known as a *tripod* or *trimalleolar fracture*.

High energy trauma affecting the front of the face can causes fractures of the maxilla. Maxillary fractures tend to follow one of three characteristic patterns, first described by the French pathologist *Le Fort* (Fig. 2). A *Le Fort II* fracture produces very heavy nasal and pharyngeal bleeding which endangers the

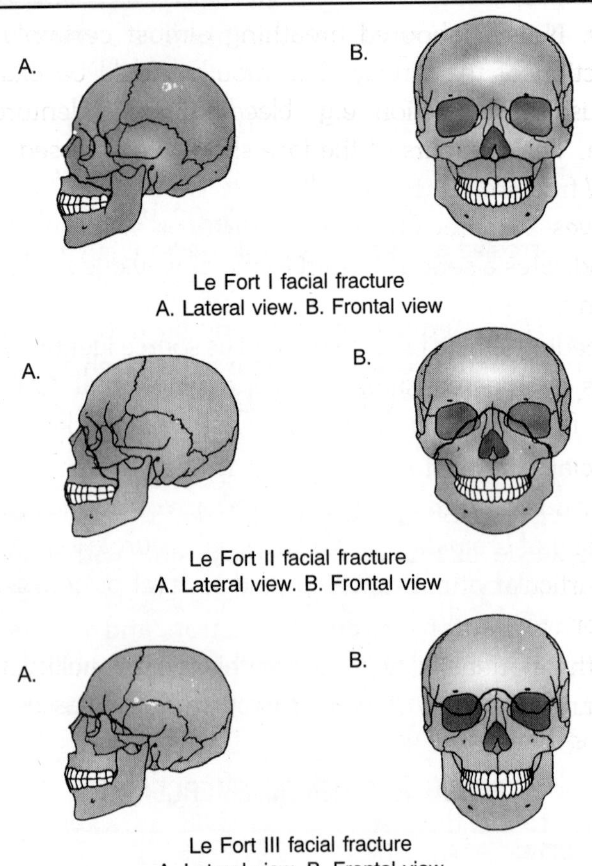

Fig. 33.2: *Patterns of fracture, Le Fort Types I-III.*

airway. A *Le Fort III* fracture commonly involves a CSF leak as there is usually an associated fracture of the cribiform plate. The airway is also at risk in a *Le Fort III* fracture because, as can be seen, the whole of the front of the face is effectively separated from the rest of the skull.

Fractures involving the mandible are associated with injury to the jaw. A midline fracture will usually be associated with a fracture of the condyles as well.

ASSESSMENT OF FACIAL INJURIES

The first priority in assessing the patient who has sustained facial trauma, as in all cases, is to assess the patency of the airway. Noisy, laboured breathing almost certainly indicates obstruction of the airway. The mouth should be examined for the cause of obstruction, e.g., bleeding, vomit, dentures and the tongue. The contours of the face should be assessed, as in a *Le Fort III* fracture the front of the face is separated from the skull and gives a characteristic 'shoved in' or dish-like appearance. This indicates a serious hazard to the airway due to the abnormal anatomy.

Bleeding should be assessed and its source identified if possible as clots of blood constitute a major airway threat. CSF should be looked for, indicating a fracture of the base of skull if found.

Facial trauma inevitably means that the brain absorbs a substantial amount of the energy involved, leading to the possibility of brain damage. A thorough neurological assessment, with particular attention being paid to level of consciousness, is therefore required.

If the patient is able to cooperate, the ability to oppose upper and lower sets of teeth correctly should be assessed. Failure to do so indicates facial bone fracture such as a *Le Fort* or mandibular fracture. Gentle palpation of the face may well allow the nurse to feel the step associated with a fracture. A complaint by the patient of double vision should alert the nurses to the possibility of a blow out fracture causing tethering of the rectus muscle that controls eye movement.

INTERVENTION

The first intervention priority is to clear and maintain the airway which is at hazard from bleeding, clots, dentures, fractured teeth, the tongue, vomit and the abnormal anatomy associated with certain fracture patterns such as a *Le Fort III fracture*.

The standard measures of mechanically clearing the oropharynx with suction and forceps (or gloved fingers), inserting an oral airway to lift the tongue forward (if tolerated), and positioning the patient on their side with the head down to aid drainage of blood, etc., should be followed immediately. Consideration should also be given to the possibility of cervical injury. In severe cases, intubation or tracheotomy may be required immediately in the A & E resuscitation room. The nurse should therefore know where the necessary equipment is located and be able to give whatever assistance is required by the medical team.

Due to the grave hazard posed to the airway by facial injuries, patients should never be left unattended or lying on their backs. Oxygen may be administered via a high concentration mask. Careful monitoring of the patient's neurological status is required due to the risk of deterioration in consciousness associated with brain trauma. A cervical collar is a wise precaution due to the risk of spinal injury.

Severe facial injuries can be very distressing to the patient, distress that can be compounded by fear of disfigurement. Psychological support from the nursing staff is therefore very important. Communication with the patient may be impeded as the injuries may interfere with normal speech. Nurses should, therefore, try to phrase questions so that the patient may answer simply yes or no.

Patients with facial fractures will usually have their fractures dealt with by wiring. They therefore need preparing for theatre in the usual way, according to hospital policy. The effectiveness of nursing intervention needs to be continuously monitored. Evaluation should concentrate on the patency of the patient's airway and also on how much bleeding is occurring, particularly from the nose and mouth where blood can be caught in a bowl and the volume measured.

DENTAL PROBLEMS

A & E departments are commonly confronted with patients in severe pain due to toothache for whom there is little we can do apart from giving them a bottle of paracetamol.

Bleeding from a tooth socket following an extraction earlier in the day is a familiar complaint seen in the evening at A & E. The presence of blood in the mouth which the patient continually has to expectorate leads to distress and anxiety, while swallowing it will cause nausea and vomiting.

The correct procedure is direct pressure to the bleeding socket applied by having the patient bite on a gauze swab. 'Intraoral bleeders can rarely be clamped and tied and electrocoagulation is of little value' is the verdict of *Anderson* and *Cosgriff*, recommending that time and effort should not be wasted on these two techniques.

Usually 20 to 30 minutes of continual pressure will control the bleeding. If this is not successful, the use of an oxidized cellulose dressing should be considered. It is helpful to ask the patient if there have been any other bleeding-related problems, as this may indicate a significant blood disorder that requires investigation. Pain associated with facial swelling and an elevated temperature is indicative of a dental abscess, usually related to non-vital or degenerative pulp, the result of advanced dental caries. The patient will often complain of having been unable to eat, drink or sleep because of the condition.

While the medical staff will probably prescribe analgesics and antibiotics (penicillin), the nursing staff should ensure that the patient understands the need for complete rest, which tablets are for pain and which are the antibiotics. This last information should be written on the tablet bottle label as patients who have been suffering from a dental abscess are often tired and distressed and may not absorb fully information given verbally. Dehydration may be present; therefore, advice should be given about the need to drink plenty of fluids. General dietary information concerning liquid nutrition may be of assistance in some cases. Such nursing interventions fit well into an Orem self-care model. In severe cases, cellulitis may develop involving the soft tissue of the whole jaw. Admission for in-patient management is required in such cases.

STUDY-QUESTIONS

1. Write a short note on the following:
   (a) Ear;
   (b) Nose;
   (c) Throat; and
   (d) Dental problems.

***

34

CHAPTER

WOMEN'S HEALTH PROBLEMS IN A & E

INTRODUCTION

In order to understand the present we often have to look at the past, and to understand the origins of many women's health problems, such an approach is essential. During the early 19th century women continued to make the transition from a rural or domestic working life into the factories of the established industrial revolution. Whilst low wages are factors of rural and urban living, the towns and cities included atmospheric pollution and a diet controlled by what was available in the shops at greater cost. *Hall*, continues by discussing the impact of higher wages upon single women which encouraged men to protect their earning potential through the unions and government policies.

Women were forced into a dependency upon men, being expected to uphold the family structure, which the moralist implied was in imminent danger of collapse. At this time, women undertook piece-work to supplement the household income. However, after the two world wars saw women being temporarily drafted into the industrial workforce and women became equated with a disposable workforce.

In parallel with the feminist movement has been a rise in the vision of education for daughters. Nevertheless, *Social Trends*, indicates that currently a quarter of women between 16 and 59 years of age have no qualifications. Educational attainment is still dependent upon the social class of the parent.

Recent economic trends have resulted in changing employment patterns. Significantly more women are in part-time employment, and have more second jobs (OPCS). In 1994, *Social Trends* indicated that a third of women were classed as economically viable with 1 in 6 recorded as unemployed. The impact of employment needs to be considered in the context of other social patterns occurring simultaneously such as changes to the family unit. Most of the women still perform the dual role of wage earner and homemaker; the conflict of this balancing act may result in stress which in turn contributes to women attending the A & E department.

STRESS AMONGEST WOMEN

Many women are now thinking and conscious of their place in society. Stress amongst women results from a diversity of internal and external factors. Society, encouraged by the media, expects certain stereotypical behaviours from 'normal' women, e.g., the housewife, mother or working woman. Rarely in these images are women seen in combined roles. Guilt and disharmony occurs as women perceive that they have failed to achieve these images. *Richardson* (1993) urges us to remember that women are more than biological reproducers and providers, but sexual, feminine individuals.

Factors which induce stress include any significant life change, e.g., divorce, separation and single parenting. Statistics provide us with the occurrence of each of these events; however, the socio-psychological impact cannot be measured although 'risk scores' of stress provide some indicators to susceptibility.

There is a strong feeling of guilt when a single mother looks at her children and sees them totally as her responsibility. There is no one to share decisions or control of the children, no one to help to decide which bills should be paid now and which can wait. It is a great burden to fall on one pair of shoulders. In 1991 there were 3 million single parents, only 1per cent of whom were lone fathers. Childcare facilities are poor: the General House-hold Survey of 1991 indicated that two-fifths of women use unpaid families or friends for childcare support.

In order to give good and appropriate care, A & E nurses should reflect upon the great stress that women have to live with, be they married or single, working or not, as a result of the tensions created by this dual role in society of woman the worker and woman the homemaker. Stress may manifest itself differently but amongst women self-poisoning (parasuicide), alcohol abuse and smoking are well-recognised signs of stress.

Alcohol abuse is by far related to social problems leading to mental and physical ill health. *Social Trends* indicates a regional variation from 6 to 14 per cent of the population which consumes alcohol to excess (over 15 units per week). According to a study carried out by *Merrill et al., Platt* and *Robinson* indicates a close association between alcohol abuse and suicide attempts.

Smoking continues to feature significantly on the health promotion agendas. Whilst smoking has decreased to 29 per cent of women, the highest usage remains amongst those of lower social groups. It is significant that deaths from lung cancer amongst women have risen by 75 per cent in twenty years.

WHO figures indicate that the incidence of parasuicide amongst women is three times greater than men. The reasons for this discrepancy may not always be clear, although it may be the culmination of a period of stress which may have been treated with antidepressants. *Hawton* and *Fagg,* indicated in their study that the incidence of self-poisoning declined in the early 1980s but increased to a rate of 711/10,0000 among 15-25 year olds by 1990. Of particular interest to the A & E nurse is the rise of paracetamol use from 14.3 per cent in 1976 to 42% in 1990.

Stress may manifest itself in physical or psychological symptoms. *Graham* described how women fail to report illness in the normal way either because they are unaware of a deterioration in their own health or by being ill they will be unable to maintain current roles within the family. Women are less able to relieve the causes of stress by walking out or going to the pub.

Whether she turns up at the GP's surgery or at the A & E department, this woman is not a malingerer nor a time waster, she has a real problem that must be recognized. The nurse should be supportive and sympathetic, not dismissive with a 'Pull yourself together, of course you can cope' attitude. Physical complaints must be accepted and investigated at their face value, even if there is a suspicion that they may be conscious or unconscious rationalizations of the woman's desire for help. Nurses do not have the right to adopt a judgemental attitude in such cases.

TRAUMA DURING PREGNANCY

Pregnancy is a state of normal health. Despite this fact, however, many A & E nurses feel very anxious when confronted by a pregnant woman who has suffered trauma because of the specific ways that trauma can affect the pregnant woman. On admission always ask for the clinic card as this will provide a wealth of information.

1. Blunt Trauma

(a) *Placental separation (abruptio placenta)*—This is the second most common cause of fetal death; maternal death is the most common. The uterus will be very painful and tense in this situation.

(b) *Uterine rupture*—Unfortunately fetal death and hysterectomy is the usual outcome.

(c) *Pelvic fractures*—This is the most common serious fracture in pregnant women.

(d) *Rupture of liver and spleen*—The gravid uterus acts as a shock absorber and protects many of the abdominal organs from trauma. However, in pregnancy the liver and spleen become distended and displaced making them more vulnerable to injury.

(e) *Placenta praevia*—Whilst not associated with specific trauma, any separation of a low-lying placenta may cause torrential blood loss and is potentially fatal for the mother.

2. Penetrating Trauma

This is usually the result of gunshot or knife wounds and therefore relatively rare in the UK. Nevertheless it is possible given that pregnancy does not exempt a woman from the risk of assault. The gravid uterus protects the woman's abdominal organs very effectively, though at the expense of the fetus.

3. Abortion and Premature Labour

Trauma may lead to a spontaneous delivery. If pregnancy is greater than 24 weeks' gestation, then neonatal assistance should be sought.

4. Maternal Shock

A woman's plasma blood volume increases by as much as 50 per cent during pregnancy with associated haemodilution. Serious bleeding with pooling in the abdominal cavity can occur, hidden by the gravid uterus. The increased blood volume of the woman means that she can lose up to a third of that volume before any signs of hypovolaemic shock appear. The normal response of compensating by shutting down the blood supply to non-vital organs means that the fetus is at great risk in maternal shock, for even in pregnancy, the uterus is non-vital.

ASSESSMENT OF THE PREGNANT WOMAN AFTER TRAUMA

The usual signs indicating abdominal trauma may be masked or complicated by pregnancy. Stretching of the abdominal wall means that guarding and rigidity are often absent. They are, therefore, unreliable indicators. The increased blood volume associated with pregnancy leads to a situation whereby hypotension and tachycardia may only become apparent when the woman has lost a third of her blood volume.

The nurse should take any complaint of pain seriously by the nurse who should ask the patient to describe the pain. Vaginal bleeding is obviously a very significant sign. Monitoring of the fetal heart rate for the tachy/bradyeardia will indicate fetal distress and the potential need for emergency delivery by Caesarean.

The psychological state of the woman, together with that of her partner or other friends and relatives, should be monitored closely throughout what may be an extremely distressing experience.

INTERVENTION

Resuscitation should proceed along the standard line described earlier, except with the addition of the basic principle that the life of the mother takes precedence over the fetus. The woman should never be kept in a supine position as the pressure from the uterus causes compression of the vena cava resulting in hypotension and fetal hypoxia. By placing the woman in the lateral position blood flow will increase to vital organs and the uterus.

The fetal heart should be monitored using a portable sonic aid. If the fetal heart is not audible then an ultrasound scan will confirm viability. Any signs of fetal distress will indicate that delivery should be precipitated immediately. The nurse should be aware of non-verbal actions as these may increase the anxiety of the woman and her partner. The woman and partner's psychological state is likely to be eased by being provided with up-to-date accurate information in an empathetic manner. The midwife on call or the maternity unit should be contacted immediately.

If spontaneous delivery does occur in A & E remember that childbirth is a perfectly normal event that women have been managing to perform successfully throughout the history of humankind. The woman should be allowed to give birth in whatever position she finds most natural, wherever she feels comfortable, i.e., chair, floor with mattress. She may or may not have made plans for delivery and anxiety will be increased with the realization that she may not attain her personal goal in the environment she had envisaged.

Most women between the menarche and the menopause experience vaginal bleeding at approximately monthly intervals. What actually happens to individuals varies enormously. For some women a normal period occurs every 3 weeks and last 8 days. For others it occurs every 8 weeks and lasts 3 days. In assessing the patient who attends A & E complaining of vaginal bleeding, the nurse needs to discover the following:

Vaginal Bleeding

1. Date of last menstrual period.
2. Normal frequency and heaviness of periods.
3. Why is this bleeding different?
4. Is there any pain, and if so, its location, type and duration.
5. Is there a possibility of pregnancy?
6. Psychological state of patient.
7. Baseline vital signs.

The interview should be conducted in strict privacy, especially the nurse is dealing with an adolescent/teenager accompanied by her parents. Pregnancy testing equipment should be available in the department.

If the pregnancy test is positive, it is usual to admit the patient are the care of the obstetric or gynaecological medical teams, depending upon the stage of the pregnancy. Keep the woman comfortable and dry. Any material passed vaginally should be kept for inspection and blood loss estimated from the number of pads used. If the patient is hypovolaemic then urgent resuscitation is required as, for example, a ruptured ectopic pregnancy can cause catastrophic bleeding.

If the pregnancy aborts in the A & E department the nurse needs to provide additional psychological support. The grieving process may have already started. Placatory comments such as 'Think of your other children' or 'There is always another chance' are inappropriate. Finally, the possibility of a criminal abortion should be borne in mind if there are any suspicious circumstances.

CONCEALED PREGNANCY

Despite general information and open discussions about pregnancy, occasionally some women are admitted to A & E complaining of acute abdominal pains only to be told they are in labour. One may assume that this occurs to teenagers who have denied the pregnancy through fear and/or ignorance. It can potentially happen to any woman who does not expect to be pregnant, particularly if menstruation is expected to be irregular, i.e., when becoming menopausal. The woman not only has to deal with the labour but has to begin the adaptation towards motherhood that would normally occur during acknowledged pregnancy. Ideally the woman should be transferred to the local maternity unit. Milst this is not always feasible, the midwife on call will usually attend. If delivery is imminent the best policy is one of hands off. Provided the fetal heart is established the woman in labour requires attendants who are friendly and calm during contractions, and usually the person, if any, who came with her.

LOST TAMPONS

This is a highly embarrassing but frequent cause of attendance at A & E, caused usually by either a faulty tampon, sexual intercourse during menstruation with the tampon in place, or an attempt to cope with a heavy period by inserting a second tampon. The result of either of these latter two events is to push the tampon high into the vagina where it cannot be retrieved.

Tact and sympathy, a Cusco's speculum, a good light source, and a pair of long-handled forceps will usually permit a female member of the nursing staff to remove the offending article promptly. In order to try to prevent a recurrence of the problem, advice should be offered about the wisdom of sexual intercourse with a tampon in place or of attempting to cope with bleeding by using two tamptons.

STUDY–QUESTIONS

1. Discuss the various type in pregnant woman.
2. Write short notes on the following
   (a) Concealed pregnancy; and
   (b) Vaginal bleeding.

35

CHAPTER MEDICAL EMERGENCY

INTRODUCTION

A medical emergency is an injury or illness that poses an immediate threat to a person's life or long term health. These emergencies may need help from another person, who should ideally be suitably qualified to do so, although some of these emergencies can be dealt with by the victim themselves. Dependant on the severity of the emergency, and the quality of any treatment given, it may require the involvement of multiple levels of care, from a first aider to an emergency physician through to specialist surgeons.

Any response to an emergency medical situation will depend strongly on the situation, the patient involved and availability of resources to help them. It will also vary depending on whether the emergency occurs whilst in hospital under medical care, or outside of any care (for instance, in the street).

CLINICAL RESPONSE IN MEDICAL EMERGENCIES

Within hospital settings, an adequate staff is generally present to deal with the average emergency situation. Emergency medicine physicians have training to deal with most medical emergencies and maintain CPR and ACLS certifications. In disasters or complex emergencies, most hospitals have protocols to summon on-site and off-site staff rapidly.

Both emergency room and inpatient medical emergencies follow the basic protocol of Advanced Cardiac Life Support. Irrespective of the nature of the emergency, adequate blood pressure and oxygenation are required before the cause of the emergency can be eliminated. Possible exceptions include the clamping of arteries in severe hemorrhage.

RESPIRATORY EMERGENCIES

AGONAL RESPIRATION

Agonal respiration is an abnormal pattern of breathing characterized by shallow, slow (3-4 per minute), irregular inspirations followed by irregular pauses. They may also be characterized as gasping, labored breathing, accompanied by strange vocalizations and myoclonus. The cause is due to cerebral ischemia, due to extreme hypoxia or even anoxia. Agonal breathing is an extremely serious medical sign requiring immediate medical attention, as the condition generally progresses to complete apnea and heralds death.

The term is sometimes (inaccurately) used to refer to labored, gasping breathing patterns accompanying organ failure (e.g. liver failure and renal failure), SIRS, septic shock, and metabolic acidosis, or in general any labored breathing, including Biot's respirations and ataxic respirations. Correct usage would restrict the term to the last breaths before death.

Agonal respirations are also commonly seen in cases of cardiac arrest, and may persist for several minutes after cessation of heartbeat. The presence of agonal respirations in these cases indicates a more favorable prognosis than in cases of cardiac arrest without agonal respirations. Agonal respiration is not the same as, and is unrelated to, the phenomenon of death rattle.

ASPHYXIA

Asphyxia is a condition of severely deficient supply of oxygen to the body that arises from being unable to breathe normally. Asphyxia causes generalized hypoxia, which primarily affects the tissues and organs most sensitive to hypoxia first, such as the brain, hence resulting in cerebral hypoxia. Asphyxia is usually characterized by air hunger, but this is not always the case; the urge to breathe is triggered by rising carbon dioxide levels in the blood rather than diminishing oxygen levels. Sometimes there is not enough carbon dioxide to cause air hunger, and victims become hypoxic without knowing it. In any case, the absence of effective remedial action will very rapidly lead to unconsciousness, brain damage, and death. The time to death is dependent on the particular mechanism of asphyxia.

Asphyxia is used to maim or kill in capital punishment, suicide, torture, and warfare. It is also used non-fatally in martial arts, combat sports, BDSM, and during sex as erotic asphyxia. Because the need to breathe is triggered by the level of carbon dioxide in the blood, some victims may not experience an urgent need to breathe and may remain unaware of the onset of hypoxia.

COMPRESSIVE ASPHYXIA

Compressive asphyxia (also called chest compression) refers to the mechanical limitation of the expansion of the lungs by compressing the torso, hence interfering with breathing. Compressive asphyxia occurs when the chest or abdomen is compressed posteriorly. In accidents, the term traumatic asphyxia or crush asphyxia is usually used to describe compressive asphyxia resulting from being crushed or pinned under a large weight or force. An example of traumatic asphyxia includes cases in which an individual has been using a car-jack to repair a car from below, only to be crushed under the weight of the vehicle when the car-jack slips. Pythons, anacondas, and other constrictor snakes kill through compressive asphyxia.

In fatal crowd disasters, contrary to popular belief, it is not the blunt trauma from trampling that causes the large part of the deaths, but rather the compressive asphyxia from being crushed against the crowd. In confined spaces, people push and lean against each other; evidence from bent steel railings in several fatal crowd accidents have shown horizontal forces over 4500 N (comparative weight approximately 460 kg). In cases where people have stacked up on each other forming a human pile, estimations have been made of around 380 kg of compressive weight in the lowest layer.

Chest compression is also featured in various grappling combat sports, where it is sometimes called wringing. Such techniques are used either to tire the opponent or as complementary or distractive moves in combination with pinning holds,or sometimes even as submission holds. Examples of chest compression include the knee-on-stomach position, or techniques such as leg scissors.

CHOKING

Choking is the mechanical obstruction of the flow of air from the environment into the lungs. Choking prevents breathing, and can be partial or complete, with partial choking allowing some, although inadequate, flow of air into the lungs. Prolonged or complete choking results in asphyxiation which leads to hypoxia and is potentially fatal. Choking can be caused by:

- Introduction of a foreign object into the airway, which becomes lodged in the pharynx, larynx or trachea.
- Respiratory diseases that involve obstruction of the airway.
- Compression of the laryngopharynx, larynx or trachea in strangles.

The type of choking most commonly recognised as such by the public is the lodging of foreign objects in the airway. This type of choking is often suffered by small children, who are unable to appreciate the hazard inherent in putting small objects in their mouth. In adults, it mostly occurs whilst the patient is eating. The symptoms and clinical signs are:

- The person cannot speak or cry out.
- The person's face turns blue (cyanosis) from lack of oxygen.
- The person desperately grabs at his or her throat.
- The person has a weak cough, and labored breathing produces a high-pitched noise.
- The person does any or all of the above, and then becomes unconscious.

Choking can be treated with a number of different procedures, with both basic techniques available for first aiders and more advanced techniques available for health professionals.

SMOKE INHALATION

Smoke inhalation is the primary cause of death in victims of indoor fires. Smoke inhalation injury refers to injury due to inhalation or exposure to hot gaseous products of combustion. This can cause serious respiratory complications.

It is estimated that "50-80 per cent of fire deaths are the result of smoke inhalation injuries rather than burns." The smoke injures or kills by a combination of thermal damage, poisoning and pulmonary irritation caused by carbon monoxide, cyanide and other combustion products. Symptoms range from coughing and vomiting to nausea, sleepiness and confusion. Burns to the nose, mouth and face; singed nostril hairs; and difficulty breathing/carbonaceous sputum (burned saliva) are also signs of smoke inhalation injury. Approximately one third of patients admitted to burns unit have pulmonary injury from smoke inhalation. The death rate of patients with both severe burns and smoke inhalation can be in excess of 50 per cent

Any person with apparent signs of smoke inhalation should be immediately evaluated by a medical professional such as a firefighter-paramedic or physician. Advanced medical care may be necessary to save the life of the patient, including mechanical ventilation, even if the person is conscious and alert. Pending advanced intervention, the patient should be brought into fresh air and given medical oxygen if available. Smoke inhalation causes three complications:

1. Impaired or reduced levels of oxygen at the tissue level: This arises due to inhalation of carbon monoxide or cyanide and is an immediate threat to life. Immediate treatment with 100 per cent oxygen is essential and is given till the level of carboxyhaemoglobin (a product formed by combining of the haemoglobin molecule with carbon monoxide; reducing the amount of haemoglobin available to transport oxygen to tissues.) falls to less than 10 per cent and the metabolic acidosis (a condition in which there is excess of acid in the body causing severe chemical imbalances and electrolyte disturbances) has resolved.
2. Thermal injury to the upper airway: Hot gases cause burns to the mucosal surfaces of the upper airway. Its complications become evident in 18-24 hours. They are: oedema, reduced ability to clear secretions, airway obstruction causing respiratory distress and noise on inspiration. In advanced stages respiratory failure can also occur. Treatment is humidified oxygen, head tilt to 30 degrees, suction to clear secretions and medicines to reduce the swelling of the mucosa. Mixtures of Helium-Oxygen (Heliox) gas may be useful to reduce laboured breathing. Endotracheal intubation may be needed to maintain airway patency especially for deep facial burns or swelling of the pharynx. Investigations include arterial blood gas analysis, fibre optic laryngoscope or bronchoscope. Tracheostomy should be avoided if possible because of an increased risk of pneumonia and sepsis.
3. Chemical injury: to the lung is due to inhalation of toxic gases and products of combustion which includes aldehydes and organic acids. It can present with symptoms of bronchospasm (narrowing of the airways), difficulty in breathing, an increased rate of breathing, wheezing and a fast heart rate initially. A day or two later, there might be swelling of the smaller airways which may start sloughing off causing airway obstruction and pneumonia in 5-7 days.

Treatment—It consists of humidified oxygen, bronchodilators, suction, endotracheal tube and chest physiotherapy. Other measures include adequate fluids and control of infection by daily sputum stains and appropriate antibiotics.

ASTHMA

Asthma is a chronic illness involving the respiratory system in which the airway occasionally constricts, becomes inflamed, and is lined with excessive amounts of mucus, often in response to one or more triggers. These episodes may be triggered by such things as exposure to an environmental stimulant (or allergen) such as cold air, warm air, moist air, exercise or exertion, or emotional stress. In children, the most common triggers are viral illnesses such as those that cause the common cold. This airway narrowing causes symptoms such as wheezing, shortness of breath, chest tightness, and coughing. The airway constriction responds to bronchodilators. Between episodes, most patients feel well but can have mild symptoms and they may remain short of breath after exercise for longer periods of time than the unaffected individual. The symptoms of asthma, which can range from mild to life threatening, can usually be controlled with a combination of drugs and environmental changes.

In some individuals asthma is characterized by chronic respiratory impairment. In others it is an intermittent illness marked by episodic symptoms that may result from a number of triggering events, including upper respiratory infection, stress, airborne allergens, air pollutants (such as smoke or traffic fumes), or exercise. Some or all of the following symptoms may be present in those with asthma: dyspnea, wheezing, stridor, coughing, an inability for physical exertion. Some asthmatics that have severe shortness of breath and tightening of the lungs never wheeze or have stridor and their symptoms may be confused with a COPD-type disease.

An acute exacerbation of asthma is referred to as an asthma attack. The clinical hallmarks of an attack are shortness of breath (dyspnea) and either wheezing or stridor. Although the former is often regarded as the sine qua non of asthma, some patients present primarily with coughing, and in the late stages of an attack, air motion may be so impaired that no wheezing may be heard. When present the cough may sometimes produce clear sputum. The onset may be sudden, with a sense of constriction in the chest, breathing becomes difficult, and wheezing occurs (primarily upon expiration, but can be in both respiratory phases).

Signs of an asthmatic episode include wheezing, rapid breathing (tachypnea), prolonged expiration, a rapid heart rate (tachycardia), rhonchous lung sounds (audible through a stethoscope), and over-inflation of the chest. During a serious asthma attack, the accessory muscles of respiration (sternocleidomastoid and scalene muscles of the neck) may be used, shown as in-drawing of tissues between the ribs and above the sternum and clavicles, and the presence of a paradoxical pulse (a pulse that is weaker during inhalation and stronger during exhalation).

During very severe attacks, an asthma sufferer can turn blue from lack of oxygen, and can experience chest pain or even loss of consciousness. Just before loss of consciousness, there is a chance that the patient will feel numbness in the limbs and palms may start to sweat. Feet may become icy cold. Severe asthma attacks, which may not be responsive to standard treatments (status asthmaticus), are life-threatening and may lead to respiratory arrest.

PNEUMOTHORAX

In medicine (pulmonology), a pneumothorax, or collapsed lung, is a potential medical emergency caused by accumulation of air or gas in the pleural cavity, occurring as a result of disease or injury.

Pneumothoraces are divided into tension and non-tension pneumathoraces. A tension pneumothorax is a medical emergency as air accumulates in the pleural space with each breath. The increase in intrathoracic pressure results in massive shifts of the mediastinum away from the affected lung compressing intrathoracic vessels. A non-tension pneumothorax by contrast is a less severe pathology because there is no ongoing accumulation of air and hence no increasing pressure on the organs within the chest. The accumulation of blood in the thoracic cavity (hemothorax) exacerbates the problem, creating a pneumohemothorax.

Signs and symptoms: Sudden shortness of breath, dry coughs, cyanosis (turning blue) and pain felt in the chest, back and/or arms are the main symptoms. In penetrating chest wounds, the sound of air flowing through the puncture hole may indicate pneumothorax, hence the term "sucking" chest wound. The flopping sound of the punctured lung is also occasionally heard.

If untreated, hypoxia may lead to loss of consciousness and coma. In addition, shifting of the mediastinum away from the site of the injury can obstruct the superior and inferior vena cava resulting in reduced cardiac preload and decreased cardiac output. Untreated, a severe pneumothorax can lead to death within several minutes.

Spontaneous pneumothoraces are reported in young people with a tall stature. As men are generally taller than women, there is a preponderance among males. The reason for this association, while unknown, is hypothesized to be the presence of subtle abnormalities in connective tissue. Some spontaneous pneumothoraces however, are results of "blebs", blister like structures on the surface of the lung, that rupture allowing the escape of air into the pleural cavity.

Pneumothorax can also occur as part of medical procedures, such as the insertion of a central venous catheter (an intravenous catheter) in the subclavian vein or jugular vein. While rare, it is considered a serious complication and needs immediate treatment. Other causes include mechanical ventilation, emphysema and rarely other lung diseases (pneumonia).

Diagnosis: The absence of audible breath sounds through a stethoscope can indicate that the lung is not unfolded in the pleural cavity. This accompanied by hyperresonance (higher pitched sounds than normal) to percussion of the chest wall is suggestive of the diagnosis. If the signs and symptoms are doubtful, an X-ray of the chest can be performed, but in severe hypoxia, emergency treatment has to be administered first.

In a supine chest X-ray the deep sulcus sign is diagnostic, which is characterized by a low lateral costophrenic angle on the affected side. In layman's terms, the place where rib and diaphragm meet appears lower on an X-ray with a deep sulcus sign and suggests the diagnosis of pneumothorax.

RESPIRATORY FAILURE

Respiratory failure is a medical term for inadequate gas exchange by the respiratory system. Respiratory failure can be indicated by observing a drop in blood oxygen level (hypoxemia) and/or a rise in arterial carbon dioxide (hypercapnia) which can be written as ($PaO_2 < 60$ mmHg, $PaCO_2 > 45$ mmHg). Classification into type I or type II relates to the absence or presence of hypercapnia respectively.

TYPES OF RESPIRATORY FAILURE

There are two types of respiratory failure:

Type 1

Type 1 respiratory failure is defined as hypoxia without hypercapnia, indeed the CO2 level may be normal or low. It is typically caused by a ventilation/perfusion mismatch; the air flowing in and out of the lungs is not matched with the flow of blood to the lungs. This type is caused by conditions that affect oxygenation like:

- Parenchymal disease
- Diseases of vasculature and shunts.

Type 2

Type 2 respiratory failure is defined build up of carbon dioxide that has been generated by the body. The underlying causes include:

- Reduced breathing effort (in the fatigued patient)
- Increased resistance to breathing (such as in asthma)
- An decrease in the area of the lung available for gas exchange (such as in emphysema).

Causes

(i) Pulmonary dysfunction:
   - Asthma
   - Emphysema
   - Chronic obstructive airway disease
   - Pneumonia
   - Pneumothorax
   - Hemothorax
   - Acute Respiratory Distress Syndrome (ARDS) is a specific and life-threatening type of respiratory failure.
   - Cystic Fibrosis

(ii) Cardiac dysfunction:
   - Pulmonary edema
   - Arrhythmia
   - Congestive heart failure
   - Valve pathology

(iii) Other
   - Fatigue due to prolonged tachypnoea in metabolic acidosis
   - Intoxication with drugs (i.e. morphine, benzo-diazepines) suppresses respiration.

Treatment

Emergency treatment follows the principles of cardio-pulmonary resuscitation. Treatment of the underlying cause is required. Mechanical ventilation may be required.

CARDIAC AND CIRCULATORY EMERGENCY

AIR EMBOLISM

An air embolism, or more generally gas embolism, is a medical condition caused by gas bubbles in the bloodstream (embolism in a medical context refers to any large moving mass or defect in the blood stream). Small amounts of air often get into the blood circulation accidentally during surgery and other medical procedures, but most of these in veins are stopped at the lungs, and a venous air embolism that shows symptoms is very rare. Death may occur if a large bubble of gas becomes lodged in the heart, stopping blood from flowing from the right ventricle to the lungs (this is similar to vapor lock in engine fuel systems). However, the amount of gas necessary for this to happen is quite variable, and also depends on a number of other factors, such as body position.

Gas embolism into an artery, termed arterial gas embolism, or AGE, is a more serious matter than in a vein, since a gas bubble in an artery may directly cause stoppage of blood flow to an area fed by the artery. The symptoms of AGE depend on the area of blood flow, and may be those of stroke or heart attack if the brain or heart (respectively) are affected.

Pathogenesis

Air embolism can occur whenever a blood vessel is open and a pressure gradient exists favoring entry of gas. Because the pressure in most arteries and veins is greater than atmospheric pressure, an air embolus does not always happen when a blood vessel is injured. In the veins above the heart, such as in the head and neck, the pressure is less than atmospheric and an injury may let air in. This is one reason why surgeons must be particularly careful when operating on the brain, and why the head of the bed is tilted down when inserting or removing a central venous catheter from the jugular or subclavian veins.

When air enters the veins, it travels to the right side of the heart, and then to the lungs. This can cause the vessels of the lung to constrict, raising the pressure in the right side of the heart. If the pressure rises high enough in a patient who is one of the 20 per cent to 30 per cent of the population with a patent foramen ovale, the gas bubble can then travel to the left side of the heart, and on to the brain or coronary arteries. Such bubbles are responsible for the most serious of gas embolic symptoms.

Trauma to the lung can also cause an air embolism. This may happen after a patient is placed on a ventilator and air is forced into an injured vein or artery, causing sudden death. Breath-holding while ascending from scuba diving may also force lung air into pulmonary arteries or veins in a similar manner, due to the pressure difference.

Air can be injected directly into the veins either accidentally or as a deliberate act. Examples include misuse of a syringe, and industrial injury resulting from use of compressed air. However, despite being employed by writers of fiction as a clandestine method of murder, amounts of air such as would be administered by a single small syringe are not likely to suddenly stop the heart, nor cause instant death. Single air bubbles in a vein do not stop the heart, due to being too small. However, such bubbles may occasionally reach the arterial system through a patent foramen ovale, as noted above, and cause random ischemic damage, depending on their route of arterial travel.

GAS EMBOLISM IN DIVING

Gas embolism is one of the diving disorders SCUBA divers sometimes suffer when they receive pressure damage to their lungs following a rapid ascent where the breath is inappropriately held against a closed glottis, allowing pressure to build up inside the lungs, relative to the blood. It is termed "gas" because the diver may be using a diving breathing gas other than air. The gas bubbles can impede the flow of oxygen-rich blood to the brain and vital organs. They can also cause clots to form in blood vessels.

Gas embolism and decompression sickness (DCS) may be difficult to distinguish, as they may have similar symptoms, especially in the central nervous system. The treatment for both is the same, because they are both the result of gas bubbles in the body. In a diving context, the two are often called decompression illness (DCI).

Treatment

Recompression is the most effective treatment of an air embolism. Normally this is carried out in a recompression chamber. This is because as pressure increases, the solubility of a gas increases.

Oxygen first aid treatment is useful for suspected gas embolism casualties or divers who have made fast ascents or missed decompression stops. Most fully closed-circuit rebreathers can deliver sustained high concentrations of oxygen-rich breathing gas and could be used as an alternative to pure open-circuit oxygen resuscitators.

BLEEDING

Bleeding, technically known as hemorrhage (American English) or haemorrhage (British English) is the loss of blood from the circulatory system. Bleeding can occur internally, where blood leaks from blood vessels inside the body or externally, either through a natural opening such as vagina, mouth or rectum, or through a break in the skin. The complete loss of blood is referred to as exsanguination and desanguination is a massive blood loss. Loss of 10-15 per cent of total blood volume can be endured without clinical sequelae in a healthy person, and blood donation typically takes 8-10 per cent of the donor's blood volume.

Causes, Prevalence, and Risk Factors

Hemorrhage generally becomes dangerous, or even fatal, when it causes hypovolemia (low blood volume) or hypotension (low blood pressure). In these scenarios various mechanisms come into play to maintain the body's homeostasis. These include the "retro-stress-relaxation" mechanism of cardiac muscle, the baroreceptor reflex and renal and endocrine responses such as the renin - angiotensin - aldosterone system (RAAS).

Certain diseases or medical conditions, such as haemophilia and low platelet count (thrombocytopenia) may increase the risk of bleeding or may allow otherwise minor bleeds to become health or life threatening. Anticoagulant medications, such as warfarin can mimic the effects of haemophilia, preventing clotting, and allowing free blood flow.

Death from hemorrhage can generally occur surprisingly quickly. This is because of 'positive feedback'. An example of this is 'cardiac repression', when poor heart contraction depletes blood flow to the heart, causing even poorer heart contraction. This kind of effect causes death to occur more quickly than expected.

First Aid

All people who have been injured should receive a thorough assessment. It should be divided into a primary and secondary survey and performed in a stepwise fashion, following the "ABCs". Notification of EMS or other rescue agencies should be performed in a timely manner and as the situation requires.

The primary survey examines and verifies that the patient's Airway is intact, that s/he is Breathing and that Circulation is working. A similar scheme and mnemonic is used as in CPR. However, during the pulse check of C, attempts should also be made to control bleeding and to assess perfusion, usually by checking capillary refill. Additionally a persons mental status should be assessed (Disability) or either an AVPU scale or via a formal Glasgow Coma Scale. In all but the most minor cases, the patient should be Exposed by removal of clothing and a secondary survey performed, examining the patient from head to toe for other injuries. The survey should not delay treatment and transport, especially if a non-correctable problem is identified.

Minor Bleeding

Minor bleeding is bleeding that falls under a Class I hemorrhage and the bleeding is easily stopped with pressure.

The largest danger in a minor wound is infection. Bleeding can be stopped with direct pressure and elevation, and the wound should be washed well with soap and water. A dressing, typically made of gauze, should be applied. Peroxide or iodine solutions (such as Betadine) can injure the cells that promote healing and may actually impair proper wound healing and delay closure.

Emergency Bleeding Control

Severe bleeding poses a very real risk of death to the casualty if not treated quickly. Therefore, preventing major bleeding should take priority over other conditions, save failure of the heart or lungs. Most protocols advise the use of direct pressure, rest and elevation of the wound above the heart to control bleeding.The use of a tourniquet is not advised in most cases, as it can lead to unnecessary necrosis or even loss of a limb. Tourniquets should rarely be used as it is usually possible to stop bleeding by the application of manual pressure.

Bleeding from Body cavities

The only minor situation is a spontaneous nosebleed, or a nosebleed caused by a slight trauma (such as a child putting his finger in his nose). Simultaneous externalised bleeding from the ear may indicate brain trauma if there has been a serious head injury. Loss of consciousness, amnesia, or fall from a height increases the likelihood that there has been a severe injury. This type of injury can also be found in motor vehicle accidents associated with death or severe injury to other passengers.

Hemoptysis, or coughing up blood, may be a sign that the person is at risk for serious bleeding. This is especially the case for patients with cancer. Hematemesis is vomiting up blood from the stomach. Often, the source of bleeding is difficult to distinguish and usually requires detailed assessment by an emergency physician.

Internal Bleeding

Internal bleeding occurs entirely within the confines of the body and can be caused by a medical condition (such as aortic aneurysm) or by trauma. Symptoms of internal bleeding include pale, clammy skin, an increased heart rate and a stupor or confused state. The most recognisable form of internal bleeding is the contusion or bruise.

Risk of Blood Contamination

Because skin is watertight, there is no immediate risk of infection to the aide from contact with blood, provided the exposed area has not been previously wounded or diseased. Before any further activity (especially eating, drinking, touching the eyes, the mouth or the nose), the skin should be thoroughly cleaned in order to avoid cross contamination.

To avoid any risk, the hands can be prevented from contact with a glove (mostly latex or nitrile rubber), or an improvised method such as a plastic bag or a cloth. This is taught as important part of protecting the rescuer in most first aid protocols.

Treatment

Before the advent of modern medicine the technique of bloodletting, or phlebotomy, was used for a number of conditions: causing bleeding intentionally to remove a controlled amount of excess or "bad" blood. Phlebotomy is still used as an extremely effective treatment for Haemochromatosis.

CARDIAC ARRHYTHMIA

Cardiac arrhythmia is any of a group of conditions in which the electrical activity of the heart is irregular or is faster or slower than normal. Some arrhythmias are life-threatening medical emergencies that can cause cardiac arrest and sudden death. Others cause aggravating symptoms, such as an awareness of a different heart beat, or palpitation, which can be annoying. Some are quite minor and can be regarded as normal. In fact, most people have felt a skip of a beat or a sudden tachycardia, which are usually not a cause for alarm. Sinus arrhythmia is the mild acceleration followed by slowing of the normal rhythm that occurs with breathing. In adults the normal resting heart rate ranges from 60 beats per minute to 100 beats per minute. The normal heart beat is controlled by a small area in the upper chamber of the heart called the sinoatrial node or sinus node. The sinus node contains specialized cells that have spontaneous electrical activity that starts each normal heart beat.

FASTER AND SLOWER ARRHYTHMIAS

In an adult, a resting heart rate faster than 100 beats/minute is considered tachycardia. This number varies with age, as the heartbeat of a younger person is naturally faster than that of an older person's. During exercise the sinus node increases its rate of electrical activity to accelerate the heart rate. Such normal fast rate that develops is called sinus tachycardia. In contrast, arrhythmias that are due to fast, abnormal electrical activity can cause tachycardias that are dangerous. If the ventricles of the heart experience one of these tachycardias for a long period of time, there can be deleterious effects. Individuals may sense a tachycardia as a pounding sensation of the heart, known as palpitations. If a tachycardia lowers blood pressure it may cause lightheadedness or dizziness, or even fainting (syncope). If the tachycardia is too fast, the pump function of the heart is impeded, and rarely may lead to sudden death.

Most tachycardias are not dangerous. Anything that increases adrenaline or its effects on the heart will increase the heart rate and potentially cause palpitations or tachycardias. Causes include stress, ingested or injected substances (ie: caffeine, amphetamines, alcohol—see Holiday heart syndrome), and an overactive thyroid gland (hyperthyroidism). Individuals who have a tachycardia are often advised to limit or remove exposure to any causative agent. However, these causative agents are not the only contributors to tachycardias and their prevalence has not been evaluated statistically.

A slow rhythm, known as bradycardia (less than 60 beats/ min), is usually not life threatening, but may cause symptoms. It may be caused by reversible causes (low oxygen, electrolyte abnormalities), or be more permanent (heart block). When it causes symptoms implantation of a permanent pacemaker may be needed. Either dysrhythmia requires medical attention to evaluate the risks associated with the arrhythmia.

FIBRILLATION

A serious variety of arrhythmia is known as fibrillation. The muscle cells of the heart normally function together, creating a single contraction when stimulated. Fibrillation occurs when the heart muscle begins a quivering motion due to a disunity in contractile cell function. Fibrillation can affect the atrium (atrial fibrillation) or the ventricle (ventricular fibrillation); ventricular fibrillation is imminently life-threatening.

Atrial fibrillation is the quivering, chaotic motion in the upper chambers of the heart, known as the atria. Atrial fibrillation is often due to serious underlying medical conditions, and should be evaluated by a physician. It is not typically a medical emergency.

Ventricular fibrillation occurs in the ventricles (lower chambers) of the heart; it is always a medical emergency. If left untreated, ventricular fibrillation (VF, or V-fib) can lead to death within minutes. When a heart goes into V-fib, effective pumping of the blood stops. V-fib is considered a form of cardiac arrest, and an individual suffering from it will not survive unless cardiopulmonary resuscitation (CPR) and defibrillation are provided immediately.

CPR can prolong the survival of the brain in the lack of a normal pulse, but defibrillation is the intervention which is most likely to restore a more healthy heart rhythm. It does this by applying an electric shock to the heart, after which sometimes the heart will revert to a rhythm that can once again pump blood.

Almost every person goes into ventricular fibrillation in the last few minutes of life as the heart muscle reacts to diminished oxygen or general blood flow, trauma, irritants, or depression of electrical impulses themselves from the brain.

Diagnosis

Cardiac dysrhythmias are often first detected by simple but nonspecific means: auscultation of the heartbeat with a stethoscope, or feeling for peripheral pulses. These cannot usually diagnose specific dysrhythmias, but can give a general indication of the heart rate and whether it is regular or irregular. Not all the electrical impulses of the heart produce audible or palpable beats; in many cardiac arrhythmias, the premature or abnormal beats do not produce an effective pumping action and are experienced as "skipped" beats.

The simplest specific diagnostic test for assessment of heart rhythm is the electrocardiogram (abbreviated ECG or EKG). A Holter monitor is an EKG recorded over a 24-hour period, to detect dysrhythmias that may happen briefly and unpredictably throughout the day.

SADS

SADS, or sudden arrhythmia death syndrome, is a term used to describe sudden death due to cardiac arrest brought on by an arrhythmia. The most common cause of sudden death in the US is coronary artery disease. Approximately 300,000 people die suddenly of this cause every year in the US. SADS can also occur from other causes. Also, there are many inherited conditions and heart diseases that can affect young people that can cause sudden death. Many of these victims have no symptoms before dying suddenly.

Causes of SADS in young people are long QT syndrome, Brugada syndrome, Catecholaminergic polymorphic ventricular tachycardia and hypertrophic cardiomyopathy and arrhythmogenic right ventricular dysplasia ("arrythmia"-causing, "right ventricle"-involving, pre-cancerous malformation).

HYPERTENSIVE EMERGENCY

Hypertensive emergency is severe hypertension with acute impairment of an organ system (especially the central nervous system, cardiovascular system and/or the renal system) and the possibility of irreversible organ-damage. In case of a hypertensive emergency, the blood pressure should be lowered aggressively over minutes to hours with an antihypertensive agent.

Several classes of antihypertensive agents are recommended and the choice for the antihypertensive agent depends on the cause for the hypertensive crisis, the severity of elevated blood pressure and the patients usual blood pressure before the hypertensive crisis. In most cases, the administration of an intravenous sodium nitroprusside injection which has an almost immediate antihypertensive effect is suitable but in many cases not readily available. In less urgent cases, oral agents like captopril, clonidine, labetalol, prazosin, which have all a delayed onset of action by several minutes compared to sodium nitroprusside, can also be used.

It is also important that the blood pressure is lowered not too abruptly, but smoothly. The initial goal in hypertensive emergencies is to reduce the pressure by no more than 25 per cent (within minutes to 1 or 2 hours) and then toward a level of 160/100 mm Hg within 2-6 hours. Excessive reductions in pressure may precipitate coronary, cerebral, or renal ischemia. The diagnosis of a hypertensive emergency is not only based on the absolute level of blood pressure, but also on the individual regular level of blood pressure before the hypertensive crisis. Individuals with a history of chronic hypertension may not tolerate a "normal" blood pressure.

ACUTE MYOCARDIAL INFARCTION

Acute myocardial infarction (AMI or MI), more commonly known as a heart attack, is a medical condition that occurs when the blood supply to a part of the heart is interrupted, most commonly due to rupture of a vulnerable plaque. The resulting ischemia or oxygen shortage causes damage and potential death of heart tissue. It is a medical emergency, and the leading cause of death for both men and women all over the world. Important risk factors are a previous history of vascular disease such as atherosclerotic coronary heart disease and/or angina, a previous heart attack or stroke, any previous episodes of abnormal heart rhythms or syncope, older age—especially men over 40 and women over 50, smoking, excessive alcohol consumption, the abuse of certain drugs, high triglyceride levels, high LDL ("Low-density lipoprotein") and low HDL ("High density lipoprotein"), diabetes, high blood pressure, obesity, and chronically high levels of stress in certain persons.

The term myocardial infarction is derived from myocardium (the heart muscle) and infarction (tissue death due to oxygen starvation). The phrase "heart attack" is sometimes used incorrectly to describe sudden cardiac death, which may or may not be the result of acute myocardial infarction.

Classical symptoms of acute myocardial infarction include chest pain (typically radiating to the left arm), shortness of breath, nausea, vomiting, palpitations, sweating, and anxiety. Patients frequently feel suddenly ill. Women often experience different symptoms from men. The most common symptoms of MI in women include shortness of breath, weakness, and fatigue. Approximately one third of all myocardial infarctions are silent, without chest pain or other symptoms.

Immediate treatment for suspected acute myocardial infarction includes oxygen, aspirin, glyceryl trinitrate and pain relief, usually morphine sulfate. The patient will receive a number of diagnostic tests, such as an electrocardiogram (ECG, EKG), a chest X-ray and blood tests to detect elevated creatine kinase or troponin levels (these are chemical markers released by damaged tissues, especially the myocardium). Further treatment may include either medications to break down blood clots that block the blood flow to the heart, or mechanically restoring the flow by dilatation or bypass surgery of the blocked coronary artery. Coronary care unit admission allows rapid and safe treatment of complications such as abnormal heart rhythms.

First Aid

As myocardial infarction is a common medical emergency, the signs are often part of first aid courses. The emergency action principles also apply in the case of myocardial infarction.

Immediate Care

When symptoms of myocardial infarction occur, people wait an average of three hours, instead of doing what is recommended: calling for help immediately. Acting immediately by calling the emergency services can prevent sustained damage to the heart.

Certain positions allow the patient to rest in a position which minimizes breathing difficulties. A half-sitting position with knees bent is often recommended. Access to more oxygen can be given by opening the window and widening the collar for easier breathing.

Aspirin can be given quickly (if the patient is not allergic to aspirin); but taking aspirin before calling the emergency medical services may be associated with unwanted delay. Aspirin has an antiplatelet effect which inhibits formation of further thrombi (blood clots) that clog arteries. Non-enteric coated or soluble preparations are preferred. If chewed or dissolved, respectively, they can be absorbed by the body even quicker. If the patient cannot swallow, the aspirin can be used sublingually.

Glyceryl trinitrate (nitroglycerin) sublingually (under the tongue) can be given if it has been prescribed for the patient. If an Automated External Defibrillator (AED) is available the rescuer should immediately bring the AED to the patient's side and be prepared to follow its instructions should the victim lose consciousness.

If possible the rescuer should obtain basic information from the victim, in case the patient is unable to answer questions once emergency medical technicians arrive (if the patient becomes unconscious). The victim's name and any information regarding the nature of the victims pain will useful to health care providers. Also the exact time that these symptoms started, what the patient was doing at the onset of symptoms, and anything else that might give clues to the pathology of the chest pain. It is also very important to relay any actions that have been taken, such as the number or dose of aspirin or nitroglycerin given, to the EMS personnel. Other general first aid principles include monitoring pulse, breathing, level of consciousness and, if possible, the blood pressure of the patient. In case of cardiac arrest, cardiopulmonary resuscitation (CPR) can be administered.

Emergency Services

Emergency Medical Services (EMS) Systems vary considerably in their ability to evaluate and treat patients with suspected acute myocardial infarction. Some provide as little as first aid and early defibrillation. Others employ highly trained paramedics with sophisticated technology and advanced protocols.Most are capable of providing oxygen, IV access, sublingual nitroglycerine, morphine, and aspirin. Some are capable of providing thrombolytic therapy in the prehospital setting.

With primary PCI emerging as the preferred therapy for ST segment elevation myocardial infarction, EMS can play a key role in reducing door to balloon intervals (the time from presentation to a hospital ER to the restoration of coronary artery blood flow) by performing a 12 lead ECG in the field and using this information to triage the patient to the most appropriate medical facility. In addition, the 12 lead ECG can be transmitted to the receiving hospital, which enables time saving decisions to be made prior to the patient's arrival. This may include a "cardiac alert" or "STEMI alert" that calls in off duty personnel in areas where the cardiac cath lab is not staffed 24 hours a day. Even in the absence of a formal alerting program, prehospital 12 lead ECGs are independently associated with reduced door to treatment intervals in the emergency department.

Treatment

A heart attack is a medical emergency which demands both immediate attention and activation of the emergency medical services. The ultimate goal of the management in the acute phase of the disease is to salvage as much myocardium as possible and prevent further complications. As time passes, the risk of damage to the heart muscle increases; hence the phrase that in myocardial infarction, "time is muscle," and time wasted is muscle lost.

The treatments itself may have complications. If attempts to restore the blood flow are initiated after a critical period of only a few hours, the result is reperfusion injury instead of amelioration. Other treatment modalities may also cause complications; the use of antithrombotics for example carries an increased risk of bleeding.

VENTRICULAR FIBRILLATION

Ventricular fibrillation (V-fib or VF) is a condition in which there is uncoordinated contraction of the cardiac muscle of the ventricles in the heart. As a result, the heart fails to adequately pump blood; hypoxia soon occurs, followed by unconsciousness within twenty to thirty seconds.

Ventricular fibrillation is a medical emergency. If the arrhythmia continues for more than a few seconds, blood circulation will cease — as evidenced by lack of pulse, blood pressure, and respiration — and eventually death will occur.

Ventricular fibrillation is a cause of cardiac arrest and sudden cardiac death. The ventricular muscle twitches randomly, rather than contracting in unison, and so the ventricles fail to pump blood into the arteries and into systemic circulation.

Ventricular fibrillation is a sudden lethal arrhythmia responsible for many deaths in the Western world, mostly brought on by ischaemic heart disease. Despite much work, the underlying nature of fibrillation is not completely understood. Most episodes of fibrillation occur in diseased hearts, but others occur in so-called normal hearts. Much work still has to be done to elucidate the mechanisms of ventricular fibrillation.

Treatment

The condition can often be reversed by the electric discharge of direct current from a defibrillator. If no defibrillator is available, a precordial thump can be delivered at the onset of VF to regain cardiac function. Antiarrhythmic agents like amiodarone or lidocaine can help, but, unlike atrial fibrillation, VF rarely reverses spontaneously in large adult mammals. Although a defibrillator is designed to correct the problem, and its effects can be dramatic, it is not always successful. In patients at high risk of ventricular fibrillation, the use of an implantable cardioverter defibrillator has been shown to be beneficial.

SHOCK

ANAPHYLAXIS

Anaphylaxis is an acute systemic (multi-system) and severe Type I *Hypersensitivity allergic reaction* in humans and other mammals. Anaphylaxis occurs when a person or animal is exposed to a trigger substance, called an allergen, to which they have already become sensitized. Minute amounts of allergens may cause a life-threatening anaphylactic reaction. Anaphylaxis may occur after ingestion, skin contact, injection of an allergen or, in rare cases, inhalation.

Anaphylactic shock, the most severe type of anaphylaxis, occurs when an allergic response triggers a quick release from mast cells of large quantities of immunological mediators (histamines, prostaglandins, leukotrienes) leading to systemic vasodilation (associated with a sudden drop in blood pressure) and edema of bronchial mucosa (resulting in bronchoconstriction and difficulty breathing). Anaphylactic shock can lead to death in a matter of minutes if left untreated.

Sign and Symptoms

Symptoms of anaphylaxis are related to the action of (IgE) and other anaphylatoxins, which act to release histamine and other mediator substances from mast cells (degranulation). In addition to other effects, histamine induces vasodilation of arterioles and constriction of bronchioles in the lungs, also known as bronchospasm (constriction of the airways).

The time between ingestion of the allergen and anaphylaxis symptoms can vary for some patients depending on the amount of allergen consumed and their reaction time. Symptoms can appear immediately, or can be delayed by half an hour to several hours after ingestion.However, symptoms of anaphylaxis usually appear very quickly once they do begin.

Causes

Anaphylaxis is a severe, whole-body allergic reaction. After an initial exposure to a substance like bee sting toxin, the person's immune system becomes sensitized to that allergen- Shocking dose. On a subsequent exposure, an allergic reaction occurs. This reaction is sudden, severe, and involves the whole body.

Tissues in different parts of the body release histamine and other substances. This causes constriction of the airways, resulting in wheezing, difficulty breathing, and gastrointestinal symptoms such as abdominal pain, cramps, vomiting, and diarrhea. Histamine causes the blood vessels to dilate (which lowers blood pressure) and fluid to leak from the bloodstream into the tissues (which lowers the blood volume). These effects result in shock. Fluid can leak into the alveoli (air sacs) of the lungs, causing pulmonary edema.

Hives and angioedema (hives on the lips, eyelids, throat, and/or tongue) often occur. Angioedema may be severe enough to block the airway. Prolonged anaphylaxis can cause heart arrhythmias.

Some drugs (polymyxin, morphine, x-ray dye, and others) may cause an "anaphylactoid" reaction (anaphylactic-like reaction) on the first exposure. This is usually due to a toxic reaction, rather than the immune system mechanism that occurs with "true" anaphylaxis. The symptoms, risk for complications without treatment, and treatment are the same, however, for both types of reactions.

Anaphylaxis can occur in response to any allergen. Common causes include insect bites/stings, horse serum (used in some vaccines), food allergies, and drug allergies. Pollens and other inhaled allergens rarely cause anaphylaxis. Some people have an anaphylactic reaction with no identifiable cause.

Anaphylaxis occurs infrequently. However, it is life-threatening and can occur at any time. Risks include prior history of any type of allergic reaction.

Emergency Treatment

Anaphylaxis is a life-threatening medical emergency because of rapid constriction of the airway, often within minutes of onset, which can lead to respiratory failure and respiratory arrest. Brain and organ damage rapidly occurs if the patient cannot breathe. Due to the severe nature of the emergency, patients experiencing or about to experience anaphylaxis require the help of advanced medical personnel. First aid measures for anaphylaxis include rescue breathing (part of CPR). Rescue breathing may be hindered by the constricted airways, but if the victim stops breathing on his or her own, it is the only way to get oxygen to him or her until professional help is available.

Another treatment for anaphylaxis is administration of epinephrine (adrenaline). Epinephrine prevents worsening of the airway constriction, stimulates the heart to continue beating, and may be life-saving. Epinephrine acts on Beta-2 adrenergic receptors in the lung as a powerful bronchodilator (i.e., it opens the airways), relieving allergic or histamine-induced acute asthmatic attack or anaphylaxis.

Clinical Care

Paramedic treatment in the field includes administration of epinephrine IM (or IV infusion in severe cases), antihistamines IM (e.g. chlorphenamine, diphenhydramine), steroids such as hydrocortisone, IV Fluid administration and in severe cases, pressor agents (which cause the heart to increase its contraction strength) such as dopamine for hypotension, administration of oxygen, and intubation during transport to advanced medical care.

In severe situations with profuse laryngeal edema (swelling of the airway), cricothyrotomy or tracheotomy may be required to maintain oxygenation. In these procedures, an incision is made through the anterior portion of the neck, over the cricoid membrane, and an endotracheal tube is inserted to allow mechanical ventilation of the victim.

The clinical treatment of anaphylaxis by a doctor and in the hospital setting aims to treat the cellular hypersensitivity reaction as well as the symptoms. Antihistamine drugs such as diphenhydramine or chlorphenamine (which inhibit the effects of histamine at histamine receptors) are continued but are usually not sufficient in anaphylaxis, and high doses of intravenous corticosteroids such as dexamethasone or hydrocortisone are often required. Hypotension is treated with intravenous fluids and sometimes vasopressor drugs. For bronchospasm, bronchodilator drugs (e.g. salbutamol, known as Albuterol in the United States) are used. In severe cases, immediate treatment with epinephrine can be lifesaving. Supportive care with mechanical ventilation may be required.

It is also possible to undergo a second reaction prior to medical attention or using an Epipen. It is suggested to seek one to two days of medical care. The possibility of biphasic reactions (recurrence of anaphylaxis) requires that patients be monitored for four hours after being transported to medical care for anaphylaxis.

CARDIOGENIC SHOCK

Cardiogenic shock is based upon an inadequate circulation of blood due to primary failure of the ventricles of the heart to function effectively.Since this is a category of shock there is insufficient perfusion of tissue (i.e. the heart) to meet the required demand for oxygen and nutrients. This leads to ce!l death from oxygen starvation, hypoxia. Because of this it may lead to cardiac arrest (or circulatory arrest) which is an acute cessation of cardiac pump function.

Cardiogenic shock is defined by sustained hypotension with tissue hypoperfusion despite adequate left ventricular filling pressure. Signs of tissue hypoperfusion include oliguria (<30 mL/h), cool extremities, and altered mentation.

Cardiogenic shock is *caused* by the failure of the heart to pump effectively. It can be due to damage to the heart muscle, most often from a large myocardial infarction. Other causes include arrhythmia, cardiomyopathy, cardiac valve problems, ventricular outflow obstruction (i.e. aortic valve stenosis, aortic dissection, systolic anterior motion (SAM) in hypertrophic cardiomyopathy), ventriculoseptal defects or medical error.

Signs and Symptoms

- Anxiety, restlessness, altered mental state due to decreased cerebral perfusion and subsequent hypoxia.
- Hypotension due to decrease in cardiac output.
- A rapid, weak, thready pulse due to decreased circulation combined with tachycardia.
- Cool, clammy, and mottled skin (cutis marmorata), due to vasoconstriction and subsequent hypoperfusion of the skin.
- Distended jugular veins due to increased jugular venous pressure.
- Oliguria (low urine output) due insufficient renal perfusion if condition persists.
- Rapid and deep respirations (hyperventilation) due to sympathetic nervous system stimulation and acidosis.
- Fatigue due to hyperventilation and hypoxia.
- Absent pulse in tachy arrhythmia.
- Pulmonary edema, involving fluid back-up in the lungs due to insufficient pumping of the heart.

DIAGNOSIS

Electrocardiogram—An electrocardiogram helps establishing the exact diagnosis and guides treatment, it may reveal:

- Cardiac arrhythmias
- Signs of cardiomyopathy

Radiology—Echocardiography may show arrhythmia, signs of PED, ventricular septal rupture (VSR), an obstructed outflow tract or cardiomyopathy.

Swan-ganz catheter—The Swan-ganz catheter or Pulmonary artery catheter may assist in the diagnosis by providing information on the hemodynamics.

Biopsy—In case of suspected cardiomyopathy a biopsy of heart muscle may be needed to make a definite diagnosis.

Treatment

In cardiogenic shock: depending on the type of myocardal infarction one can infuse fluids or in shock refractory to infusing fluids inotropica. In case of cardiac arrhythmia several anti-arrhythmic agents may be administered, i.e. adenosine, verapamil, amiodarone, ß-blocker. Positive inotropic agents, which enhance the heart's pumping capabilities, are used to improve the contractility and correct the hypotension. Should that not suffice an intra-aortic balloon pump (which reduces workload for the heart, and improves perfusion of the coronary arteries) can be considered or a left ventricular assist device (which augments the pump-function of the heart).

HYPOVOLEMIA

In physiology and medicine, hypovolemia (also hypovolaemia) is a state of decreased blood volume; more specifically, decrease in volume of blood plasma.

Common causes of hypovolemia can be dehydration, bleeding, severe burns and drugs such as diuretics or vasodilators typically used to treat hypertensive individuals. Rarely, it may occur as a result of a blood donation.

Effects—Severe hypovolemia leads to hypovolemic shock. A low blood volume can result in multiple organ failure, kidney damage and failure, brain damage, coma and death (desanguination).

Diagnosis

Clinical symptoms may not present until 10-20 per cent of total whole-blood volume is lost. Hypovolemia can be recognized by elevated pulse, diminished blood pressure, and the absence of perfusion as assessed by skin signs (skin turning pale) and/or capillary refill on forehead, lips and nail beds. The patient may feel dizzy, faint, nauseated, or very thirsty. These signs are also characteristic of most types of shock.

Note that in children, compensation can result in an artificially high blood pressure despite hypovolemia. This is another reason (aside from initial lower blood volume) that even the possibility of internal bleeding in children should always be treated aggressively.

Also look for obvious signs of external bleeding while remembering that people can bleed to death internally without any external blood loss. Also consider possible mechanisms of injury (especially the steering wheel and/or use/non-use of seat belt in motor vehicle accidents) that may have caused internal bleeding such as ruptured or bruised internal organs. If trained to do so and the situation permits, conduct a secondary survey and check the chest and abdominal cavities for pain, deformity, guarding or swelling. (Injuries to the pelvis and bleeding into the thigh from the femoral artery can also be life-threatening.)

Treatment

Minor hypovolemia from a known cause that has been completely controlled (such as a blood transfusion from a healthy patient who is not anemic) may be countered with initial rest for up to half an hour, oral fluids including moderate sugars (apple juice is good) and the advice to the donor to eat good solid meals with proteins for the next few days. Typically, this would involve a fluid volume of less than one liter (1000 ml), although this is highly dependent on body weight. Larger people can tolerate slightly more blood loss than smaller people. More serious hypovolemia should be assessed by a nurse or doctor. When in doubt, treat hypovolemia aggressively.

First Aid

External bleeding should be controlled by direct pressure. If direct pressure fails, other techniques such as elevation and pressure points should be considered. The tourniquet should be used in the case of massive hemorrhage i.e. arterial bleeds, such as the femoral artery. If a first-aider recognizes internal bleeding, the life-saving measure to take is to immediately call for emergency assistance.

Hospital Treatment

If the hypovolemia was caused by medication, the administration of antidotes may be appropriate but should be carefully monitored to avoid shock or the emergence of other pre-existing conditions. Blood transfusions coupled with surgical repair are the definitive treatment for hypovolemia caused by trauma.

NEUROGENIC SHOCK

Neurogenic shock is shock caused by the sudden loss of the sympathetic nervous system signals to the smooth muscle in vessel walls. This can result from severe central nervous system (brain and spinal cord) damage. With the sudden loss of background sympathetic stimulation, the vessels suddenly relax resulting in a sudden decrease in peripheral vascular resistance and decreased blood pressure.

Signs and symptoms—hypotension, bradycardia, warm, dry extremities, peripheral, vasodilation,venous pooling, poikilothermia, decreased cardiac output (with cervical or high thoracic injury)

Treatment

- Large volumes of fluid may be needed to restore normal hemodynamics.
- Vasopressors (Norepinephrine).
- Atropine (speeds up heart rate and Cardiac Output).

UROLOGICAL, ANDROLOGICAL, GYNECOLOGIC, AND OBSTETRIC

ECLAMPSIA

Eclampsia is a serious complication of pregnancy and is characterised by convulsions. Usually eclampsia occurs after the onset of pre-eclampsia though sometimes no pre-eclamptic symptoms are recognisable. The convulsions may appear before, during or after labour, though cases of eclampsia after just 20 weeks of pregnancy have been recorded.

Signs and Symptoms

The majority of cases are heralded by pregnancy-induced hypertension and proteinuria but the only true sign of eclampsia is an eclamptic convulsion, of which there are four stages. Patients with edema and oliguria may develop renal failure or pulmonary edema.

- Premonitory stage— This stage is usually missed unless constantly monitored, the woman rolls her eyes while her facial and hand muscles twitch slightly.
- Tonic stage—Soon after the premonitory stage the twitching turns into clenching. Sometimes the woman may bite her tongue as she clenches her teeth, while the arms and legs go rigid. The respiratory muscles also spasm, causing the woman to stop breathing. This stage continues for around 30 seconds.
- Clonic stage—The spasm stops but the muscles start to jerk violently. Frothy, slightly bloodied saliva appears on the lips and can sometimes be inhaled. After around two minutes the convulsions stop, leading into a temporary unconscious stage.
- Comatose stage — The woman falls deeply unconscious, breathing noisily. This can last only a few minutes or may persist for hours.

Epidemiology

Eclampsia is usually treated well in the majority of cases

with just under one in 50 affected women and one in 14 fetuses of affected women developing complications.

Treatment

The treatment of seizures in eclampsia consists of:

- Prevention of convulsion
- Control the blood pressure
- Delivery of fetus

Prevention of convulsion is usually done using magnesium sulfate with a loading of Magnesium sulfate 20 per cent solution, 4 g IV over 5 minutes. Then maintain with 1 g magnesium sulfate (10 per cent solution) in 1000 ml fluid drip 1g/hr.

The blood pressure may be controlled by hydralazine 5 mg IV slowly every 5 minutes until blood pressure is lowered. Repeat hourly as needed or give hydralazine 12.5 mg IM every 2 hours as needed.

Delivery should take place as soon as the woman's condition has stabilized. Delaying delivery to increase fetal maturity is unsafe for both the woman and the fetus, after delivery the womans health relative to the condition is improved drastically. Delivery should occur regardless of the gestational age.

In severe pre-eclampsia, delivery should occur within 24 hours of the onset of symptoms. In eclampsia, delivery should occur within 12 hours of the onset of convulsions. If vaginal delivery is not anticipated within 12 hours (for eclampsia) or 24 hours (for severe pre-eclampsia), deliver by caesarean section.

ECTOPIC PREGNANCY

An ectopic pregnancy is a complication of pregnancy in which the fertilized ovum is implanted in any tissue other than the uterine wall. Most ectopic pregnancies occur in the Fallopian tube (so-called tubal pregnancies), but implantation can also occur in the cervix, ovaries, and abdomen. The fetus produces enzymes that allow it to implant in varied types of tissues, and thus an embryo implanted elsewhere than the uterus can cause great tissue damage in its efforts to reach a sufficient supply of blood.

In a normal pregnancy, the fertilized egg enters the uterus and settles into the uterine lining where it has plenty of room to divide and grow. About 1 per cent of pregnancies are in an ectopic location with implantation not occurring inside of the womb, and of these 98 per cent occur in the Fallopian tubes.

In a typical ectopic pregnancy, the embryo does not reach the uterus, but instead adheres to the lining of the Fallopian tube. The implanted embryo burrows actively into the tubal lining. Most commonly this invades vessels and will cause bleeding. This bleeding expels the implantation out of the tubal end as a tubal abortion. Some women thinking they are having a miscarriage are actually having a tubal abortion. There is no inflammation of the tube in ectopic pregnancy. The pain is caused by prostaglandins released at the implantation site, and by free blood in the peritoneal cavity, which is locally irritant. Sometimes the bleeding might be heavy enough to threaten the health or life of the woman. Usually this degree of bleeding is due to delay in diagnosis, but sometimes, especially if the implantation is in the proximal tube (just before it enters the uterus), it may invade into the nearby Sampson artery, causing heavy bleeding earlier than usual.

If left untreated, about half of ectopic pregnancies will resolve without treatment. These are the tubal abortions. The advent of methotrexate treatment for ectopic pregnancy has reduced the need for surgery; however, surgical intervention is still required in cases where the Fallopian tube has ruptured or is in danger of doing so. This intervention may be laparoscopic or through a larger incision, known as a laparotomy.

Causes

The causes of ectopic pregnancy are unknown. After fertilization of the oocyte in the peritoneal cavity, the egg takes about nine days to migrate down the tube to the uterine cavity at which time it implants. Wherever the embryo finds itself at that time, it will begin to implant.

There are some speculative specific causes or associations. Smoking, advanced maternal age and prior tubal damage of any origin are well shown risk factors for ectopic pregnancy.

Diagnosis

An ectopic pregnancy has to be suspected in any woman with lower abdominal pain or unusual bleeding who is or might be sexually active and whose pregnancy test is positive. An abnormal rise in blood ßhCG levels may also indicate an ectopic pregnancy. The threshold of discrimination of intrauterine pregnancy today is around 3000 IU/ml of β-human chorionic gonadotropin (βhCG). A high resolution, vaginal ultrasound scan showing no intrauterine pregnancy is presumptive evidence that an ectopic pregnancy is present if the threshold of discrimination for βhCG has been reached.

An empty uterus with levels lower than 3000 IU/ml may be evidence of an ectopic pregnancy, but may also be consistent with an intrauterine pregnancy which is simply too small to be seen on ultrasound. If the diagnosis is uncertain, it may be necessary to wait a few days and repeat the blood work and ultrasound. If the βhCG falls on repeat examination, this strongly suggests an abortion or rupture.

An ultrasound showing a gestational sac with fetal heart in the fallopian tube is clear evidence of ectopic pregnancy. Free fluid which is non-echogenic is a normal finding in the late menstrual cycle and early normal pregnancy. This is a transudate and is not presumptive evidence of bleeding. Echogenic free fluid suggests the presence of blood clot and is suggestive of free blood in the peritoneum.

A laparoscopy or laparotomy can also be performed to visually confirm an ectopic pregnancy. Often if a tubal abortion has occurred, or a tubal rupture has occurred, it is hard actually to find the pregnancy tissue. Laparoscopy in very early ectopic pregnancy may rarely show a normal looking fallopian tube.

Treatment

(i) *Nonsurgical treatment*—Early treatment of an ectopic pregnancy with the antimetabolite methotrexate has proven to be a viable alternative to surgical treatment.

(ii) *Surgical treatment*— If hemorrhaging has already occurred, surgical intervention may be necessary if there is evidence of ongoing blood loss. However, as already stated, about half of ectopics result in tubal abortion and are self limiting. The option to go to surgery is thus often a difficult decision to make in an obviously stable patient with minimal evidence of blood clot on ultrasound.

Surgeons use laparoscopy or laparotomy to gain access to the pelvis and can either incise the affected Fallopian and remove only the pregnancy (salpingostorny) or remove the affected tube with the pregnancy (salpingectomy). The first successful surgery for an ectopic pregnancy was performed by Robert Lawson Tait in 1883.

Chances of Future Pregnancy

The chance of future pregnancy depends on the status of the adnexa left behind. The chance of recurrent ectopic pregnancy is about 10 per cent and is independent of whether the affected tube was repaired (salpingostomy) or removed (salpingectomy). Successful pregnancy rates vary widely between different centres, and appear to be operator dependent. Pregnancy rates with successful methotrexate treatment compare favourably with the highest reported pregnancy rates. Often, patients may have to resort to in vitro fertilisation to achieve a successful pregnancy. The use of in vitro fertilisation does not preclude further ectopic pregnancies, but the likelihood is reduced.

Complications

The most common complication is rupture with internal bleeding that leads to shock. Death from rupture is rare. Infertility occurs in 10 - 15 per cent of women who have had an ectopic pregnancy.

TESTICULAR TORSION

In testicular torsion the spermatic cord that provides the blood supply to a testicle is twisted, cutting off the blood supply, often causing orchalgia. Prolonged testicular torsion will result in the death of the testicle and surrounding tissues. It is also believed that torsion occurring during fetal development can lead to the so-called neonatal torsion or vanishing testis, and is one of the causes of an infant being born with monorchism.

In most males, the testicles are attached to the inner lining of the scrotum. Males whose attachment is higher up are at risk of testicular torsion. This condition is known as a bell clapper deformity (as in the central piece of a bell) and is a major cause of testicular torsion. A male who notices the ability of either or both testicles to freely rotate within the scrotum should be aware that he is at risk of testicular torsion. Testicles that are in a much lower position and/or in a slightly rotated position in the scrotal sack are a visual indicator of this risk.

Torsions are sometimes called "winter syndrome". This is because they often happen in winter, when it is cold outside. The scrotum of a man who has been lying in a warm bed is relaxed. When he arises, his scrotum is exposed to the colder room air. If the spermatic cord is twisted while the scrotum is loose, the sudden contraction that results from the abrupt temperature change can trap the testicle in that position. The result is a testicular torsion.

Diagnosis

Emergency testing for torsion may be indicated when the onset of pain is sudden and/or severe, or the test results available during the initial examination do not enable a diagnosis of urethritis or urinary tract infection to be made. A doppler ultrasound scan of the scrotum, if available, is of immense help in the diagnosis by showing the presence or absence of blood flow to the testicle. Dizziness and nausea are often present when there is an absence of blood supply to the testicle, as well as a tremendous amount of pain. If the diagnosis is questionable, an expert should be consulted immediately, because testicular viability may be compromised. If physical examination suggests a compromised blood supply and the patient has had such symptoms for a significant period of time, medical personnel may choose to bring the patient directly to surgery without an ultrasound since the time required for ultrasound testing could affect testicular viability.

Color Doppler sonography is used to identify the absence of blood flow typically found in a twisted testicle, which distinguishes the condition from epididymitis.

Urinalysis (analyzing chemical composition of urine) can be used to rule out bacterial infections.

Surgical exploration may be necessary if diagnosis cannot be made using other methods. If there is the slightest hint of a torsion of the testicle, then doctors will perform surgery; even if the testicle turns out not to have twisted, they will still protect it by attaching the testicle to the scrotum wall.

Treatment

With prompt diagnosis and treatment the testicle can be saved in a high number of cases.Testicular torsion is a medical emergency that needs immediate treatment. If treated within 6 hours, there is nearly a 100 per cent chance of saving the testicle. Within 12 hours this rate decreases to 70 per cent, within 24 hours is 20 per cent, and after 24 hours the rate approaches 0. (eMedicineHealth) Once the testicle is dead it must be removed to prevent gangrenous infection.

ACUTE RENAL FAILURE (ARF)

Acute renal failure (ARF), also known as acute kidney failure or acute kidney injury, is a rapid loss of renal function due to damage to the kidneys, resulting in retention of nitrogenous (urea and creatinine) and non-nitrogenous waste products that are normally excreted by the kidney. Depending on the severity and duration of the renal dysfunction, this accumulation is accompanied by metabolic disturbances, such as metabolic acidosis (acidification of the blood) and hyperkalaemia (elevated potassium levels), changes in body fluid balance, and effects on many other organ systems. It can be characterised by oliguria or anuria (decrease or cessation of urine production), although nonoliguric ARF may occur. It is a serious disease and treated as a medical emergency.

Causes

Acute renal failure is usually categorised (as in the flowchart below) according to pre-renal, renal and post-renal causes.

(i) Pre-renal (causes in the blood supply):

- hypovolemia (decreased blood volume), usually from shock or dehydration and fluid loss or excessive diuretics use.
- hepatorenal syndrome in which renal perfusion is compromised in liver failure.
- vascular problems, such as atheroembolic disease and renal vein thrombosis (which can occur as a complication of the nephrotic syndrome).

(ii) Renal (damage to the kidney itself):

- infection usually sepsis (systemic inflammation due to infection),rarely of the kidney itself, termed pyelonephritis.
- toxins or medication (e.g. some NSAIDs, aminoglycoside antibiotics, iodinated contrast, lithium).
- rhabdomyolysis (breakdown of muscle tissue) - the resultant release of myoglobin in the blood affects the kidney; it can be caused by injury (especially crush injury and extensive blunt trauma), statins, stimulants and some other drugs.
- hemolysis (breakdown of red blood cells) - the hemoglobin damages the tubules; it may be caused by various conditions such as sickle-cell disease, and lupus erythematosus.

- multiple myeloma, either due to hypercalcemia or "cast nephropathy" (multiple myeloma can also cause chronic renal failure by a different mechanism).
- acute glomerulonephritis which may be due to a variety of causes, such as anti glomerular basement membrane disease/Goodpasture's syndrome, Wegener's granulomatosis or acute lupus nephritis with systemic lupus erythematosus.

(iii) Post-renal (obstructive causes in the urinary tract) due to:

- medication interfering with normal bladder emptying.
- benign prostatic hypertrophy or prostate cancer.
- kidney stones.
- due to abdominal malignancy (e.g. ovarian cancer, colorectal cancer).
- obstructed urinary catheter.

Diagnosis

Renal failure is generally diagnosed either when creatinine or blood urea nitrogen tests are markedly elevated in an ill patient, especially when oliguria is present. Previous measurements of renal function may offer comparison, which is especially important if a patient is known to have chronic renal failure as well. If the cause is not apparent, a large amount of blood tests and examination of a urine specimen is typically performed to elucidate the cause of acute renal failure, medical ultrasonography of the renal tract is essential to rule out obstruction of the urinary tract. Consensus criteria for the diagnosis of ARF are:

- *Risk*: serum creatinine increased 1.5 times OR urine production of <0.5 ml/kg body weight for 6 hours.
- *Injury*: creatinine 2.0 times OR urine production <0.5 ml/kg for 12 h.
- *Failure*: creatinine 3.0 times OR creatinine >355 μmol/l (with a rise of >44) or urine output below 0.3 ml/kg for 24h.

- *Loss*: persistent ARF or more than four weeks complete loss of kidney function.

Kidney biopsy may be performed in the setting of acute renal failure, to provide a definitive diagnosis and sometimes an idea of the prognosis, unless the cause is clear and appropriate screening investigations are reassuringly negative.

Treatment

Acute renal failure may be reversible if treated promptly and appropriately. Resuscitation to normotension and a normal cardiac output is key. The main interventions are monitoring fluid intake and output as closely as possible; insertion of a urinary catheter is useful for monitoring urine output as well as relieving possible bladder outlet obstruction, such as with an enlarged prostate. In the absence of fluid overload, administering intravenous fluids is typically the first step to improve renal function. Fluid administration may be monitored with the use of a central venous catheter to avoid over or under replacement of fluid. If the cause is obstruction of the urinary tract, relief of the obstruction (with a nephrostomy or urinary catheter) may be necessary. Metabolic acidosis and hyperkalemia, the two most serious biochemical manifestations of acute renal failure, may require medical treatment with sodium bicarbonate administration and antihyperkalemic measures, unless dialysis is required.

Should hypotension prove a persistent problem in the fluid replete patient, inotropes such as norepinephrine and/or dobutamine may be given to improve cardiac output and hence renal perfusion. Whilst a useful pressor, there is no evidence dopamine is of any specific benefit.[3], and at least a suggestion of possible harm. A Swan-Ganz catheter may be used, to measure pulmonary artery occlusion pressure to provide a guide to left atrial pressure (and thus left heart function) as a target for inotropic support.

The use of diuretics such as furosemide, whilst widespread and sometimes convenient in ameliorating fluid overload, does not reduce the risk of complications and death.[4].In practice diuretics may simply mask things, making it more difficult to judge the adequacy of resuscitation. Lack of improvement with fluid resuscitation, therapy-resistant hyperkalemia, metabolic acidosis or fluid overload may necessitate artificial support in the form of dialysis or hemofiltration. Depending on the cause, a proportion of patients will never regain full renal function, thus having end stage renal failure requiring lifelong dialysis or a kidney transplant.

CHRONIC KIDNEY DISEASE (CKD)

Chronic kidney disease (CKD), also known as chronic renal disease, is a progressive loss of renal function over a period of months or years through five stages. Each stage is a progression through an abnormally low and progressively worse glomerular filtration rate, which is usually determined indirectly by the creatinine level in blood serum. Stage 1 CKD is mildly diminished renal function, with few overt symptoms. Stage 5 CKD is a severe illness and requires some form of renal replacement therapy (dialysis or renal transplant). Stage 5 CKD is also called end-stage renal disease (ESRD). ESRD is how the US Centers for Medicare and Medicaid Services and US federal legislation reference this stage of illness. Stage 5 CKD is also known as chronic kidney failure (CKF) or chronic renal failure (CRF).

Signs and Symptoms

Initially it is without specific symptoms and can only be detected as an increase in serum creatinine or protein in the urine. As the kidney function decreases:

- Blood pressure is increased due to fluid overload and production of vasoactive hormones leading to hypertension and congestive heart failure.
- Urea accumulates, leading to azotemia and ultimately uremia (symptoms ranging from lethargy to pericarditis and encephalopathy).
- Potassium accumulates in the blood (known as hyperkalemia with symptoms ranging from malaise to fatal cardiac arrhythmias).

- Erythropoietin synthesis is decreased (leading to anemia causing fatigue).
- Fluid volume overload - symptoms may range from mild edema to life-threatening pulmonary edema
- Hyperphosphatemia - due to reduced phosphate excretion, associated with hypocalcemia (due to vitamin D3 deficiency).
- Later this progresses to tertiary hyperparathyroidism, with hypercalcaemia, renal osteodystrophy and vascular calcification.
- Metabolic acidosis, due to decreased generation of bicarbonate by the kidney, is one of the most life threatening consequences of renal failure. Causes altered enzyme activity by excess acid acting on enzymes and also depression of the CNS by excess acid interfering with neuronal excitability.

People with CKD suffer from accelerated atherosclerosis and have higher incidence of cardiovascular disease, with a poorer prognosis.

Diagnosis

In many CKD patients, previous renal disease or other underlying diseases are already known. A small number presents with CKD of unknown cause. In these patients, a cause is occasionally identified retrospectively.

It is important to differentiate CKD from acute renal failure (ARF) because ARF can be reversible. Abdominal ultrasound is commonly performed, in which the size of the kidneys are measured. Kidneys with CKD are usually smaller (< 9 cm) than normal kidneys with notable exceptions such as in diabetic nephropathy and polycystic kidney disease. Another diagnostic clue that helps differentiate CKD and ARF is a gradual rise in serum creatinine (over several months or years) as opposed to a sudden increase in the serum creatinine (several days to weeks). If these levels are unavailable (because the patient has been well and has had no blood tests) it is occasionally necessary to treat a patient briefly as having ARF until it has been established that the renal impairment is irreversible.

Numerous uremic toxins (see link) are accumulating in chronic renal failure patients treated with standard dialysis. These toxins show various cytotoxic activities in the serum, have different molecular weights and some of them are bound to other proteins, primarily to albumin. Such toxic protein bound substances are receiving the attention of scientists who are interested in improving the standard chronic dialysis procedures used today.

DIALYSIS

In medicine, dialysis is primarily used to provide an artificial replacement for lost kidney function (renal replacement therapy) due to renal failure. Dialysis may be used for very sick patients who have suddenly but temporarily, lost their kidney function (acute renal failure) or for quite stable patients who have permanently lost their kidney function (stage 5 chronic kidney disease). When healthy, the kidneys maintain the body's internal equilibrium of water and minerals (sodium, potassium, chloride, calcium, phosphorus, magnesium, sulfate) and the kidneys remove from the blood the daily metabolic load of fixed hydrogen ions. The kidneys also function as a part of the endocrine system producing erythropoietin and 1,25-dihydroxycholecalciferol (calcitriol). Dialysis treatments imperfectly replace some of these functions through the diffusion (waste removal) and convection (fluid removal). Dialysis is an imperfect treatment to replace kidney function because it does not correct the endocrine functions of the kidney.

URINARY RETENTION

Urinary retention also known as ischuria is a lack of ability to urinate. It is a common complication of benign prostatic hypertrophy (also known as benign prostatic hyperplasia or BPH), although anticholinergics may also play a role, and requires a catheter. Various medications (e.g. some antidepressants) and recreational use of amphetamines and opiates are notorious for this.

Signs and Symptoms

Urinary retention is characterised by poor urinary stream with intermittance, straining, a sense of incomplete voiding and urgency. As the bladder remains full, it may lead to incontinence, nocturia (need to urinate at night) and high frequency. Retention is a medical emergency, as the bladder may distend (stretch) to enormous sizes and possibly tear if not dealt with quickly. If the bladder distends enough it will begin to become painful. The water can also pass back up the ureters and get into the kidneys, causing kidney failure. You should go straight to your emergency department as soon as possible if you are unable to urinate and you have a painfully full bladder. In the longer term, obstruction of the urinary tract may cause:

- Bladder stones.
- Loss of detrusor muscle tone (atonic bladder is an extreme form).
- Hydronephrosis (congestion of the kidneys).
- Hypertrophy of detrusor muscle.
- Diverticula in the bladder wall (leads to stones and infection).

Causes

- Benign prostatic hypertrophy.
- Prostate cancer and other pelvic malignancies.
- Congenital urtheral valve abnormalities.
- Detrusor muscle dyssynergia.
- Circumcision.
- Damage to the Bladder.
- Obstruction in the urethra, for example a metastasis or a precipitated pseudogout crystal in the urine.
- Paruresis ("shy bladder syndrome") in extreme cases, urinary retention can result.

Diagnostic Tests

Uroflowmetry may aid in establishing the type of micturition abnormality. A post-void residual scan may show the amount of urine retained. Determination of the serum prostate-specific antigen (PSA) may aid in diagnosing or ruling out prostate cancer. Urea and creatinine determinations may be necessary to rule out backflow kidney damage.

Treatment

One study describes five men who suffered acute urinary retention and who were all advised by their urologists that they must undergo surgery (transurethral resection of the prostate, TURP). Instead all five men were treated with catheter removal followed by repetitive prostatic massage, extensive microbial diagnosis, and antibiotics, as well as alpha-blockers, and in two cases finasteride. During treatment, statistically significant improvements occurred in global symptom severity scores, urethral white blood cell (WBC) counts, WBC counts of the expressed prostatic secretions (EPS), EPS red blood cell (RBC) counts, urinary WBC counts, and urinary RBC counts. The treatment enabled catheter removal in all 5 men (100 per cent) as well as successful urination in all 5 men (100 per cent). Surgery was able to be postponed indefinitely in all five men.

In acute urinary retention, urinary catheterization or suprapubic cystostomy instantly relieves the retention. In the longer term, treatment depends on the cause. Benign prostatic hypertrophy may respond to alpha blocker and 5-alpha-reductase inhibitor therapy, or surgically with prostatectomy or transurethral resection of the prostate (TURP).

A simple and minor surgery will correct and prevent testicular torsion. It can be done in an emergency situation after determination that the testicle is cut off from blood supply or as an outpatient procedure for patients who have experienced frequent episodes with testicular torsion. If necessary, the surgeon will first untwist the testicle(s). The surgeon will then permanently suture the testicles to the inner lining of the scrotum. If only one testicle has been problematic, the surgeon may suture both testicles as a preventative effort.

Paraphimosis

Paraphimosis is a medical condition where the foreskin becomes trapped behind the glans penis, and cannot be pulled back to its normal flaccid position covering the glans penis. If the condition persists for several hours or there is any sign of a lack of blood flow, paraphimosis should be treated as a medical emergency, as it can result in gangrene or other serious complications.

Paraphimosis can often be reduced by manipulation. This involves compressing the glans and moving the foreskin back to its normal position, perhaps with the aid of a lubricant. If this fails, the foreskin may need to be cut (dorsal slit procedure) or removed by circumcision. An alternate method, the Dundee technique, entails placing multiple punctures in the swollen foreskin with a fine needle, and then expressing the edema fluid by manual pressure.

Prevention of recurrence is through education of the patient and his caregivers on the need to pull back the foreskin over the glans after it has been retracted (for example, when cleaning the glans or passing a Foley catheter), or through elective circumcision or preputioplasty.

NEUROLOGICAL AND PSYCHIATRIC

SUICIDE

Suicide is the act of intentionally terminating one's own life. Suicide occurs for a number of reasons such as depression, substance abuse, shame, avoiding pain, financial difficulties or other undesirable situations.

In schizophrenia suicide can be triggered by either the depression that is common with this disorder, or in response to command auditory hallucinations. Suicide among people suffering from bipolar disorder is often an impulse, which is due to the sufferer's extreme mood swings (one of the main symptoms of bipolar disorder). Severe depression is considered a terminal illness due to the likelihood of suicide when left untreated.

Modern medicine treats suicide as a mental health issue. Overwhelming or persistent suicidal thoughts are considered a medical emergency. Medical professionals advise that people who have expressed plans to kill themselves be encouraged to seek medical attention immediately. This is especially relevant if the means (weapons, drugs, or other methods) are available, or if the patient has crafted a detailed plan for executing the suicide. Medical personnel frequently receive special training to look for suicidal signs in patients. Individuals suffering from depression are considered a high-risk group for suicidal behavior. Suicide hotlines are widely available for people seeking help. However, the negative and often too clinical reception that many suicidal people receive after relating their feelings to health professionals (e.g. threats of institutionalization, increased dosages of medication, the social stigma) may cause patients to remain more guarded about their mental health history or suicidal urges and ideation.

STROKE OR CEREBROVASCULAR ACCIDENT (CVA)

Stroke or cerebrovascular accident (CVA) is the clinical designation for a rapidly developing loss of brain function due to a disturbance in the blood vessels supplying blood to the brain. This phenomenon can be due to ischemia (lack of blood supply) caused by thrombosis or embolism, or due to a hemorrhage.

Stroke is a medical emergency and can cause permanent neurological damage, complications and death if not promptly diagnosed and treated. It is the third leading cause of death and the leading cause of adult disability in the United States and Europe. It is predicted that stroke will soon become the leading cause of death worldwide. Risk factors for stroke include advanced age, hypertension (high blood pressure), previous stroke or transient ischaemic attack (TIA, see below), diabetes, high cholesterol, cigarette smoking, atrial fibrillation, migraine with aura, and thrombophilia (a tendency to thrombosis). In clinical practice, blood pressure is the most important modifiable risk factor of stroke.

Stroke symptoms typically develop rapidly (seconds to minutes). The symptoms of a stroke are related to the anatomical location of the damage; nature and severity of the symptoms can therefore vary widely. On the basis of the history and neurological examination, as well as the presence of risk factors, a doctor can rapidly diagnose the anatomical nature of the stroke (i.e. which part of the brain is affected), even if the exact cause is not yet known.

The traditional definition of stroke, devised by the World Health Organisation in the 1970s, is of a "neurological deficit of cerebrovascular cause that persists beyond 24 hours or is interrupted by death within 24 hours". This definition was supposed to reflect the reversibility of tissue damage and was devised for the purpose, with the time frame of 24 hours being chosen arbitrarily. It divides stroke from TIA, which is a related syndrome of stroke symptoms that resolve completely within 24 hours. With the availability of treatments that, when given early, can reduce stroke severity, many now prefer alternative concepts, such as brain attack and acute ischemic cerebrovascular syndrome (modeled after heart attack and acute coronary syndrome respectively), that reflect the urgency of stroke symptoms and the need to act swiftly.

Treatment of stroke is occasionally with thrombolysis ("clot buster"), but usually with supportive care (physiotherapy and occupational therapy) and secondary prevention with antiplatelet drugs (aspirin and often dipyridamole), blood pressure control, statins and anticoagulation (in selected patients).

CONVULSION OR SEIZURE

A seizure is a temporary abnormal electro-physiologic phenomenon of the brain, resulting in abnormal synchronization of electrical neuronal activity. It can manifest as an alteration in mental state, tonic or clonic movements, convulsions, and various other psychic symptoms. It is caused by a temporary abnormal electrical activity of a group of brain cells. The medical syndrome of recurrent, unprovoked seizures is termed epilepsy, but some seizures may occur in people who do not have epilepsy.The treatment of epilepsy is a subspecialty of neurology; the study of seizures is part of neuroscience.

Signs and Symptoms

Seizures can cause involuntary changes in body movement or function, sensation, awareness, or behavior. A seizure can last from a few seconds to status epilepticus, a continuous seizure that will not stop without intervention. Seizure is often associated with a sudden and involuntary contraction of a group of muscles. However, a seizure can also be as subtle as marching numbness of a part of the body, a brief loss of memory, sparkling or flashes, sensing an unpleasant odor, a strange epigastric sensation or a sensation of fear. Therefore seizures are typically classified as motor, sensory, autonomic, emotional or cognitive.

In some cases, the full onset of a seizure event is preceded by some of the sensations described above. These sensations can serve as a warning to the sufferer that a full tonic-clonic seizure is about to occur. These "warning sensations" are cumulatively called an aura.

Symptoms experienced by a person during a seizure depend on where in the brain the disturbance in electrical activity occurs. Recent studies show that seizures happen in sleep more often than was thought. A person having a tonic-clonic seizure may cry out, lose consciousness and fall to the ground, and convulse, often violently. A person having a complex partial seizure may appear confused or dazed and will not be able to respond to questions or direction. Some people have seizures that are not noticeable to others. Sometimes, the only clue that a person is having an absence seizure is rapid blinking or a few seconds of staring into space.

It is commonly thought among healthcare providers that many seizures, especially in children, are preceded by tachycardia that frequently persists throughout the seizure. This early increase in heart rate may supplement an aura as a physiological warning sign of an imminent seizure.

Diagnosis

(i) Determining whether a seizure occurred
(ii) Physical examination
(iii) Serum prolactin level
(iv) EEG: An isolated abnormal electrical activity recorded by an electroencephalography examination without a clinical presentation is called subclinical seizure. They may identify background epileptogenic activity, as well as help identify particular causes of seizures.
(v) Investigation of underlying cause: Additional diagnostic methods include CT Scanning and MRI imaging or angiography. These may show structural lesions within the brain, but the majority of those with epilepsy show nothing unusual.

As seizures have a differential diagnosis, it is common for patients to be simultaneously investigated for cardiac and endocrine causes. Checking glucose levels, for example, is a mandatory action in the management of seizures as hypoglycemia may cause seizures, and failure to administer glucose would be harmful to the patient. Other causes typically considered are syncope and cardiac arrhythmias, and occasionally panic attacks and cataplexy. For more information, see non-epileptic seizures.

Management

The first aid for a seizure depends on the type of seizure occurring. Generalized seizures will cause the person to fall, which may result in injury. A tonic-clonic seizure results in violent movements that cannot and should not be suppressed. The person should never be restrained, nor should there be any attempt to put something in the mouth. Potentially sharp or dangerous objects should also be moved from the vicinity, so that the individual is not hurt. After the seizure if the person is not fully conscious and alert, they should be placed in the recovery position.

It is not necessary to call an ambulance if the person is known to have epilepsy, if the seizure is shorter than five minutes and is typical for them, if it is not immediately followed by another seizure, and if the person is uninjured. Otherwise, or if in any doubt, medical assistance should be sought. A seizure longer than five minutes is a medical emergency. Relatives and other caregivers of those known to have epilepsy often carry medicine such as rectal diazepam or buccal midazolam in order to rapidly end the seizure.

MENINGITIS

Meningitis is the inflammation of the protective membranes covering the central nervous system, known collectively as the meninges. Meningitis may develop in response to a number of causes, including infectious agents, physical injury, cancer, or certain drugs. While some forms of meningitis are mild and resolve on their own, meningitis is a potentially serious condition owing to the proximity of the inflammation to the brain and spinal cord. The potential for serious neurological damage or even death necessitates prompt medical attention and evaluation. Infectious meningitis, the most common form, is typically treated with antibiotics and requires close observation.

Signs and Symptoms

Headache is the most common symptom of meningitis (87 percent) followed by nuchal rigidity ("neck stiffness", 83 percent). The classic triad of diagnostic signs consists of nuchal rigidity (being unable to flex the neck forward), fever and altered mental status. All three features are present in only 44 per cent of all cases of infectious meningitis. Other signs commonly associated with meningitis are photophobia (inability to tolerate bright light), phonophobia (inability to tolerate loud noises), irritability and delirium (in small children) and seizures (in 20-40 per cent of cases). In infants (0-6 months), swelling of the fontanelle (soft spot) may be present.

Nuchal rigidity is typically assessed with the patient lying supine, and both hips and knees flexed. If pain is elicited when the knees are passively extended (Kernig's sign), this indicates nuchal rigidity and meningitis. In infants, forward flexion of the neck may cause involuntary knee and hip flexion (Brudzinski's sign). Although commonly tested, the sensitivity and specificity of Kernig's and Brudzinski's tests are uncertain.

In "meningococcal" meningitis (i.e. meningitis caused by the bacteria Neisseria meningitidis), a rapidly-spreading petechial rash is typical, and may precede other symptoms. The rash consists of numerous small, irregular purple or red spots on the trunk, lower extremities, mucous membranes, conjunctiva, and occasionally on the palms of hands and soles of feet.

Diagnosis

The suspicion of meningitis is generally based on the nature of the symptoms and findings on physical examination. Meningitis is a medical emergency, and referral to hospital is indicated. If meningitis is suspected based on clinical examination, early administration of antibiotics is recommended, as the condition may deteriorate rapidly. In the hospital setting, initial management consists of stabilization (e.g. securing the airway in a depressed level of consciousness, administration of intravenous fluids in hypotension or shock), followed by antibiotics if not already administered.

Investigations include blood tests (electrolytes, liver and kidney function, inflammatory markers and a complete blood count) and usually X-ray examination of the chest. The most important test in identifying or ruling out meningitis is analysis of the cerebrospinal fluid (fluid that envelops the brain and the spinal cord) through lumbar puncture (LP). However, if the patient is at risk for a cerebral mass lesion or elevated intracranial pressure (recent head injury, a known immune system problem, localizing neurological signs, or evidence on examination of a raised ICP), a lumbar puncture may be contraindicated because of the possibility of fatal brain herniation. In such cases a CT or MRI scan is generally performed prior to the lumbar puncture to exclude this possibility. Otherwise, the CT or MRI should be performed after the LP, with MRI preferred over CT due to its superiority in demonstrating areas of cerebral edema, ischemia, and meningeal inflammation.

During the lumbar puncture procedure, the opening pressure is measured. A pressure of over 180 mmH2O is indicative of bacterial meningitis.

The cerebrospinal fluid (CSF) sample is examined for white blood cells (and which subtypes), red blood cells, protein content and glucose level. Gram staining of the sample may demonstrate bacteria in bacterial meningitis, but absence of bacteria does not exclude bacterial meningitis; microbiological culture of the sample may still yield a causative organism. The type of white blood cell predominantly present predicts whether meningitis is due to bacterial or viral infection. Other tests performed on the CSF sample include latex agglutination test, limulus lysates, or polymerase chain reaction (PCR) for bacterial or viral DNA. If the patient is immunocompromised, testing the CSF for toxoplasmosis, Epstein-Barr virus, cytomegalovirus, JC virus and fungal infection may be performed.

FAINTING

Fainting, also called *syncope* is a sudden, and generally momentary, loss of consciousness, or blacking out caused by the Central Ischaemic Response, because of a lack of sufficient blood and oxygen in the brain. The first symptoms a person feels before fainting are dizziness; a dimming of vision, or brownout; tinnitus; and feeling hot. Moments later, the person's vision turns black, and he or she drops to the floor (or slumps if seated in a chair). If the person is unable to slump from the position to a near horizontal position, he or she risks dying of the Suspension trauma effect.

Factors that influence fainting are taking in too little food and fluids, low blood pressure, hypoglycemia, growth spurts, physical exercise in excess of the energy reserve of the body, emotional distress, and lack of sleep. Even standing up too quickly or being in too hot a room can cause fainting. Recommended treatment is to allow the person to lie on the ground with his or her legs slightly elevated. As the dizziness and the momentary blindness passes, the person may experience visual disturbances in the form of small bright dots (phosphene). These will also pass within a few minutes. If fainting happens frequently, or if there is no obvious explanation, it is important to see a doctor about it.

More serious causes of fainting include cardiac (heart-related) causes such as an abnormal heart rhythm (an arrhythmia), where the heart beats too slowly, too rapidly or too irregularly to pump enough blood to the brain. Some arrhythmias can be life-threatening. Other important cardio-vascular conditions that can be manifested by syncope include subclavian steal syndrome and aortic stenosis.

Clinical Symptoms

If the patient states, "I felt dizzy with blurry vision, muscle weakness, during the fall I bumped my knee, hit my head and passed out," then it is not syncope, it is termed pre or near-syncope. If the patient states, "I felt dizzy, shadows came over my eyes, and when I woke up I was lying on the floor," then it is diagnosed as syncope. Patients who experience a syncoptic episode do not remember falling.

METABOLIC EMERGENCIES

DEHYDRATION

Dehydration (hypohydration) is the removal of water (hydro in ancient Greek) from an object. Medically, it is a condition in which the body contains an insufficient volume of water for normal functioning.

Causes

In humans, dehydration can be caused by a wide range of diseases and states that impair water homeostasis in the body. These include:

(i) External or stress-related causes;

- Prolonged physical activity without consuming adequate water, especially in a hot and/or humid environment
- Prolonged exposure to dry air, e.g., in high-flying airplanes (5-15 per cent r.h.)
- Survival situations, especially desert survival condi-tions
- Blood loss or hypotension due to physical trauma
- Diarrhea
- Hyperthermia
- Shock (hypovolemic)
- Vomiting
- Burns
- Lacrimation

(ii) Infectious diseases:

- Cholera
- Gastroenteritis
- Shigellosis
- Yellow fever

(iii) Malnutrition:

- Electrolyte disturbance
- Hypernatremia (also caused by dehydration)
- Hyponatremia, especially from restricted salt diets
- Consumption of alcohol, caffeine or other diuretic substances.
- Fasting
- Recent rapid weight loss may reflect progressive depletion of fluid volume. (The loss of 1 L of fluid results in a weight loss of 1 kg, or 2.2 lb.)

- Patient refusal of nutrition and hydration

(iv) Other causes of obligate water loss:

- Severe hyperglycemia, especially in Diabetes mellitus
- Glycosuria.

Symptoms and Prognosis

Symptoms may include headaches similar to what is experienced during a hangover, a sudden episode of visual snow, decreased blood pressure (hypotension), and dizziness or fainting when standing up due to orthostatic hypotension. Untreated dehydration generally results in delirium, unconsciousness, swelling of the tongue and in extreme cases death.

Dehydration symptoms generally become noticeable after 2 per cent of one's normal water volume has been lost. Initially, one experiences thirst and discomfort, possibly along with loss of appetite and dry skin. This can be followed by constipation. Athletes may suffer a loss of performance of up to 30 per cent[2], and experience flushing, low endurance, rapid heart rates, elevated body temperatures, and rapid onset of fatigue.

Symptoms of mild dehydration include thirst, decreased urine volume, abnormally dark urine, unexplained tiredness, lack of tears when crying, headache, dry mouth, and dizziness when standing due to orthostatic hypotension.

In moderate to severe dehydration, there may be no urine output at all. Other symptoms in these states include lethargy or extreme sleepiness, seizures, sunken fontanel (soft spot) in infants, fainting, and sunken eyes.

The symptoms become increasingly severe with greater water loss. One's heart and respiration rates begin to increase to compensate for decreased plasma volume and blood pressure, while body temperature may rise because of decreased sweating. Around 5 per cent to 6 per cent water loss, one may become groggy or sleepy, experience headaches or nausea, and may feel tingling in one's limbs (paresthesia). With 10 per cent to 15 per cent fluid loss, muscles may become spastic, skin may shrivel and wrinkle, vision may dim, urination will be greatly reduced and may become painful, and delirium may begin. Losses greater than 15 per cent are usually fatal.

Treatment

The best treatment for minor dehydration is drinking water and stopping fluid loss. Water is preferable to sport drinks and other commercially-sold rehydration fluids, as the balance of electrolytes they provide may not match the replacement requirements of the individual. To stop fluid loss from vomiting and diarrhea, avoid solid foods and drink only clear liquids.

In more severe cases, correction of a dehydrated state is accomplished by the replenishment of necessary water and electrolytes (rehydration, through oral rehydration therapy or intravenous therapy). Even in the case of serious lack of fresh water (e.g., at sea or in a desert), drinking seawater or urine does not help, nor does the consumption of alcohol. It is often thought that the sudden influx of salt into the body from seawater will cause the cells to dehydrate and the kidneys to overload and shut down but it has been calculated that an average adult can drink up to 0.2 liters of seawater per day before the kidneys start to fail.

When dehydrated, unnecessary sweating should be avoided, as it wastes water. If there is only dry food, it is better not to eat, as water is necessary for digestion. For severe cases of dehydration where fainting, unconsciousness, or other severely inhibiting symptom is present (the patient is incapable of standing or thinking clearly), emergency attention is required. Fluids containing a proper balance of replacement electrolytes are given orally or intravenously with continuing assessment of electrolyte status; complete resolution is the norm in all but the most extreme cases.

Avoiding Dehydration

Dehydration is best avoided by drinking plenty of water. The greater the amount of water lost through perspiration, the more water must be consumed to replace it and avoid dehydration. Since the body cannot tolerate large deficits or excesses in total body water, consumption of water must be roughly concurrent with the loss (in other words, if one is perspiring, one should also be drinking water frequently). Drinking water slightly beyond the needs of the body entails no risk, since the kidneys will efficiently remove any excess water through the urine with a large margin of safety.

A person's body, during an average day in a temperate climate such as the United Kingdom, loses approximately 2.5 litres of water. This can be through the lungs as water vapor, through the skin as sweat, or through the kidneys as urine. Some water (a less significant amount, in the absence of diarrhea) is also lost through the bowels. In warm or humid weather or during heavy exertion, however, the water loss can increase by an order of magnitude or more through perspiration;all of which must be promptly replaced. In extreme cases, the losses may be great enough to exceed the body's ability to absorb water from the gastrointestinal tract; in these cases, it is not possible to drink enough water to stay hydrated, and the only way to avoid dehydration is to reduce perspiration (through rest, a move to a cooler environment, etc.).

A useful rule of thumb for avoiding dehydration in hot or humid environments or during strenuous activity involves monitoring the frequency and character of urination. If one develops a full bladder at least every 3-5 hours and the urine is only lightly colored or colorless, chances are that dehydration is not occurring; if urine is deeply colored, or urination occurs only after many hours or not at all, water intake may not be adequate to maintain proper hydration.

When large amounts of water are being lost through perspiration and concurrently replaced by drinking, maintaining proper electrolyte balance becomes an issue Drinking fluids that are hypertonic or hypotonic with respect to perspiration may have grave consequences (hyponatremia or hypernatremia, principally) as the total volume of water turnover increases.

If water is being lost through abnormal mechanisms such as vomiting or diarrhea, an imbalance can develop very quickly into a medical emergency. In fact, the main mechanisms through which diseases such as infantile diarrhea and cholera kill their victims are dehydration and loss of electrolytes. During sports events, water stops and water breaks are provided to avoid dehydration of athletes.

DIABETIC COMA

Diabetic coma is a medical emergency in which a person with diabetes mellitus is comatose (unconscious) because of one of the acute complications of diabetes:

(i) Severe diabetic hypoglycemia

(ii) Diabetic ketoacidosis advanced enough to result in unconsciousness from a combination of severe hyperglycemia, dehydration and shock, and exhaustion

(iii) Hyperosmolar nonketotic coma in which extreme hyperglycemia and dehydration alone are sufficient to cause unconsciousness.

In most medical contexts, the term diabetic coma refers to the diagnostic dilemma posed when a physician is confronted with an unconscious patient about whom nothing is known except that he has diabetes. An example might be a physician working in an emergency department who receives an unconscious patient wearing a medical identification tag saying DIABETIC. Paramedics may be called to rescue an unconscious person by friends who identify him as diabetic. Brief descriptions of the three major conditions are followed by a discussion of the diagnostic process used to distinguish among them, as well as a few other conditions which must be considered.

An estimated 2 to 15 percent of people with diabetes will suffer from at least one episode of diabetic coma in their lifetimes as a result of severe hypoglycemia.

SEVERE HYPOGLYCEMIA

People with type 1 diabetes mellitus who must take insulin in full replacement doses are most vulnerable to episodes of hypoglycemia. It is usually mild enough to reverse by eating or drinking carbohydrates, but blood glucose occasionally can fall fast enough and low enough to produce unconsciousness before hypoglycemia can be recognized and reversed. Hypoglycemia can be severe enough to cause unconsciousness during sleep. Predisposing factors can include eating less than usual, prolonged exercise earlier in the day, and heavy drinking. Some people with diabetes can lose their ability to recognize the symptoms of early hypoglycemia.

Unconsciousness due to hypoglycemia can occur within 20 minutes to an hour after early symptoms and is not usually preceded by other illness or symptoms. Twitching or convulsions may occur. A person unconscious from hypoglycemia is usually pale, has a rapid heart beat, and is soaked in sweat: all signs of the adrenaline response to hypoglycemia. The individual is not usually dehydrated and breathing is normal or shallow. A meter or laboratory glucose at the time of discovery is usually low, but not always severely, and in some cases may have already risen from the nadir that triggered the unconsciousness. Unconsciousness due to hypoglycemia is treated by raising the blood glucose with intravenous glucose or injected glucagon.

ADVANCED DIABETIC KETOACIDOSIS

Diabetic ketoacidosis (DKA), if it progresses and worsens without treatment, can eventually cause unconsciousness, from a combination of severe hyperglycemia, dehydration and shock, and exhaustion. Coma only occurs at an advanced stage, usually after 36 hours or more of worsening vomiting and hyperventilation.

In the early to middle stages of ketoacidosis, patients are typically flushed and breathing rapidly and deeply, but visible dehydration, pallor from diminished perfusion, shallower breathing, and rapid heart rate are often present when coma is reached. However these features are variable and not always as described.

If the patient is known to have diabetes, the diagnosis of DKA is usually suspected from the appearance and a history of 1-2 days of vomiting. The diagnosis is confirmed when the usual blood chemistries in the emergency department reveal hyperglycemia and severe metabolic acidosis.

Treatment of DKA consists of isotonic fluids to rapidly stabilize the circulation, continued intravenous saline with potassium and other electrolytes to replace deficits, insulin to reverse the ketoacidosis, and careful monitoring for complications.

NONKETOTIC HYPEROSMOLAR COMA

Nonketotic hyperosmolar coma usually develops more insidiously than DKA because the principal symptom is lethargy progressing to obtundation, rather than vomiting and an obvious illness. Extreme hyperglycemia is accompanied by dehydration due to inadequate fluid intake. Coma from NKHC occurs most often in patients who develop type 2 or steroid diabetes and have an impaired ability to recognize thirst and drink. It is classically a nursing home condition but can occur in all ages.

The diagnosis is usually discovered when a chemistry screen performed because of obtundation reveals extreme hyperglycemia (often above 1800 mg/dl (100 mM)) and dehydration. The treatment consists of insulin and gradual rehydration with intravenous fluids.

Causes of Diabetic Coma

Diabetic coma was a more significant diagnostic problem before the late 1970s, when glucose meters and rapid blood chemistry analyzers became universally available in hospitals. In modern medical practice, it rarely takes more than a few questions, a quick look, and a glucose meter to determine the cause of unconsciousness in a patient with diabetes. Laboratory confirmation can usually be obtained in half an hour or less. Also, the astute physician remembers that other conditions can cause unconsciousness in a person with diabetes: stroke, uremic encephalopathy, alcohol, drug overdose, head injury, or seizure.

Fortunately, most episodes of diabetic hypoglycemia, DKA, and extreme hyperosmolarity do not reach unconsciousness before a family member or caretaker seeks medical help.

Treatment

Ketoacidotic Diabetic Coma: intravenous fluids, insulin and administration of potassium and sodium.

Hyperosmolar Diabetic Coma: plenty of intravenous fluids, insulin, potassium and sodium given as soon as possible.

Hypoglycaemic Diabetic Coma: administration of the hormone glucagon to reverse the effects of insulin, or glucose given intravenously.

ELECTROLYTE DISTURBANCE

Electrolytes play a vital role in maintaining homeostasis within the body. They help to regulate myocardial and neurological function, fluid balance, oxygen delivery, acid-base balance and much more. Electrolyte imbalances can develop by the following mechanisms: excessive ingestion; diminished elimination of an electrolyte; diminished ingestion or excessive elimination of an electrolyte. The most common cause of electrolyte disturbances is renal failure. The most serious electrolyte disturbances involve abnormalities in the levels of sodium, potassium, and/or calcium. Other electrolyte imbalances are less common, and often occur in conjunction with major electrolyte changes. Chronic laxative abuse or severe diarrhea or vomiting can lead to electrolyte disturbances along with dehydration. People suffering from bulimia or anorexia are at especially high risk for an electrolyte imbalance.

Electrolytes are important because they are what your cells (especially nerve, heart, muscle) use to maintain voltages across their cell membranes and to carry electrical impulses (nerve impulses, muscle contractions) across themselves and to other cells. Your kidneys work to keep the electrolyte concentrations in your blood constant despite changes in your body. For example, when you exercise heavily, you lose electrolytes in your sweat, particularly sodium and potassium. These electrolytes must be replaced to keep the electrolyte concentrations of your body fluids constant.

Electrolyte Abnormalities and ECG Changes

The most notable feature of hyperkalemia is the "tent shaped" or "peaked" T wave. Delayed ventricular depolarization leads to a widened QRS complex and the P wave becomes wider and flatter. When hyperkalemia becomes severe, the ECG resembles a sine wave as the P wave disappears from view. In contrast, hypokalemia is associated with flattenting of the T wave and the appearance of a U wave. When untreated, hypokalemia may lead severe arrhythmias.

The fast ventricular depolarization and repolarization associated with hypercalcemia lead to a characteristic shortening of the QT interval. Hypocalcemia has the opposite effect, lengthening the QT interval.

ACIDOSIS

Acidosis is an increased acidity (i.e. an increased hydrogen ion concentration). If not further qualified, it refers to acidity of the blood plasma. Acidosis is said to occur when arterial pH falls below 7.35, while its counterpart (alkalosis) occurs at a pH over 7.45. Arterial blood gas analysis and other tests are required to separate the main causes.

The term acidemia describes the state of low blood pH, while acidosis is used to describe the processes leading to these states. Nevertheless, physicians sometimes use the terms interchangeably. The distinction may be relevant where a patient has factors causing both acidosis and alkalosis, where the relative severity of both determines whether the result is a high or a low pH.

The rate of cellular metabolic activity affects and, at the same time, is affected by the pH of the body fluids. In mammals, the normal pH of arterial blood lies between 7.35 and 7.50 depending on the species (e.g. healthy human-arterial blood pH varies between 7.35 and 7.45). Blood pH values compatible with life in mammals are limited to a pH range between 6.8 and 7.8. Changes in the pH of arterial blood (and therefore the extracellular fluid) outside this range result in irreversible cell damage.

RESPIRATORY ACIDOSIS

Respiratory acidosis results from a build-up of carbon dioxide in the blood (hypercapnia) due to hypoventilation. It is most often caused by pulmonary problerns, although head injuries, drugs (especially anaesthetics and sedatives), and brain tumors can also bring it on. Pneumothorax, emphysema, chronic bronchitis, asthma, severe pneumonia, and aspiration are among the most frequent causes. It can also occur as a compensatory response to chronic metabolic alkalosis.

One key to distinguish between respiratory and metabolic acidosis is that in respiratory acidosis, the CO_2 is increased while the bicarbonate is either normal (uncompensated) or increased (compensated). Compensation occurs if respiratory acidosis is present, and a chronic phase is entered with partial buffering of the acidosis through renal bicarbonate retention.

However, in cases where chronic illnesses which compromise pulmonary function persist, such as late-stage emphysema and certain types of muscular dystrophy, compensatory mechanisms will be unable to reverse this acidotic conditon. As metabolic bicarbonate production becomes exhausted, and extraeneous bicarbonate infusion can no longer reverse the extreme buildup of carbon dioxide associated with uncompensated respiratory acidosis, mechanical ventilation will usually be applied.

METABOLIC ACIDOSIS

Metabolic acidosis is an increased production of metabolic acids, usually resulting from disturbances in the ability to excrete acid via the kidneys. Renal acidosis is associated with an accumulation of urea and creatinine as well as metabolic acid residues of protein catabolism.

An increase in the production of other acids may also produce metabolic acidosis. For example, lactic acidosis may occur from (i) severe (PaO_2 <36 mm Hg) hypoxemia causing a fall in the rate of oxygen diffusion from arterial blood to tissues, or (ii) hypoperfusion (e.g. hypovolemic shock) causing an inadequate blood delivery of oxygen to tissues. A rise in lactate out of proportion to the level of pyruvate, e.g. in mixed venous blood, is termed "excess lactate", and may also be an indicator of fermention due to anaerobic metabolism occurring in muscle cells, as seen during strenuous exercise. Once oxygenation is restored, the acidosis clears quickly. Another example of increased production of acids occurs in starvation and diabetic acidosis. It is due to the accumulation of ketoacids (ketosis) and reflects a severe shift from glycolysis to lipolysis for energy needs.

Acid consumption from poisoning, elevated levels of iron in the blood, and chronically decreased production of bicarbonate may also produce metabolic acidosis. Metabolic acidosis is compensated for in the lungs, as increased exhalation of carbon dioxide promptly shifts the buffering equation to reduce metabolic acid. This is a result of stimulation to chemoreceptors which increases alveolar ventilation, leading to respiratory compensation, otherwise known as Kussmaul breathing (a specific type of hyperventilation). Should this situation persist the patient is at risk for exhaustion leading to respiratory failure.

Mutations to the V-ATPase 'a4' or 'B1' isoforms result in distal renal tubular acidosis, a condition that leads to metabolic acidosis, in some cases with sensorineural deafness.

Arterial blood gasses will indicate low pH, low blood HCO_3, and normal or low $PaCO_2$. In addition to arterial blood gas, an anion gap can also differentiate between possible causes.

The Henderson-Hasselbalch equation is useful for calculating blood pH, because blood is a buffer solution. The amount of metabolic acid accumulating can also be quantitated by using buffer base deviation, a derivative estimate of the metabolic as opposed to the respiratory component. In hypovolemic shock for example, approximately 50 per cent of the metabolic acid accumulation is lactic acid, which disappears as blood flow and oxygen debt are corrected.

Treatment

Treatment of uncompensated metabolic acidosis is focused upon correcting the underlying problem. When metabolic acidosis is severe and can no longer be compensated for adequately by the lungs, neutralizing the acidosis with infusions of bicarbonate may be required.

CONSTIPATION

Constipation, costiveness, or irregularity, is a condition of the digestive system where a person (or animal) experiences hard feces that are difficult to egest. It may be extremely painful, and in severe cases (fecal impaction) lead to symptoms of bowel obstruction. The term obstipation is used for severe constipation. Causes of constipation may be dietary, hormonal, anatomical, a side effect of medications (e.g. some painkillers), or an illness or disorder. Treatments consist of changes in dietary and exercise habits, the use of laxatives, and other medical interventions depending on the underlying cause.

Constipation is one of the most common digestive complaints. It varies greatly between different people, as each person's bowel movements differ. Rate of defecation is not in itself a problem, as infrequent defecation without problems is not abnormal. Constipation is most common in children and older people, and affects women more than men. In children, constipation can lead to soiling (enuresis and encopresis).

In common constipation, the stool is hard and difficult and painful to pass. Usually, there is an infrequent urge to void. Straining to pass stool may cause hemorrhoids and anal fissures, which are themselves painful. In later stages of constipation, the abdomen may become distended and diffusely tender and crampy, occasionally with enhanced bowel sounds.

Diagnosis

The diagnosis is essentially made from the patient's description of the symptoms. Bowel movements that are difficult to pass, very firm, or made up of small rabbit-like pellets qualify as constipation, even if they occur every day. Other symptoms related to constipation can include bloating, distention, abdominal pain, or a sense of incomplete emptying.

Inquiring about dietary habits may reveal a low intake of dietary fiber or inadequate amounts of fluids. Constipation as a result of poor ambulation or immobility should be considered in the elderly. Constipation may arise as a side effect of medications (especially antidepressants and opiates). Rarely, other symptoms suggestive of hypothyroidism may be elicited.

During physical examination, scybala (manually palpable lumps of stool) may be detected on palpation of the abdomen. Rectal examination gives an impression of the anal sphincter tone and whether the lower rectum contains any feces or not; if so, then suppositories or enemas may be considered. Otherwise, oral medication may be required. Rectal examination also gives information on the consistency of the stool, presence of hemorrhoids, admixture of blood and whether any tumors or abnormalities are present.

X-rays of the abdomen, generally only performed on hospitalized patients or if bowel obstruction is suspected, may reveal impacted fecal matter in the colon, and confirm or rule out other causes of similar symptoms.

Chronic constipation (symptoms present for more than 3 months at least 3 days per month) associated with abdominal discomfort is often diagnosed as irritable bowel syndrome (IBS) when no obvious cause is found. Physicians caring for patients with chronic constipation are advised to rule out obvious causes through normal testing.

Causes

The main causes of constipation include:

- Hardening of the feaces:
  - Improper mastication (chewing) of food.
  - Insufficient intake of dietary fiber.
  - Dehydration from any cause or inadeqūate fluid intake.
  - Medication, e.g. diuretics and those containing iron, calcium, aluminium.
- Paralysis or slowed transit, where peristaltic action is diminished or absent, so that feces are not moved along:
  - Hypothyroidism (slow-acting thyroid gland)
  - Hypokalemia
  - Injured anal sphincter (patulous anus)
  - Medications, such as loperamide, opioids (e.g., codeine and morphine) and certain tricyclic antidepressants
  - Severe illness due to other causes
  - Acute porphyria (a rare inherited condition)
  - Lead poisoning
- Dyschezia (usually the result of suppressing defecation)
- Constriction, where part of the intestine or rectum is narrowed or blocked, not allowing feces to pass:
  - Stenosis (Strictures).
  - Diverticula.
  - Tumors, either of the bowel or surrounding tissues.
  - Retained foreign body or a bezoar.
- Psychosomatic constipation, based on anxiety or unfamiliarity with surroundings.
  - Functional constipation.
  - Constipation-predominant irritable bowel syndrome, characterized by a combination of constipation and abdominal discomfort and/or pain.
- Smoking cessation (nicotine has a laxative effect)·
- Abdominal surgery, other types of surgery, childbirth.

Treatment

In people without medical problems, the main intervention is to increase the intake of fluids (preferably water) and dietary fiber. The latter may be achieved by consuming more vegetables and fruit and whole meal bread, and by adding linseeds to one's diet. The routine non-medical use of laxatives is to be discouraged as this may result in bowel action becoming dependent upon their use. Enemas can be used to provide a form of mechanical stimulation. In alternative and traditional medicine, colonic irrigation, enemas, exercise, diet and herbs are used to treat constipation.

LIVER DIALYSIS

Liver dialysis is a detoxification treatment for liver failure and has shown promise for patients with hepatorenal syndrome. It is similar to hemodialysis and based on the same principles. Like a bioartificial liver device, it is a form of artificial extracorporeal liver support.

A critical issue of the clinical syndrome in liver failure is the accumulation of toxins not cleared by the failing liver. Based on this hypothesis, the removal of lipophilic, albumin-bound substances such as bilirubin, bile acids, metabolites of aromatic amino acids, medium-chain fatty acids and cytokines should be beneficial to the clinical course of a patient in liver failure. This led to the development of artificial filtration and adsorption devices. Hemodialysis is used for renal failure and primarily removes water soluble toxins, however it does not remove toxins bound to albumin that accumulate in liver failure.

LIVER TRANSPLANTATION

Liver transplantation or hepatic transplantation is the replacement of a diseased liver with a healthy liver allograft. The most commonly used technique is orthotopic transplantation, in which the native liver is removed and the donor organ is placed in the same anatomic location as the original liver. Liver transplantation nowadays is a well accepted treatment option for end-stage liver disease and acute liver failure.

HEPATITIS

Hepatitis (plural hepatitides) implies injury to liver characterised by presence of inflammatory cells in the liver tissue. The condition can be self limiting, healing on its own or can progress to scarring of the liver. Acute hepatitis is when it lasts less than 6 months and chronic hepatitis is when it persists longer. A group of viruses known as the hepatitis viruses cause most cases of liver damage worldwide. Hepatitis can also be due to toxins (notably alcohol), other infections or from autoimmune process. It may run a subclinical course when the affected person may not feel ill. The patient becomes unwell and symptomatic when the disease impairs liver functions that include, among other things, screening of harmful substances, regulation of blood composition, and production of bile to help digestion.

Causes

Acute Hepatitis

- Viral Hepatitis: Hepatitis A to E (more than 95 per cent of viral cause), Herpes simplex, Cytomegalovirus, Epstein-Barr, yellow fever virus, adenoviruses.
- Non viral infection: toxoplasma, Leptospira, Q fever, rocky mountain spotted fever.
- Alcohol.
- Toxins: Amanita toxin in mushrooms, Carbon tetrachloride, asafetida.
- Drugs: Paracetamol, amoxycillin, anti tuberculosis medicines, minocycline and many others.
- Circulatory insufficiency
- Pregnancy
- Auto immune conditions e.g. Systemic Lupus Erythematosus (SLE).
- Metabolic diseases e.g. Wilson's disease.

Chronic Hepatitis

- Viral Hepatitis: Hepatitis B with or without hepatitis D, Hepatitis C (Hepatitis A and E do not lead to chronic disease).
- Autoimmune: Autoimmune hepatitis.
- Alcohol.
- Drugs: Methyl-dopa, nitrofurantoin, isoniazide, ketoconazole.
- Non-alcoholic steatohepatitis.
- Heredity: Wilson's disease, alpha 1-antitrypsin deficiency.
- Primary biliary cirrhosis and primary sclerosing cholangitis occasionally mimic chronic hepatitis.

Signs and symptoms

Acute Hepatitis

Clinically, the course of acute hepatitis varies widely from mild symptoms requiring no treatment to fulminant hepatic failure needing liver transplantation. Acute viral hepatitis are more likely to be asymptomatic in younger people. Symptomatic individuals may present after convalescent stage of 7 to 10 days, with the total illness lasting 2 to 6 weeks.

Initial features are of nonspecific flu-like symptoms, common to almost all acute viral infections and may include malaise, muscle and joint aches, fever, nausea or vomiting, diarrhea, and headache. More specific symptoms, which can be present in acute hepatitis from any cause are: profound loss of appetite, aversion to smoking among smokers, dark urine, yellowing of the eyes and skin (i.e. jaundice) and abdominal discomfort. Physical findings are usually minimal, apart from jaundice (33 per cent) and tender hepatomegaly (10 per cent). There can be occasional lymphadenopathy (5 per cent) or splenomegaly (5 per cent).

Chronic Hepatitis

Majority of patients will remain asymptomatic or mildly symptomatic, abnormal blood tests being the only manifestation. Features may be related to extent of liver damage or the cause of hepatitis. Many experience return of symptoms related to acute hepatitis. Jaundice can be a late feature and may indicate extensive damage. Other features include abdominal fullness from enlarged liver or spleen, low grade fever and fluid retention (ascites). Extensive damage and scarring of liver i.e. cirrhosis leads to weight loss, easy bruising and bleeding tendencies. Acne, abnormal menstruation, lung scarring, inflammation of the thyroid gland and kidneys may be present in women with autoimmune hepatitis. Findings on clinical examination are usually those of cirrhosis or are related to aetiology.

Types of Hepatitis

Most cases of acute hepatitis are due to viral infections:

- Hepatitis A
- Hepatitis B
- Hepatitis C
- Hepatitis B with D
- Hepatitis E
- Hepatitis F (existence unknown)
- Hepatitis G
- In addition to the hepatitis viruses (please note that the hepatitis viruses are not all related). Other viruses can also cause hepatitis, including cytomegalovirus, Epstein-Barr virus, yellow fever, etc.

Hepatitis A

Hepatitis A or infectious jaundice is caused by a picornavirus. It is transmitted by the orofecal route, transmitted to humans through methods such as contaminated food. It causes an acute form of hepatitis and does not have a chronic stage. The patient's immune system makes antibodies against hepatitis A that confer immunity against future infection. People with hepatitis A are advised to rest, stay hydrated and avoid alcohol. A vaccine is available that will prevent infection from hepatitis A for life. Hepatitis A can be spread through personal contact, consumption of raw sea food or drinking contaminated water. This occurs primarily in third world countries. Strict personal hygiene and the avoidance of raw and unpeeled foods can help prevent an infection. Infected people excrete the hepatitis A virus with their faeces two weeks before and one week after the appearance of jaundice. The time between the infection and the start of the illness can run from 15 to 45 days, and approximately 15 per cent of sufferers may experience relapsing symptoms from six months to a year following initial diagnosis.

Hepatitis B

Hepatitis B is caused by a hepadnavirus, which can cause both acute and chronic hepatitis. Chronic hepatitis develops in the 15 per cent of patients who are unable to eliminate the virus after an initial infection. Identified methods of transmission include blood (blood transfusion, now rare), tattoos (both amateur and professionally done), sexually (through sexual intercourse or through contact with blood or bodily fluids), or via mother to child by breast feeding (minimal evidence of transplacental crossing). However, in about half of cases the source of infection cannot be determined. Blood contact can occur by sharing syringes in intravenous drug use, shaving accessories such as razor blades, or touching wounds on infected persons. Needle-exchange programmes have been created in many countries as a form of prevention. Patients with chronic hepatitis B have antibodies against hepatitis B, but these antibodies are not enough to clear the infection that establishes itself in the DNA of the affected liver cells. The continued production of virus combined with antibodies is a likely cause of immune complex disease seen in these patients. A vaccine is available that will prevent infection from hepatitis B for life. Hepatitis B infections result in 500,000 to 1,200,000 deaths per year worldwide due to the complications of chronic hepatitis, cirrhosis, and hepatocellular carcinoma. Hepatitis B is endemic in a number of (mainly South-East Asian) countries, making cirrhosis and hepatocellular carcinoma big killers. There are six FDA-approved treatment options available for persons with a chronic hepatitis B infection: alpha-interferon, pegylated interferon adefovir, entecavir, telbivudine and lamivudine. About 45 per cent of persons on treatment achieve a sustained response.

Hepatitis C

Hepatitis C (originally "non-A non-B hepatitis") is caused by a Flavivirus. It can be transmitted through contact with blood (including through sexual contact where the two parties' blood is mixed) and can also cross the placenta. Hepatitis C may lead to a chronic form of hepatitis, culminating in cirrhosis. It can remain asymptomatic for 10-20 years. Patients with hepatitis C are susceptible to severe hepatitis if they contract either hepatitis A or B, so all hepatitis C patients should be immunized against hepatitis A and hepatitis B if they are not already immune. The virus can cause cirrhosis of the liver. HCV viral levels can be reduced to undetectable levels by a combination of interferon and the antiviral drug ribavirin. The genotype of the virus determines the rate of response to this treatment regimen. Genotype 1 is more resistant to interferon therapy than other HCV genotypes.

Hepatitis D

Hepatitis D is considered a subviral satellite, as it can only propagate in the presence of the Hepatitis B virus.

Hepatitis E

Hepatitis E produces symptoms similar to hepatitis A, although it can take a fulminant course in some patients, particularly pregnant women; it is more prevalent in the Indian subcontinent.

Hepatitis F

Hepatitis F is a hypothetical virus linked to hepatitis. Several hepatitis F candidates emerged in the 1990s; none of these reports have been substantiated.

Hepatitis G

Another type of hepatitis, hepatitis G, has been identified, and is probably spread by blood and sexual contact.There is, however, doubt about whether it causes hepatitis, or is just associated with hepatitis, as it does not appear to be primarily replicated in the liver. Other viral infections can cause hepatitis (inflammation of the liver):

- Mumps virus
- Rubella virus
- Cytomegalovirus
- Epstein-Barr virus
- Other herpes viruses.

Alcoholic Hepatitis

Ethanol, mostly in alcoholic beverages, is a significant cause of hepatitis. Usually alcoholic hepatitis comes after a period of increased alcohol consumption. Alcoholic hepatitis is characterized by a variable constellation of symptoms, which may include feeling unwell, enlargement of the liver, development of fluid in the abdomen ascites, and modest elevation of liver blood tests. Alcoholic hepatitis can vary from mild with only liver test elevation to severe liver inflammation with development of jaundice, prolonged prothrombin time, and liver failure. Severe cases are characterized by either obtundation (dulled consciousness) or the combination of elevated bilirubin levels and prolonged prothrombin time; the mortality rate in both categories is 50 per cent within 30 days of onset.

Alcoholic hepatitis is distinct from cirrhosis caused by long term alcohol consumption. Alcoholic hepatitis can occur in patients with chronic alcoholic liver disease and alcoholic cirrhosis. Alcoholic hepatitis by itself does not lead to cirrhosis, but cirrhosis is more common in patients with long term alcohol consumption. Patients who drink alcohol to excess are also more often than others found to have hepatitis C. The combination of hepatitis C and alcohol consumption accelerates the development of cirrhosis in Western countries.

MALNUTRITION

Malnutrition is a general term for a medical condition caused by an improper or insufficient diet. It most often refers to undernutrition resulting from inadequate consumption, poor absorption, or excessive loss of nutrients, but the term can also encompass overnutrition, resulting from overeating or excessive intake of specific nutrients. An individual will experience malnutrition if the appropriate amount of, or quality of nutrients comprising a healthy diet are not consumed for an extended period of time. An extended period of malnutrition can result in starvation, disease, and infection.

Malnutrition is the lack of sufficient nutrients to maintain healthy bodily functions and is typically associated with extreme poverty in economically developing countries. It is a common cause of reduced intelligence in parts of the world affected by famine. Malnutrition as the result of inappropriate dieting, overeating or the absence of a "balanced diet" is often observed in economically developed countries (eg. as indicated by increasing levels of obesity).

Most commonly, malnourished people either do not have enough calories in their diet, or are eating a diet that lacks protein, vitamins, or trace minerals. Medical problems arising from malnutrition are commonly referred to as deficiency diseases. Scurvy is a well-known and now rare form of malnutrition, in which the victim is deficient in vitamin C.

Common forms of malnutrition include protein-energy malnutrition (PEM) and micronutrient malnutrition. PEM refers to inadequate availability or absorption of energy and proteins in the body. Micronutrient malnutrition refers to inadequate availability of some essential nutrients such as vitamins and trace elements that are required by the body in small quantities. Micronutrient deficiencies lead to a variety of diseases and impair normal functioning of the body. Deficiency in micronutrients such as Vitamin A reduces the capacity of the body to resist diseases. Deficiency in iron, iodine and vitamin A is widely prevalent and represent a major public health challenge. An array of afflictions ranging from stunted growth, reduced intelligence and various cognitive abilities, reduced sociability, reduced leadership and assertiveness, reduced activity and energy, reduced muscle growth and strength, and poorer health overall are directly implicated to nutrient deficiencies. Also, another, although rare, effect of malnutrition is black spots appearing on the skin.

Hunger is the normal psychological response brought on by the physiological condition of needing food. Hunger can also affect the mental state of a person, and is often used as a metonym for general undernourishment.

STUDY QUESTIONS

Write short notes on the following:

(a) Pneumothorax

(b) Asthma

(c) Bleeding

(d) Cardiac arrhythmia

(e) Ectopic pregnancy

(f) Diabetic coma

(g) Dialysis

(h) Meningitis

(i) Metabolic Emergencies.

***

36

CHAPTER

COMMON MEDICAL PROBLEMS

APPENDICITIS

The appendix or ermiform appendix is near the junction of the small intestine and the large intestine. It is connected to the cecum from which it develop embryologically.The term "vermiform" comes from Latin and means "wormlike in appearance".

The most common diseases of the appendix (in humans) are *appendicitis* or epityphlitis. It is a condition characterized by inflammation of the appendix. While mild cases may resolve without treatment, most require removal of the inflamed appendix, either by laparotomy or laparoscopy. Untreated, mortality is high, mainly due to peritonitis and shock.

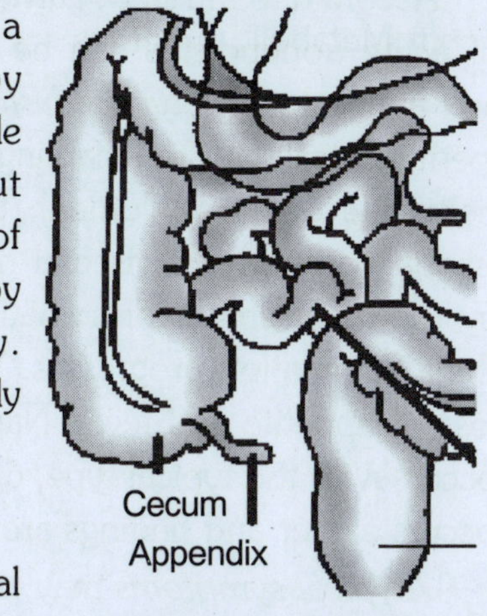

Fig. 36.1: *Appendix*

CAUSES

Obstruction of the appendiceal lumen has been attributed to a number of common sources including from fecaliths (a hard mass of fecal matter), normal stool, viral induced ulcers, or lymphoid hyperplasia. When such obstruction occurs the appendix subsequently becomes filled with mucus and distends, increasing intraluminal and intramural pressures, resulting in thrombosis and occlusion of the small vessels, and stasis of lymphatic flow. As these progress, the appendix becomes ischemic and then necrotic.

Rarely, spontaneous recovery can occur at this point. As bacteria begin to leak out through the dying walls, pus forms within and around the appendix (suppuration). The end result of this cascade is appendiceal rupture causing peritonitis, which may lead to septicemia and eventually death. A number of environmental factors involving diet and hygiene have been proposed to be alternate causes of appendicitis, none of which has been studied in detail. According to the Medical Journal of Australia, "Dietary theories, notably an inadequate fibre intake, have been advanced to account for the geography of the disease, but it is clear that diet can not fully explain the epidemiology."

SYMPTOMS

Accordin to the study carried out by Hobler K., the symptoms of acute appendicitis can be classified into two types, typical and atypical . The *typical history* includes pain starting centrally (periumbilical) before localising to the right iliac fossa (the lower right side of the abdomen); this is due to the poor localizing (spatial) property of visceral nerves from the mid-gut, followed by the involvement of somatic nerves (parietal peritoneum) as the inflammation progresses. The pain is usually associated with loss of appetite and fever. Nausea or vomiting may or may not occur. With the typical type, diagnosis is easier to make, surgery occurs earlier and findings are often less severe.

Atypical symptoms may include pain beginning in the right lower quadrant, diarrhea and a more prolonged, smoldering course. Being more difficult to diagnose, CT scans and ultrasound tests are more useful. Surgical findings are more apt to be severe (suppuration, abscess, perforation, etc.

In either type of history, physical findings of appendicitis usually include localized findings in the right lower quadrant suggesting peritonitis. The abdominal wall becomes very sensitive to gentle pressure (palpation)and tapping (percussion). Coughing causes point tenderness in this area (McBurney's Point) and this is the least painful way to localize the inflamed appendix. If the abdomen on palpation is also involuntarily guarded (rigid), there should be a strong suspicion of peritonitis requiring urgent surgical intervention.

DIAGNOSIS

Diagnosis is based on historical proven action in human examination locally abuse stomach and physical examination backed by an elevation of neutrophilic white cells. Atypical histories often requires ultrasound and/or CT scanning.

The classical history in appendicitis is diffuse pain in the periumbilical region which then localizes as pain and tenderness at McBurney's point (associated with an inflamed appendix coming in contact with the surrounding parietal peritoneum). This point is located on the right-hand side of the abdomen one-third of the distance between the anterior superior iliac spine and the navel. Here, on gentle palpation, the abdominal muscles often feel firm to rigid because of involuntary spasm, and a cough also produces a localized soreness.

Other physical findings include right-side tenderness on a digital rectal examination. Since the appendix normally lies on the right, if a finger is inserted into the rectum and there may be tenderness when pressure is applied toward the right indicating an increased likelihood that the patient has a pelvic appendix. Other signs used in the diagnosis of appendicitis are the psoas sign (useful in retrocecal appendicitis), the obturator sign (specifically the obturator internus muscle), Blumberg's sign, and Rovsing's sign.

Ultrasonography and Doppler sonography also provide useful means to detect appendicitis, especially in children. In some cases (15 per cent approximately), however, ultrasonography of the iliac fossa does not reveal any abnormalities despite the presence of appendicitis. This is especially true of early appendicitis before the appendix has become significantly distended and in adults where larger amounts of fat and bowel gas make actually seeing the appendix technically difficult. Despite these limitations, in experienced hands sonographic imaging can often distinguish between appendicitis and other diseases with very similar symptoms such as inflammation of lymph nodes near the appendix or pain originating from other pelvic organs such as the ovaries or fallopian tubes.

In places where it is readily available, CT scan has become the diagnostic test of choice, especially in adults whose diagnosis is not obvious on history and physical. The use of CT in pregnant women and children is significantly limited, however, by concerns regarding radiation exposure. A properly performed CT scan with modern equipment has a detection rate (sensitivity) of over 95 per cent and a similar specificity.

Signs of appendicitis on CT scan include lack of contrast (oral dye) in the appendix and direct visualization of appendiceal enlargement (greater than 6 mm in diameter on cross section). The inflammation caused by appendicitis in the surrounding peritoneal fat (so called "fat stranding") can also be observed on CT, providing a mechanism to detect early appendicitis and a clue that appendicitis may be present even when the appendix is not well seen. Thus, diagnosis of appendicitis by CT is made more difficult in very thin patients and in children, both of whom tend to lack significant fat within the abdomen. The utility of CT scanning is made clear, however, by the impact it has had on negative appendectomy rates.

TREATMENT

The treatment begins by keeping the patient from eating or drinking anything, even water, in preparation for surgery. An intravenous drip is used to hydrate the patient. Antibiotics given intravenously such as cefuroxime and metronidazole may be administered early to help kill bacteria and thus reduce the spread of infection in the abdomen and postoperative complications in the abdomen or wound. Equivocal cases may become more difficult to assess with antibiotic treatment and benefit from serieal examinations. If the stomach is empty (no food in the past six hours) general anaesthesia is usually used. Otherwise, spinal anaesthesia may be used.

The surgical procedure for the removal of the appendix is called an *appendicectomy* (also known as an *appendectomy*). Often now the operation can be performed via a laparoscopic approach, or via three small incisions with a camera to visualize the area of interest in the abdomen. If the findings reveal suppurative appendicitis with complications such as rupture, abscess, adhesions, etc., conversion to open laparotomy may be necessary. An open laparotomy incision if required most often centers on the area of maximum tenderess, McBurney's Point, in the right lower quadrant. A transverse or a gridiron diagonal incision is used most commonly.

PROGNOSIS

When timely proper treatment is given, most appendicitis patients recover easily, but complications can occur if treatment is delayed or if peritonitis occurs. Recovery time depends on age, condition, complications, and other circumstances, including the amount of alcohol consumption, but usually is between 10 and 28 days. For young children (around 10 years old) the recovery takes three weeks.

The real possibility of life-threatening peritonitis is the reason why acute appendicitis warrants speedy evaluation and treatment. The patient may have to undergo a medical evacuation. Appendectomies have occasionally been performed in emergency conditions (i.e., outside of a proper hospital), when a timely medical evaluation was impossible.

Typical acute appendicitis responds quickly to appendectomy and occasionally will resolve spontaneously. If appendicitis resolves spontaneously, it remains controversial whether an elective interval appendectomy should be performed to prevent a recurrent episode of appendicitis. Atypical appendicitis (associated with suppurative appendicitis) is more difficult to diagnose and is more apt to be complicated even when operated early. In either condition prompt diagnosis and appendectomy yield the best results with full recovery in two to four weeks usually. Mortality and severe complications are unusual but do occur, especially if peritonitis persists and is untreated.

DRUG OVERDOSE

The term drug overdose (or simply overdose or OD) describes the ingestion or application of a drug or other substance in quantities greater than are recommended or generally practiced. An overdose is widely considered harmful and dangerous as it can result in death.

The word "overdose" implies that there is a safe dosage; therefore, the term is commonly only applied to drugs, not poison. Drug overdoses are sometimes caused intentionally to commit suicide or as self-harm, but many drug overdoses are accidental and are usually the result of either irresponsible behavior or the misreading of product labels. Other causes of overdose include use of multiple drugs with counter indications simultaneously (for instance, heroin/certain prescription pain medications and cocaine/amphetamines/alcohol) and use after a period of abstinence or unexpected purity of the drug consumed.

A common unintentional overdose in young children involves multi-vitamins containing iron. Iron is a component of the hemoglobin molecule in blood, used to transport oxygen to living cells. When taken in small amounts, iron allows the body to replenish hemoglobin, but in large amounts it causes severe pH imbalances in the body. If this overdose is not treated with chelation therapy, it can lead to death or permanent coma.

MISCONCEPTIONS

Deaths caused by adulterated drugs, most commonly heroin, are often incorrectly attributed to overdose.

SYMPTOMS

Symptoms of overdose occur in various forms:

- Exaggerated form of normal action (e.g., sleepiness on antiepileptics, hypoglycemia on insulin).
- Other effects due to chemical properties of the medication (e.g., metabolic acidosis in aspirin, liver failure due to paracetamol)
- Non-specific symptoms due to central nervous system irritation (e.g., confusion, vertigo, nausea, vomiting, delirium, seizures)

DIAGNOSIS

Diagnosis of an overdosed patient becomes easy when if the drug is known. However, it can be very difficult if the patient cannot (or refuses to) state what drug they have overdosed on. At times, certain symptoms and signs exhibited by the patient, or blood tests, can reveal the drug in question. Even without knowing the drug, most patients can be treated with general supportive measures.

In some instances, antidotes may be administered if there is sufficient indication that the patient has overdosed on a particular type of medication. Naloxone in opioids and flumazenil in benzodiazepines, are specific receptor antagonists and they reverse completely the effect of the poisoning drug.

FIRST AID

(i) Depressants

First aid can prevent a death from overdose of depressants, as it may take several hours for someone to die in these cases. The common drugs in this category include opiates (ie. heroin, morphine and methadone), alcohol, and certain prescription drugs (such as Benzodiazepines). Signs of overdose are those of a depressed central nervous system — slow, infrequent or shallow breathing, blue lips or fingernails, cold or pale skin, slow or faint pulse, snoring or gurgling noises, and the inability to be aroused from nodding off (unresponsiveness).

- The first step is to stay calm and try to get a response from the person by pinching the back of their arm, calling their name, or rubbing your knuckles against their chest.
- If there is no response, check to make sure their airway is not blocked and see if they are breathing.
- If breathing or pulse are not detectable, commence cardiopulmonary resuscitation. If these signs are present, roll the person in question on his/her side into the recovery position.
- Call an ambulance. Ideally, someone should call an ambulance immediately while another person evaluates the patient and performs CPR if necessary.

(ii) Stimulants

People can overdose on stimulants, such as amphetamines, and cocaine, with symptoms such as rapid heartbeat, muscle cramps, seizures, paranoia, psychosis, confusion, loss of control of movement, vomiting, lack of consciousness, and possibly cardiac arrest. It can lead to an often fatal condition known as excited delirium.

First aid in these cases involves staying with the person and helping them to remain calm. Move them to a quiet area, and where possible, apply a wet cloth to their neck or forehead. If unconscious, place them in the recovery position and call an ambulance.

BOWEL OBSTRUCTION

Bowel obstruction is a mechanical or functional obstruction of the intestines, preventing the normal transit of the products of digestion. It can occur at any level distal to the duodenum of the small intestine and is a medical emergency. Although many cases are not treated surgically, it is a surgical problem.

CAUSES

(i) Small bowel obstruction

Causes of small bowel obstruction include:

- Adhesions from previous abdominal surgery.
- Hernias containing bowel.
- Crohn's disease causing adhesions or inflammatory structures.
- Neoplasms, benign or malignant.
- Intussusception in children.
- Volvulus.
- Ischaemic strictures.
- Foreign bodies (e.g., gallstones in gallstone ileus, swallowed objects).
- Intestinal atresia.
- Carcinoid rare, preferred location: ileum.

(ii) Large bowel obstruction

Causes of large bowel obstruction include:

- Neoplasms.
- Hernias.
- Inflammatory bowel disease.
- Colonic volvulus (sigmoid, caecal, transverse colon).
- Faecal impaction.
- Colon atresia.
- Benign strictures (Diverticular Disease).

DIFFERENTIAL DIAGNOSIS

Differential diagnoses of bowel obstruction include:

- Ileus.
- Pseudo-obstruction or Ogilvie's syndrome.
- Intra-abdominal sepsis.
- Pneumonia or other systemic illness.

SIGNS AND SYMPTOMS

Depending on the level of obstruction, bowel obstruction can present with abdominal pain, abdominal distension, vomiting, fecal vomiting, and constipation. Obstruction may be due to causes within the bowel lumen, within the wall of the bowel, or external to the bowel (such as compression, entrapment or volvulus).

Bowel obstruction may be complicated by dehydration and electrolyte abnormalities due to vomiting; respiratory compromise from pressure on the diaphragm by a distended abdomen, or aspiration of vomitus; bowel ischaemia or perforation from prolonged distension or pressure from a foreign body.

In small bowel obstruction the pain tends to be colicky (cramping and intermittent) in nature, with spasms lasting a few minutes. The pain tends to be central and mid-abdominal. Vomiting occurs before constipation.

In large bowel obstruction the pain is felt lower in the abdomen and the spasms last longer. Constipation occurs earlier and vomiting may be less prominent. Proximal obstruction of the large bowel may present as small bowel obstruction.

DIAGNOSIS

The main diagnostic tools are blood tests, X-rays of the abdomen, CT scanning and/or ultrasound. If a mass is identified, biopsy may determine the nature of the mass. Radiological signs of bowel obstruction include bowel distension and the presence of multiple (more than six) gas-fluid levels on supine and erect abdominal radiographs. Contrast enema or small bowel series or CT scan can be used to define the level of obstruction, whether the obstruction is partial or complete, and to help define the cause of the obstruction.

TREATMENT

Some causes of bowel obstruction may resolve spontaneously; many require operative treatment. In adults, frequently the need for surgical intervention and the treatment of the causative lesion is required. In malignant large bowel obstruction, endoscopically placed self-expanding metal stents may be used to temporarily relieve the obstruction as a bridge to surgery; or as palliation.

(i) Small Bowel Obstruction

In the management of small bowel obstructions it is often said that "never let the sun rise or set on small-bowel obstruction"because they are sometimes fatal if treatment is delayed. Treatment for a small bowel obstruction is both non-surgical (conservative) and surgical.

Conservative treatment involves insertion of a nasogastric tube, correction of dehydration and electrolyte abnormalities. Opioid pain relievers may be used for patients with severe pain. Antiemetics may be administered if the patient is vomiting. Adhesive obstructions often settle without surgery. If obstruction is complete a surgery is required.

Small bowel obstruction caused by Crohn's disease, peritoneal carcinomatosis, sclerosing peritonitis, radiation enteritis and postpartum bowel obstruction are typically treated conservatively, i.e. without surgery. Conversely, a small bowel obstruction in a "virgin abdomen" (an abdomen that has not seen an operation) is almost never treated conservatively.

(ii) Bowel Obstruction in Children

Fetal and neonatal bowel obstructions are often caused by an intestinal atresia where there is a narrowing or absence of a part of the intestine. These atresias are often discovered before birth via a sonogram and treated with using laparotomy after birth. If the area affected is small then the surgeon may be able to remove the damaged portion and join the intestine back together. In instantances where the narrowing is longer, or the area is damaged and cannot be used for a period of time, a temporary stoma may be placed.

HEADACHE

In medical terminology headache is called *cephalgia* A headache is a condition of pain in the head; sometimes neck or upper back pain may also be interpreted as a headache. It ranks amongst the most common local pain complaints.

The vast majority of headaches are benign and self-limiting. Common causes are tension, migraine, eye strain, dehydration, low blood sugar, and sinusitis. Much rarer are headaches due to life-threatening conditions such as meningitis, encephalitis, cerebral aneurysms, extremely high blood pressure, and brain tumors. When the headache occurs in conjunction with a head injury the cause is usually quite evident. A large percentage of headaches among females are caused by ever-fluctuating estrogen during menstrual years. This can occur prior to, during or even midcycle menstruation.

Treatment of uncomplicated headache is usually symptomatic with over-the-counter painkillers such as aspirin, paracetamol (acetaminophen), or ibuprofen, although some specific forms of headaches (e.g., migraines) may demand other, more suitable treatment. It may be possible to relate the occurrence of a headache to other particular triggers such as stress or particular foods, which can then be avoided.

The brain in itself is not sensitive to pain, because it lacks pain-sensitive nerve fibers. Several areas of the head can hurt, including a network of nerves which extend over the scalp and certain nerves in the face, mouth, and throat. The meninges and the blood vessels do have pain perception. Headaches often result from traction to or irritation of the meninges and blood vessels. The muscles of the head may similarly be sensitive to pain.

TYPES OF HEADACHE

There are five types of headache: vascular, myogenic (muscle tension), cervicogenic, traction, and inflammatory.

(i) *Vascular*—The most common type of vascular headache is migraine. Migraine headaches are usually characterized by severe pain on one or both sides of the head, an upset stomach, and, for some people, disturbed vision. It is more common in women. While vascular changes are evident during a migraine, the cause of the headache is neurologic, not vascular. After migraine, the most common type of vascular headache is the "toxic" headache produced by fever. Other kinds of vascular headaches include cluster headaches, which cause repeated episodes of intense pain, and headaches resulting from high blood pressure (rare).

(ii) *Muscular/myogenic*—Muscular (or myogenic) headaches appear to involve the tightening or tensing of facial and neck muscles; they may radiate to the forehead. Tension headache is the most common form of myogenic headache.

(iii) *Cervicogenic*—Cervicogenic headaches occurs due to disorders of the neck, including the anatomical structures innervated by the cervical roots C1–C3. Cervical headache is often precipitated by neck movement and/or sustained awkward head positioning. It is often accompanied by restricted cervical range of motion, ipsilateral neck, shoulder, or arm pain of a rather vague non-radicular nature or, occasionally, arm pain of a radicular nature.

(iv) *Traction and Inflammatory*—Traction and inflammatory headaches are symptoms of other disorders, ranging from stroke to sinus infection. A headache may also be a symptom of sinusitis. Like other types of pain, headaches can serve as warning signals of more serious disorders. This is particularly true for headaches caused by inflammation, including those related to meningitis as well as those resulting from diseases of the sinuses, spine, neck, ears, and teeth.

DIAGNOSIS

While, statistically, headaches are most likely to be harmless and self-limiting, some specific headache syndromes may demand specific treatment or may be warning signals of more serious disorders. Some headache subtypes are characterized by a specific pattern of symptoms, and no further testing may be necessary, while others may prompt further diagnostic tests.

Headache associated with specific symptoms may warrant urgent medical attention, particularly sudden, severe headache or sudden headache associated with a stiff neck; headaches associated with fever, convulsions or accompanied by confusion or loss of consciousness; headaches following a blow to the head, or associated with pain in the eye or ear; persistent headache in a person with no previous history of headaches; and recurring headache in children.

The most important step in diagnosing a headache is for the physician to take a careful history and to examine the patient. In the majority of cases the diagnosis will be a "primary headache" which means that the headache, whilst unpleasant is not a occurring as a manifestation of a more serious condition. The main types of primary headache are tension headache, migraine and the trigeminal autonomic cephalgias of which cluster headache is an example. As it is often difficult for patients to recall the precise details regarding each headache, it is often useful for the sufferer to fill-out a "headache diary" detailing the characteristics of the headache. When the headache does not clearly fit into one of the recognized primary headache syndromes or when atypical symptoms or signs are present then further investigations are justified. Computed tomography (CT/CAT) scans of the brain or sinuses are commonly performed, or magnetic resonance imaging (MRI) in specific settings. Blood tests may help narrow down the differential diagnosis, but are rarely confirmatory of specific headache forms.

TREATMENT

Most of the headaches do not require medical attention, and respond with simple analgesia (painkillers) such as paracetamol/acetaminophen or members of the NSAID class such as aspirin/acetylsalicylic acid or ibuprofen.

In recurrent unexplained headaches, healthcare professionals may recommend keeping a "headache diary" with entries on type of headache, associated symptoms, precipitating and aggravating factors. This may reveal specific patterns, such as an association with medication, menstruation or absenteeism or with certain foods. It was reported in March 2007 by two separate teams of researchers that stimulating the brain with implanted electrodes appears to help ease the pain of cluster headaches.

MIGRAINE

Migraine is a neurological disease that can cause a wide range of symptoms during an attack. The most commonly thought of symptom is headache.

It is widespread in the population. In the U.S., 18 per cent of women and 6 per cent of men report having had at least one migraine episode in the previous year, with seriousness ranging from an annoyance to a life-threatening and/or daily experience. Treatments are typically expensive. Periodic or unpredictable disability can cause poverty due to patients' inability to hold down a job.

Usually migraine causes episodes of severe or moderate headache which is often one-sided and pulsating lasting from several hours to three days, accompanied by gastrointestinal upsets, such as nausea and vomiting, and a heightened sensitivity to bright lights (photophobia) and noise (phonophobia). Approximately one third of people who experience migraine get a preceding aura. The word migraine is French in origin and comes from the Greek hemicrania, as does the Old English term megrim. Literally, hemicrania means "half (the) head".

Migraines' secondary characteristics are inconsistent. Triggers precipitating a particular episode of migraine vary widely. The efficacy of the simplest treatment, applying warmth or coolness to the affected area of the head, varies between persons, sometimes worsening the migraine. A particular migraine rescue drug may sometimes work and sometimes not work in the same patient. Some migraine types don't have pain or may manifest symptoms in parts of the body other than the head.

TYPES OF MIGRAIN

There are several types of migrain which are mentioned below:

(i) *Defining Severity of Pain*—In addition to classifying the type of headache, intensity of pain on a verbal 4 point scale:

- 0 no pain
- 1 mild pain 'does not interfere with usual activities'
- 2 moderate pain 'inhibits, but does not wholly prevent usual activities'
- 3 severe pain 'prevents all activities'

(ii) *Migraine Without Aura*—This is the most commonly seen form of migraine; patients who primarily suffer from migraine without aura may also have attacks of migraine with aura. It is a recurrent headache disorder manifesting in attacks lasting 4-72 hours. Typical characteristics of the headache are unilateral location, pulsating quality, moderate or severe intensity, aggravation by routine physical activity and association with nausea and/or photophobia and phonophobia.

(iii) *Migraine With Aura*—This is the second most commonly seen form of migraine: patients who primarily suffer from migraine with aura may also have attacks of migraine without aura. It is a recurrent disorder manifesting in attacks of reversible focal neurological symptoms that usually develop gradually over 5-20 minutes and last for less than 60 minutes.

(iv) *Basilar Type Migraine*—Basilar type migraine (BTM), formerly known as basilar artery migraine (BAM) or basilar migraine (BM), is an uncommon type of complicated migraine with symptoms that result from brainstem dysfunction. Serious episodes of BTM can lead to stroke, coma, or even death. The use of triptans and other vasoconstrictors as abortive treatments in BTM is contraindicated. Abortive treatments for BTM often focus on vasodilation and restoration of normal blood flow to the vertebrobasilar territory and subsequent return of normal brainstem function.

(v) *Familial Hemiplegic Migraine*—Familial hemiplegic migraine 'FHM' is a type of migraine with a possible polygenetic component. These migraine attacks may last 4-72 hours and are apparently caused by ion channel mutations, three types of which have been identified to date. Patients who experience this syndrome have relatively typical migraine headaches preceded and/or accompanied by reversible limb weakness on one side as well as visual, sensory or speech difficulties. A non-familial form exists as well, "sporadic hemiplegic migraine" (SHM). It is often difficult to make the diagnosis between basilar-type migraine and hemiplegic migraine. When making the differential diagnosis is difficult, the deciding symptom is often the motor weakness or unilateral paralysis which can occur in FHM or SHM. While basilar-type migraine can present with tingling or numbness, true motor weakness and/or paralysis occur only in hemiplegic migraine.

(vi) *Abdominal Migraine*—Abdominal migraine is a recurrent disorder of unknown origin which occurs mainly in children. It is characterised by episodes of moderate to severe central abdominal pain lasting 1-72 hours. There is usually associated nausea and vomiting but the child is entirely well between attacks. Most children with abdominal migraine will develop migraine headache later in life and the two may co-exist during adolescence.

(vii) *Acephalgic Migraine*—Acephalgic migraine is a neurological syndrome. It is a variant of migraine in which the patient may experience aura symptoms such as scintillating scotoma, nausea, photophobia, hemiparesis and other migraine symptoms but does not experience headache. Acephalgic migraine is also referred to as amigrainous migraine, ocular migraine, or optical migraine. Sufferers of acephalgic migraine are more likely than the general population to develop classical migraine with headache. The prevention and treatment of acephalgic migraine is broadly the same as for classical migraine. However, because of the absence of "headache", diagnosis of acephalgic migraine is apt to be significantly delayed and the risk of misdiagnosis significantly increased.

SIGNS AND SYMPTOMS

The signs and symptoms of migraine vary among patients. Therefore, what a patient experiences before, during and after an attack cannot be defined exactly. The four phases of a migraine attack listed below are common but not necessarily experienced by all migraine sufferers. Additionally, the phases experienced and the symptoms experienced during them can vary from one migraine attack to another in the same migraineur:

(i) *Prodrome Phase* — Prodromal symptoms occur in 40 to 60 per cent of migraineurs. This phase may consist of altered mood, irritability, depression or euphoria, fatigue, yawning, excessive sleepiness, craving for certain food (e.g., chocolate), stiff muscles (especially in the neck), constipation or diarrhea, increased urination, and other vegetative symptoms. These symptoms usually precede the headache phase of the migraine attack by several hours or days, and experience teaches the patient or observant family how to detect that a migraine attack is near.

(ii) *Aura Phase* — For the 20-30 per cent of migraineurs who suffer migraine with aura, this aura comprises focal neurological phenomena that precede or accompany the attack. They appear gradually over 5 to 20 minutes and generally last fewer than 60 minutes. The headache phase of the migraine attack usually begins within 60 minutes of the end of the aura phase, but it is sometimes delayed up to several hours, and it can be missing entirely. Symptoms of migraine aura can be visual, sensory, or motor in nature. Visual aura is the most common of the neurological events. There is a disturbance of vision consisting usually of unformed flashes of white and/or black or rarely of multicolored lights (photopsia) or formations of dazzling zigzag lines (scintillating scotoma; often arranged like the battlements of a castle, hence the alternative terms "fortification spectra" or "teichopsia"). Some patients complain of blurred or shimmering or cloudy vision, as though they were look□ing through thick or smoked glass, or, in some cases, tunnel vision and hemianopsia. The somatosensory aura of migraine consists of digitolingual or cheiro-oral paresthesias, a feeling of pins-and-needles experienced in the hand and arm as well as in the ipsilateral nose-mouth area. Paresthesia migrate up the arm and then extend to involve the face, lips and tongue. Other symptoms of the aura phase can include auditory or olfactory hallucinations, temporary dysphasia, vertigo, tingling or numbness of the face and extremities, and hypersensitivity to touch.

(iii) *Pain Phase* —The typical migraine headache is unilateral, throbbing, moderate to severe and can be aggravated by physical activity. Not all of these features are necessary. The pain may be bilateral at the onset or start on one side and become generalized, and usually alternates sides from one attack to the next. The onset is usually gradual. The pain peaks and then subsides, and usually lasts between 4 and 72 hours in adults and 1 and 48 hours in children. The frequency of attacks is extremely variable, from a few in a lifetime to several times a week, and the average migraineur experiences from one to three headaches a month. The head pain varies greatly in intensity. The pain of migraine is invariably accompanied by other features. Nausea occurs in almost 90 percent of patients, while vomiting occurs in about one third of patients. Many patients experience sensory hyperexcitability manifested by photophobia, phonophobia, osmophobia and seek a dark and quiet room. Blurred vision, nasal stuffiness, diarrhea, polyuria, pallor or sweating may be noted during the headache phase. There may be localized edema of the scalp or face, scalp tenderness, prominence of a vein or artery in the temple, or stiffness and tenderness of the neck. Impairment of concentration and mood are common. Lightheadedness, rather than true vertigo and a feeling of faintness may occur. The extremities tend to be cold and moist.

(iv) *Postdrome Phase* —The patient may feel tired, "washed out", irritable, or listless and may have impaired concentration, scalp tenderness or mood changes. Some people feel unusually refreshed or euphoric after an attack, whereas others note depression and malaise. Often, some of the minor headache phase symptoms may continue, such as loss of appetite, photophobia, and lightheadedness.

DIAGNOSIS

Migraines are underdiagnosedand misdiagnosed.The International Headache Society, points out that the diagnosis of migraine without aura can be made following criteria, the "5, 4, 3, 2, 1 criteria":

- 5 or more attacks
- 4 hours to 3 days in duration
- 2 or more of - unilateral location, pulsating quality, moderate to severe pain, aggravation by or avoidance of routine physical activity
- 1 or more accompanying symptoms - nausea and/or vomiting,photophobia, phonophobia

For migraine with aura, only two attacks are required to justify the diagnosis.

The mnemonic POUNDing (Pulsating, duration of 4-72 hOurs, Unilateral, Nausea, Disabling) can help diagnose migraine.

If 4 of the 5 criteria are met, then the positive likelihood ratio for diagnosing migraine is 24. The presence of either disability, nausea or sensitivity, can diagnose migraine with: sensitivity of 81 per cent, specificity of 75 per cent.

TRIGGERS

Triggers may be categorized as behavioral, environmental, infectious, dietary, chemical, or hormonal. In the medical literature, these factors are known as 'precipitants.' Migraine attacks may be triggered by:

- Allergic reactions
- Bright lights, loud noises, and certain odors or perfumes
- Physical or emotional stress
- Changes in sleep patterns
- Smoking or exposure to smoke
- Skipping meals
- Alcohol or caffeine
- Menstrual cycle fluctuations, birth control pills
- Tension headaches
- Foods containing tyramine (red wine, aged cheese, smoked fish, chicken livers, figs, and some beans), monosodium glutamate (MSG), or nitrates (like bacon, hot dogs, and salami)
- Other foods such as chocolate, nuts, peanut butter, avocado, banana, citrus, onions, dairy products, and fermented or pickled foods.·

Many people report that one or more dietary, physical, hormonal, emotional, or environmental factors precipitate their migraines. The most-often reported triggers include: pesticides (sprayed fruits/vegetables), perfumes or fragrances (30 per cent of sufferers) stress, over-illumination or glare, alcohol, foods, too much or too little sleep, and weather. Some women experience migraines in conjunction with monthly menstrual cycles.

WEATHER

Several studies have found some migraines are triggered by

changes in weather. Temperature mixed with humidity. High humidity plus high or low temperature was the biggest cause.

Hair Wash Headache

Another trigger for Migraine has been proposed by Dr.K.Ravishankar, a neurologist and headache specialist from India. He reported an unusual trigger for migraine seen among women, Hair Wash Headache. It is described as a migraine headache that originates with a head bath while sitting on the floor, or hanging the head downwards for an extended period of time.

TREATMENT

Conventional treatment focuses on three areas: trigger avoidance, symptomatic control, and preventive drugs. Patients who experience migraines often find that the recommended treatments are not 100 per cent effective at preventing migraines, and sometimes may not be effective at all. Children and adolescents, are often first given drug treatment, but the value of diet modification should not be overlooked. The simple task of starting a diet journal to help modify the intake of trigger foods like hot dogs, chocolate, cheese and ice cream could help alleviate symptoms.

PHYSICAL THERAPY

Most of the physicians believe that the frequency of migraines can be reducing by doing exercise for 15-20 minutes per day. Massage therapy and physical therapy are often very effective forms of treatment to reduce the frequency and intensity of migraines. However, it is important to be treated by a well-trained therapist who understands the pathophysiology of migraines. Deep massage can 'trigger' a migraine attack in a person who is not used to such treatments. It is advisable to start sessions as short in duration and then work up to longer treatments. Frequent migraines can leave the sufferer with a stiff neck which can cause stress headaches that can then exacerbate the migraines.

TOOTHACHE

In medical terminology toothache is also known as *odontalgia.* Toothache is an aching pain in or around a tooth. In most cases toothaches are caused by problems in the tooth or jaw, such as cavities, gum disease, the emergence of wisdom teeth, a cracked tooth, jaw disease, or exposed tooth root. Causes of a toothache may also be a symptom of diseases of the heart, such as angina or a myocardial infarction, due to referred pain. After having one or more teeth extracted a condition known as dry socket can develop, leading to extreme pain. The severity of a toothache can range from a mild discomfort to excruciating pain, which can be experienced either chronically or sporadically. This pain can often be aggravated somewhat by chewing or by hot or cold temperatures. An oral examination complete with X-rays can help discover the cause. Severe pain may be considered a dental emergency.

Atypical odontalgia is a type of toothache present in apparently normal teeth. The pain, generally dull, often moves from one tooth to another for a period of 4 months to several years. This is most commonly occurs in middle-aged women.

COMMON COLD (ACUTE VIRAL NASOPHARYNGITIS)

Acute viral nasopharyngitis, or acute coryza, usually known as the common cold, is a highly contagious, viral infectious disease of the upper respiratory system, primarily caused by picornaviruses or coronaviruses.

Common symptoms are sore throat, runny nose, nasal congestion, sneezing and cough; sometimes accompanied by muscle aches, fatigue, malaise, headache, muscle weakness, or loss of appetite. Fever and extreme exhaustion are more usual in influenza. The symptoms of a cold usually resolve after about one week, but can last up to 14 days. Symptoms may be more severe in infants and young children. Although the disease is generally mild and self-limiting, patients with common colds often seek professional medical help, use over-the-counter drugs, and may miss school or work days. No vaccines are available: the primary method to prevent infection is hand-washing to minimize person-to-person transmission of the virus. There are no antiviral drugs approved to treat or cure the infection.

VIRUS

Common colds are most often caused by infection by a rhinovirus, a type of picornavirus. Other viruses causing colds are coronavirus, human parainfluenza viruses, human respiratory syncytial virus, adenoviruses, enteroviruses, or metapneumovirus.

TRANSMISSION

The common cold virus is transmitted between people by one of two ways:

- in aerosol form generated by coughing, sneezing, or
- from contact with the saliva or nasal secretions of an infected person, either directly or from contaminated surfaces.

The infectious period (time during which an infected person can infect others) begins about one day before symptoms begin, and continues for the first five days of the illness. Symptoms, however, are not necessary for viral shedding or transmission, as a percentage of asymptomatic subjects exhibit viruses in nasal swabs.

The virus enters the cells of the lining of the nasopharynx (the area between the nose and throat), and rapidly multiplies. The major entry point is normally the nose, but can also be the eyes (in this case drainage into the nasopharynx would occur through the Nasolacrimal duct).

SIGN AND SYMPTOMS

After initial infection, the viral replication cycle begins within 8 to 12 hours. Symptoms can occur shortly thereafter, and usually begin within 2 to 5 days after infection, although occasionally in as little as 10 hours after infection. The initial indication of a cold is often a sore or scratchy throat. Other common symptoms are runny nose, congestion, sneezing and cough. Sometimes muscle aches, fatigue, malaise, headache, weakness, or loss of appetite also occur. Colds occasionally cause fever and can sometimes lead to extreme exhaustion. (However, these symptoms are more usual in influenza, and can differentiate the two infections.) The symptoms of a cold usually resolve after about one week, but can last up to 14 days, with a cough lasting longer than other symptoms. Symptoms may be more severe in infants and young children, and may include fever and hives.

TREATMENT

Treatment is limited to symptomatic supportive options, maximizing the comfort of the patient, and limiting complications and harmful sequelae. The most reliable treatment is a combination of fluids and plenty of rest.

The common cold is self-limiting, and the host's immune system effectively deals with the infection. Within a few days, the body's humoral immune response begins producing specific antibodies that can prevent the virus from infecting cells. Additionally, as part of the cell-mediated immune response, leukocytes destroy the virus through phagocytosis and destroy infected cells to prevent further viral replication. In healthy, immunocompetent individuals, the common cold resolves in seven days on average.

ANTIBIOTICS

Antibiotics do not work effectively in common cold. Their use in cases of common cold infection is ineffective and may contribute to antibiotic resistance of bacteria present in the patient's body.

HERBAL REMEDIES

Herbal teas, such as chamomile tea, or lemon or ginger root tisanes may soothe some symptoms and comfort the patient. Liquorice and garlic preparations have been suggested as treatments for the common cold, although efficacy is unproven.

BACK PAIN

Back pain (also known "dorsalgia") is pain felt in the back that may originate from the muscles, nerves, bones, joints or other structures in the spine.

The pain may be have a sudden onset or it can be a chronic pain, it can be felt constantly or intermittently, stay in one place or refer or radiate to other areas. It may be a dull ache, or a sharp or piercing or burning sensation. The pain may be felt in the neck (and might radiate into the arm and hand), in the upper back, or in the low back, (and might radiate into the leg or foot), and may include symptoms other than pain, such as weakness, numbness or tingling.

Back pain is one of humanity's most frequent complaints. In the U.S., acute low back pain (also called lumbago) is the fifth most common reason for all physician visits. About nine out of ten adults experience back pain at some point in their life, and five out of ten working adults have back pain every year.

The spine is a complex interconnecting network of nerves, joints, muscles, tendons and ligaments, and all are capable of producing pain. Large nerves that originate in the spine and go to the legs and arms can make pain radiate to the extremities.

ASSOCIATED CONDITIONS

Back pain can be a sign of a serious medical problem, although this is not most frequently the underlying cause:

- Typical warning signs of a potentially life-threatening problem are bowel and/or bladder incontinence or progressive weakness in the legs. Patients with these symptoms should seek immediate medical care.
- Severe back pain (such as pain that is bad enough to interrupt sleep) that occurs with other signs of severe illness (e.g. fever, unexplained weight loss) may also indicate a serious underlying medical condition.

- Back pain that occurs after a trauma, such as a car accident or fall, should also be promptly evaluated by a medical professional to check for a fracture or other injury.
- Back pain in individuals with medical conditions that put them at high risk for a spinal fracture, such as osteoporosis or multiple myeloma, also warrants prompt medical attention.

In general, however, back pain does not usually require immediate medical intervention. The vast majority of episodes of back pain are self-limiting and non-progressive. Most back pain syndromes are due to inflammation, especially in the acute phase, which typically lasts for two weeks to three months.

UNDERLYING CAUSES

Transient back pain is likely one of the first symptoms of *influenza. Muscle strains* (pulled muscles) are commonly identified as the cause of back pain, as are muscle imbalances. Pain from such an injury often remains as long as the muscle imbalances persist. The muscle imbalances cause a mechanical problem with the skeleton, building up pressure at points along the spine, which causes the pain.

Another cause of acute low back pain is a *Meniscoid Occlusion.* The more mobile regions of the spine, such as the facet joints, have invaginations of their synovial membranes that act as a cushion to help the bones move over each other smoothly. The synovial membrane is well supplied with blood and nerves. When these become pinched or trapped sudden severe pain may result. The pinching causes the membrane to become inflamed, causing greater pressure and ongoing pain. Symptoms include severe low back pain that may be accompanied by muscle spasm, pain with walking, concentration of pain to one side, but no radiculopathy (radiating pain down buttock and leg). Relief should be felt with flexion (bending forward),and exacerbated with extension (bending backward).

When back pain lasts more than three months, or if there is more radicular pain (sciatica) than back pain, a more specific diagnosis can usually be made. There are several common causes of back pain: for adults under age 50, these include spinal disc herniation and degenerative disc disease or isthmic spondylolisthesis; in adults over age 50, common causes also include osteoarthritis (degenerative joint disease) and spinal stenosis,trauma, cancer, infection, fractures, and inflammatory disease. Non-anatomical factors can also contribute to or cause back pain, such as stress,repressed anger,or depression. Even if there is an anatomical cause for the pain, if depression is present it should also be treated concurrently.

TREATMENT

In the treatment of backpain, the main focus should be on maximal reduction in pain intensity as rapidly as possible; restoring the individual's ability to function in everyday activities; helping the patient cope with residual pain; assessing`for side-effects of therapy; and facilitating the patient's passage through the legal and socioeconomic impediments to recovery. For many, the goal is to keep the pain to a manageable level to progress with rehabilitation, which then can lead to long term pain relief. Also, for some people the goal is to use non-surgical therapies to manage the pain and avoid major surgery, while for others surgery may be the quickest way to feel better.

Not all treatments work for all conditions or for all individuals with the same condition, and many find that they need to try several treatment options to determine what works best for them. The present stage of the condition (acute or chronic) is also a determining factor in the choice of treatment. Only a minority of back pain patients (most estimates are 1per cent - 10 per cent) require surgery.

CONSERVATIVE TREATMENT

- Heat therapy is useful for back spasms or other conditions. A meta-analysis of studies by the Cochrane Collaboration concluded that heat therapy can reduce symptoms of acute and sub-acute low-back pain. Some patients find that moist heat works best (e.g., a hot bath or whirlpool) or continuous low-level heat (e.g., a heat wrap that stays warm for 4 to 6 hours). Cold therapy (e.g., ice or cold pack application) may be effective at relieving back pain in some cases.

- Use of medications, such as muscle relaxants, narcotics, non-steroidal anti-inflammatory drugs (NSAIDs/NSAIAs) or paracetamol (acetaminophen). A meta-analysis of randomized controlled trials by the Cochrane Collaboration found that injection therapy, usually with corticosteroids, does not appear to help regardless of whether the injection is facet joint, epidural or a local injection.
- Herbal analgesics may also be effective.
- Exercises can be an effective approach, particularly when done under supervision of a professional such as a physical therapist. Generally, some form of consistent stretching and exercise is believed to be an essential component of most back treatment programs. However, one study found that exercise is also effective for chronic back pain, but not for acute pain. According to another study back-mobilizing exercises in acute settings are less effective than continuation of ordinary activities as tolerated.
- Physical therapy and exercise, including stretching and strengthening (with specific focus on the muscles which support the spine), often learned with the help of a health professional, such as a physical therapist. Physical therapy may be especially effective when part of a 'work hardening' program, or 'back school'.
- Massage therapy, especially from an experienced therapist, may help. Acupressure or pressure point massage may be more beneficial than classic (Swedish) massage.

- Body Awareness Therapy such as the Feldenkrais Method has been studied in relation to Fibromyalgia and chronic pain and studies have indicated positive effects. Organized exercise programs using these therapies have been developed.
- Manipulation, as provided by an appropriately trained and qualified chiropractor, osteopath, physical therapist, or a physiatrist. Studies of the effect of manipulation suggest that this approach has a small benefit similar to other therapies and superior to placebo.
- Acupuncture has a small benefit for chronic back pain. The Cochrane Collaboration concluded that "for chronic low-back pain, acupuncture is more effective for pain relief and functional improvement than no treatment or sham treatment immediately after treatment and in the short-term only. Acupuncture is not more effective than other conventional and alternative treatments."
- Education, and attitude adjustment to focus on psychological or emotional causes - respondent-cognitive therapy and progressive relaxation therapy can reduce chronic pain.
- Most people will benefit from assessing any ergonomic or postural factors that may contribute to their back pain, such as improper lifting technique, poor posture, or poor support from their mattress or office chair, etc. Although this recommendation has not been tested, this intervention is a part of many 'back schools' which do help.

SURGERY

Surgery may sometimes be appropriate for patients with:

- Lumbar disc herniation or degenerative disc disease;
- Spinal stenosis from lumbar disc herniation, degenerative joint disease, or spondylolisthesis;
- Scoliosis;
- Compression fracture.

TRAVEL SIKCNESS

Motion sickness or kinetosis is a condition in which a disagreement exists between visually perceived movement and the vestibular system's sense of movement. Depending on the cause it can also be referred to as seasickness, carsickness, simulation sickness, airsickness, or space sickness.

The most common symptoms of motion sickness are dizziness, fatigue, and nausea. Sopite syndrome is also a side effect of motion sickness. In fact, nausea in Greek means seasickness (naus means ship). If the motion causing nausea is not resolved, the sufferer will frequently vomit. Unlike ordinary sickness, vomiting in motion sickness tends not to relieve the nausea.

About 33 per cent of people are susceptible to motion sickness even in mild circumstances such as being on a boat in calm water, although nearly 66 per cent of people are susceptible in more severe conditions. Approximately 50 per cent of the astronauts in the U.S. space program have suffered from space sickness.

Motion sickness on the sea can result from being in the berth of a rolling boat without being able to see the horizon. Sudden jerky movements tend to be worse for provoking motion sickness than slower smooth ones, because they disrupt the fluid balance more.[citation needed] A "corkscrewing" boat will upset more people than one that is gliding smoothly across the oncoming waves. Cars driving rapidly around winding roads or up and down a series of hills will upset more people than cars that are moving over smooth, straight roads. Looking down into one's lap to consult a map or attempting to read a book while a passenger in a car may also bring on motion sickness.

The most common hypothesis for the cause of motion sickness is that it evolved as a defense mechanism against neurotoxins.[6] The area postrema in the brain is responsible for inducing vomiting when poisons are detected, and for resolving conflicts between vision and balance. When feeling motion but not seeing it (for example, in a ship with no windows), the inner ear transmits to the brain that it senses motion, but the eyes tell the brain that everything is still. As a result of the disconcordance, the brain will come to the conclusion that one of them is hallucinating and further conclude that the hallucination is due to poison ingestion. The brain responds by inducing vomiting, to clear the supposed toxin.

KINDS OF TRAVEL SICKNESS

(i) *Airsickness*—Airsickness is a sensation which is induced by air travel. It is a specific form of motion sickness, and is considered a normal response in healthy individuals. Airsickness occurs when the central nervous system receives conflicting messages from the body (including the inner ear, eyes and muscles) affecting balance and equilibrium.

(ii) *Sea-sickness*—Seasickness is a form of motion sickness characterized by a feeling of nausea and, in extreme cases, vertigo experienced after spending time on a craft on water. It is typically brought on by the rocking motion of the craft.

(iii) *Simulation Sickness*—Simulation sickness, or simulator sickness, is a condition where a person exhibits symptoms similar to motion sickness caused by playing computer/simulation/video games.

The most common theory for the cause of simulation sickness is that the illusion of motion created by the virtual world, combined with the absence of motion detected by the inner ear, causes the area postrema in the brain to infer that one is hallucinating and further conclude that the hallucination is due to poison ingestion. The brain responds by inducing nausea and vomiting, to clear the supposed toxin.

(iii) *Space Sicknesss*— Space sickness was effectively unknown during the earliest spaceflights, as these were undertaken in very cramped conditions; it seems to be aggravated by being able to freely move around, and so is more common in larger spacecraft. Around 60% of all Space Shuttle astronauts currently experience it on their first flight; the first case is now suspected to be Gherman Titov, in August, 1961 onboard Vostok 2, who reported dizziness and nausea. However, the first significant cases were in early Apollo flights; Frank Borman on Apollo 8 and Rusty Schweickart on Apollo 9. Both experienced identifiable and reasonably severe symptoms — in the latter case causing the mission plan to be modified

TREATMENT

Several methods of cures and prevention for motion sickness have been proposed.

Natural Method

One common suggestion is to simply look out of the window of the moving vehicle and to gaze toward the horizon in the direction of travel. This helps to re-orient the inner sense of balance by providing a visual reaffirmation of motion.

In the night, or in a ship without windows, it is helpful to simply close one's eyes, or if possible, take a nap. This resolves the input conflict between the eyes and the inner ear. Napping also helps prevent psychogenic effects (i.e. the effect of sickness being magnified by thinking about it). Fresh, cool air can also relieve motion sickness slightly, although it is likely this is related to avoiding foul odors which can worsen nausea.

Chemical Method

Over-the-counter and prescription medications are readily available, such as Dramamine (dimenhydrinate) and Bonine/ Antivert (meclizine). Scopolamine is effective and is sometimes used in the form of transdermal patches (1.5 mg) or as a newer tablet form (0.4 mg).

Interestingly, many pharmacological treatments which are effective for nausea and vomiting in some medical conditions may not be effective for motion sickness. Ginger root is a mild anti-emetic and sucking on crystallized ginger or sipping ginger tea can help to relieve the nausea.

HERNIA

A hernia occurs when an organ or tissue squeezes through a hole or a weak spot in a surrounding muscle or connective tissue called fascia. The hernia has three parts: the *orifice* through which it herniates, the *hernial sac*, and its *contents*.

A hernia may be likened to a failure in the sidewall of a pneumatic tire. The tire's inner tube behaves like the organ and the side wall like the body cavity wall providing the restraint. A weakness in the sidewall allows a bulge to develop, which can become a split, allowing the inner tube to protrude, and leading to the eventual failure of the tire. By far most hernias develop in the abdomen, when a weakness in the abdominal wall evolves into a localized hole, or "defect", through which adipose tissue, or abdominal organs covered with peritoneum, may protrude. Another common hernia involves the intervertebral disc, and causes back pain or sciatica.

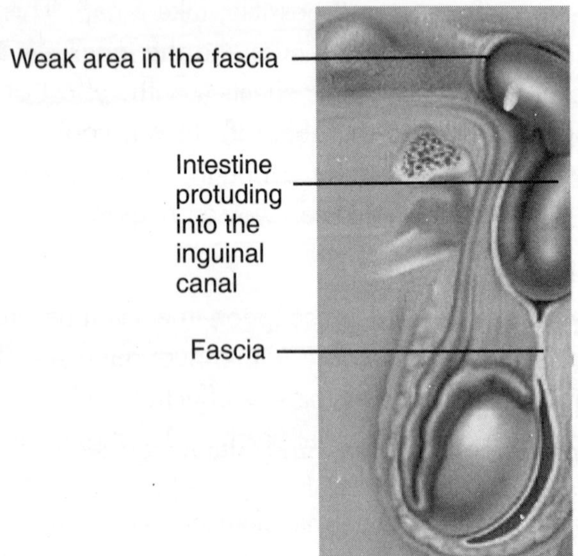

Fig. 36.2: *Hernia.*

Hernias may present either with pain at the site, a visible or palpable lump, or in some cases by more vague symptoms resulting from pressure on an organ which has become "stuck" in the hernia, sometimes leading to organ dysfunction. Fatty tissue usually enters a hernia first, but it may be followed by or accompanied by an organ. Most of the time, hernias develop when pressure in the compartment of the residing organ is increased, and the boundary is weak or weakened.

- Weakening of containing membranes or muscles is usually *congenital* (which explains part of the tendency of hernias to run in families), and increases with *age* (for example, degeneration of the annulus fibrosus of the intervertebral disc), but it may be on the basis of other *illnesses*, such as Ehlers-Danlos syndrome or Marfan syndrome, *stretching* of muscles during pregnancy, losing weight in obese people, etc., or because of *scars* from previous surgery.
- Many conditions chronically increase intra-abdominal pressure, (pregnancy, ascites, COPD, dyschezia, benign prostatic hypertrophy) and hence abdominal hernias are very frequent. Increased intracranial pressure can cause parts of the brain to herniate through narrowed portions of the cranial cavity or through the foramen magnum. Increased pressure on the intervertebral discs, as produced by heavy lifting or lifting with improper technique, increases the risk of herniation.

CLASSIFICATION OF HERNIA

Hernias can be classified according to their anatomical location. These are:

(i) abdominal hernias
(ii) diaphragmatic hernias and hiatal hernias (for example, paraesophageal hernia of the stomach)
(iii) pelvic hernias, for example, obturator hernia
(iv) hernias of the nucleus pulposus of the intervertebral discs
(v) intracranial hernias

Each of the above hernias may be characterised by several aspects:

- Congenital or acquired—congenital hernias occur prenatally or in the first year(s) of life, and are caused by a congenital defect, whereas acquired hernias develop later on in life. However, this may be on the basis of a locus minoris resistentiae (Lat. place of least resistance) that is congenital, but only becomes symptomatic later on in life, when degeneration and increased stress (for example, increased abdominal pressure from coughing in COPD) provoke the hernia.
- Complete or incomplete—for example, the stomach may partially herniate into the chest, or completely.
- Internal or external—external ones herniate to the outside world, whereas internal hernias protrude from their normal compartment to another (for example, mesenteric hernias).
- Intraparietal hernia—hernia that does not reach all the way to the subcutis, but only to the musculoaponeurotic layer. An example is a Spigelian hernia. Intraparietal hernias may produces less obvious bulging, and may be less easily detected on clinical examination.
- Bilateral—in this case, simultaneous repair may be considered, sometimes even with a giant prosthetic reinforcement.
- Reducible or irreducible (also known as incarcerated)—the hernial contents can or cannot be returned to their normal site with simple manipulation. If irreducible, hernias can develop several complications (hence, they can be complicated or uncomplicated):
- Strangulation—pressure on the hernial contents may compromise blood supply (especially veins, with their low pressure, are sensitive, and venous congestion often results) and cause ischemia, and later necrosis and gangrene, which may become fatal.
- Obstruction—for example, when a part of the bowel herniates, bowel contents can no longer pass the obstruction.

This results in cramps, and later on vomiting, ileus, absence of flatus and absence of defecation. These signs mandate urgent surgery. Another complication arises when the herniated organ itself, or surrounding organs start dysfunctioning (for example, sliding hernia of the stomach causing heartburn, lumbar disc hernia causing sciatic nerve pain, etc.).

Other Types of Hernia

The most common types are inguinal, incisional, femoral, umbilical and hiatal.

(i) Individual hernias—A sportman's hernia is a syndrome characterized by chronic groin pain in athletes and a dilated superficial ring of the inguinal canal, although a true hernia is not present.

(ii) Inguinal hernia—By far the most common hernias (up to 75 per cent of all abdominal hernias) are the so-called inguinal hernias. For a thorough understanding of inguinal hernias, much insight is needed in the anatomy of the inguinal canal. Inguinal hernias are further divided into the more common indirect inguinal hernia (2/3, depicted here), in which the inguinal canal is entered via a congenital weakness at its entrance (the internal inguinal ring), and the direct inguinal hernia type (1/3), where the hernia contents push through a weak spot in the back wall of the inguinal canal. Inguinal hernias are more common in men than women while femoral hernias are more common in women.

(iii) Femoral hernia—Femoral hernias occur just below the inguinal ligament, when abdominal contents pass into the weak area at the posterior wall of the femoral canal. They can be hard to distinguish from the inguinal type (especially when ascending cephalad): however, they generally appear more rounded, and, in contrast to inguinal hernias, there is a strong female preponderance in femoral hernias. The incidence of strangulation in femoral hernias is high. Repair techniques are similar for femoral and inguinal hernia.

(iv) Umbilical hernia—Umbilical hernias are especially common in infants of African descent, and occur more in boys. They involve protrusion of intraabdominal contents through a weakness at the site of passage of the umbilical cord through the abdominal wall. These hernias often resolve spontaneously. Umbilical hernias in adults are largely acquired, and are more frequent in obese or pregnant women. Abnormal decussation of fibers at the linea alba may contribute.

(v) Incisional hernia—An incisional hernia occurs when the defect is the result of an incompletely healed surgical wound. When these occur in median laparotomy incisions in the linea alba, they are termed ventral hernias. These can be the most frustrating and difficult to treat, as the repair utilizes already attenuated tissue.

(vi) Diaphragmatic hernia—Higher in the abdomen, an (internal) "diaphragmatic hernia" results when part of the stomach or intestine protrudes into the chest cavity through a defect in the diaphragm.

A hiatus hernia is a particular variant of this type, in which the normal passageway through which the esophagus meets the stomach (esophageal hiatus) serves as a functional "defect", allowing part of the stomach to (periodically) "herniate" into the chest. Hiatus hernias may be either "*sliding*," in which the gastroesophageal junction itself slides through the defect into the chest, or non-sliding (also known as *para-esophageal*), in which case the junction remains fixed while another portion of the stomach moves up through the defect. Non-sliding or para-esophageal hernias can be dangerous as they may allow the stomach to rotate and obstruct.

Complications

Complications may arise post-operation, including rejection of the mesh that is used to repair the hernia. In the event of a mesh rejection, the mesh will very likely need to be removed. Mesh rejection can be detected by obvious, sometimes localised swelling and pain around the mesh area. Continuous discharge from the scar is likely for a while after the mesh has been removed.

An untreated hernia may complicate by:

- Inflammation
- Irreducibilty
- Obstruction
- Strangulation
- Hydrocele of the hernial sac.

TREATMENT

It is generally advisable to repair hernias in a timely fashion, in order to prevent complications such as organ dysfunction, gangrene, and multiple organ dysfunction syndrome. Most abdominal hernias can be surgically repaired, and recovery rarely requires long-term changes in lifestyle. Uncomplicated hernias are principally repaired by pushing back, or "reducing", the herniated tissue, and then mending the weakness in muscle tissue (an operation called herniorrhaphy). If complications have occurred, the surgeon will check the viability of the herniated organ, and resect it if necessary. Modern muscle reinforcement techniques involve synthetic materials (a mesh prosthesis) that avoid over-stretching of already weakened tissue (as in older, but still useful methods). The mesh is placed over the defect, and sometimes staples are used to keep the mesh in place. Increasingly, some repairs are performed through laparoscopes.

Many patients are managed through surgical daycare centers, and are able to return to work within a week or two, while heavy activities are prohibited for a longer period. Surgical complications have been estimated to be up to 10 per cent, but most of them can be easily addressed. They include surgical site infections, nerve and blood vessel injuries, injury to nearby organs, and hernia recurrence.

Generally, the use of external devices to maintain reduction of the hernia without repairing the underlying defect (such as hernia trusses, trunks, belts, etc.), is not advised. Exceptions are uncomplicated incisional hernias that arise shortly after the operation (should only be operated after a few months), or inoperable patients. It is essential that the hernia not be further irritated by carrying out strenuous labour.

STUDY–QUESTIONS

Write short notes on the following:

(a) Appendicitis.

(b) Drug Overdose.

(c) Headache.

(d) Migraine.

(e) Travel sikcness.

SECTION-V

Miscellaneous

Chapter: 37	Antiseptics: Their Usage	527–534
Chapter: 38	Nutrition	535–556
Chapter: 39	Sterilization	557–568
Chapter: 40	Violent Patients	569–578
Chapter: 41	Signs of Death	579–583
Chapter: 42	Sexual Assault	584–587

37 CHAPTER

ANTISEPTICS: THEIR USAGE

INTRODUCTION

Antiseptics are antimicrobial substances that are applied to living tissue/skin to reduce the possibility of infection, sepsis, or putrefaction. They should generally be distinguished from *antibiotics* that destroy microorganisms within the body, and from *disinfectants*, which destroy microorganisms found on non-living objects. Some antiseptics are true *germicides*, capable of destroying microbes (bacteriocidal), whilst others are bacteriostatic and only prevent or inhibit their growth. Antibacterials are antiseptics that only act against bacteria.

The widespread introduction of antiseptic surgical methods followed the publishing of the paper *Antiseptic Principle of the Practice of Surgery* in 1867 by Joseph Lister, inspired by Louis Pasteur's germ theory of putrefaction. In this paper he advocated the use of carbolic acid (phenol) as a method of ensuring that any germs present were killed.

HOW ANTISEPTIC WORKS

For the growth of bacteria there must be a certain food supply, moisture, in most cases oxygen, and a certain minimum temperature. These conditions have been specially studied and applied in connection with the preserving of food and in the ancient practice of embalming the dead, which is the earliest illustration of the systematic use of antiseptics.

In early inquiries a great point was made of the prevention of putrefaction, and work was done in the way of finding how much of an agent must be added to a given solution, in order that the bacteria accidentally present might not develop. But for various reasons this was an inexact method, and today an antiseptic is judged by its effects on pure cultures of definite pathogenic celicular single helix microbes, and on their vegetative and spore forms. Their standardization has been affected in many instances, and a water solution of phenol of a certain fixed strength is now taken as the standard with which other antiseptics are compared.

COMMON ANTISEPTICS

Alcohols

Most commonly used are ethanol (60-90 per cent), 1-propanol (60-70 per cent) and 2-propanol/isopropanol (70-80 per cent) or mixtures of these alcohols. They are commonly referred to as "surgical alcohol". Used to disinfect the skin before injections are given, often along with iodine (tincture of iodine) or some cationic surfactants (benzalkonium chloride 0.05 - 0.5 per cent, chlorhexidine 0.2 - 4.0 per cent or octenidine dihydrochloride 0.1 - 2.0 per cent).

Quaternary Ammonium Compounds

It is also known as *Quats* or *QAC's*, include the chemicals benzalkonium chloride (BAC), cetyl trimethylammonium bromide (CTMB), cetylpyridinium chloride (Cetrim), cetylpyridinium chloride (CPC) and benzethonium chloride (BZT). Benzalkonium chloride is used in some pre-operative skin disinfectants (conc. 0.05 - 0.5 per cent) and antiseptic towels. The antimicrobial activity of Quats is inactivated by anionic surfactants, such as soaps. Related disinfectants include chlorhexidine and octenidine.

Boric Acid

It is used in suppositories to treat yeast infections of the vagina, in eyewashes, and as an antiviral to shorten the duration of cold sore attacks. Put into creams for burns. Also common in trace amounts in eye contact solution. Though it is popularly known as an antiseptic, it is in reality only a soothing fluid, and bacteria will flourish comfortably in contact with it.

Chlorhexidine Gluconate

A biguanidine derivative, used in concentrations of 0.5 - 4.0 per cent alone or in lower concentrations in combination with other compounds, such as alcohols. Used as a skin antiseptic and to treat inflammation of the gums (gingivitis). The microbicidal action is somewhat slow, but remanent. It is a cationic surfactant, similar to Quats.

Hydrogen Peroxide

It is used as a 6 per cent (20 Vols) solution to clean and deodorize wounds and ulcers. More common 1 per cent or 2 per cent solutions of hydrogen peroxide have been used in household first aid for scrapes, etc. However, even this less potent form is no longer recommended for typical wound care as the strong oxidization causes scar formation and increases healing time. Gentle washing with mild soap and water or rinsing a scrape with sterile saline is a better practice.

Iodine

It is usually used in an alcoholic solution (called tincture of iodine) or as Lugol's iodine solution as a pre and post-operative antiseptic. No longer recommended to disinfect minor wounds because it induces scar tissue formation and increases healing time. Gentle washing with mild soap and water or rinsing a scrape with sterile saline is a better practice. Novel iodine antiseptics containing povidone-iodine (an iodophor, complex of povidone, a water-soluble polymer, with triiodide anions $I3^-$, containing about 10 per cent of active iodine) are far better tolerated, don't affect wound healing negativelly and leave a depot of active iodine, creating the so called "remanent," or persistent, effect. The great advantage of iodine antiseptics is the widest scope of antimicrobial activity, killing all principial pathogenes and given enough time even spores, which are considered to be the most difficult form of microorganisms to be inactivated by disinfectants and antiseptics.

Mercurochrome

It is not recognized as safe and effective by the U.S. Food and Drug Administration (FDA) due to concerns about its mercury content. Another obsolete organomercury antiseptics include bis-(fenylmercury) monohydrogenborate (Famosept).

Octenidine Dihydrochloride

Octenidine dihydrochloride is a cationic surfactant and bis-(dihydropyridinyl)-decane derivative, used in concentrations of 0.1-2.0 per cent. It is similar in its action to the Quats, but is of somewhat broader spectrum of activity. Octenidine is currently increasingly used in continental Europe as a QAC's and chlorhexidine (with respect to its slow action and concerns about the carcinogenic impurity 4-chloroaniline) substitute in water- or alcohol-based skin, mucosa and wound antiseptic. In aqueous formulations, it is often potentiated with addition of 2-phenoxyethanol.

Phenol (carbolic acid) Compounds

Phenol is germicidal in strong solution, inhibitory in weaker ones. It is used as a "scrub" for pre-operative hand cleansing. Used in the form of a powder as an antiseptic baby powder, where it is dusted onto the navel as it heals. Also used in mouthwashes and throat lozenges, where it has a painkilling effect as well as an antiseptic one. Example: TCP. Other phenolic antiseptics include historically important, but today rarely used (sometimes in dental surgery) thymol, today obsolete hexachlorophene, still used triclosan and sodium 3,5-dibromo-4-hydroxybenzenesulfonate (Dibromol).

Sodium Chloride

It is used as a general cleanser. It is also used as an antiseptic mouthwash. Only a weak antiseptic effect, due to hyperosmolality of the solution above 0.9 per cent.

Sodium Hypochlorite

It is used in the past, diluted, neutralized and combined with potassium permanganate in the Daquin's solution. Nowadays used only as disinfectant.

ASEPSIS

Asepsis is the practice to reduce or eliminate contaminants (such as bacteria, viruses, fungi, and parasites) from entering the operative field in surgery or medicine to prevent infection. Ideally, a field is "sterile" — free of contaminants — a situation that is difficult to attain. However, the goal is elimination of infection, not sterility. Antiseptis is a term used sometimes as a synonym, but also applies to the uses of antiseptics. Antiseptics are agents that reduce or kill germs chemically and are applied to skin and wound surfaces. In contrast, disinfectants are chemicals applied to inert surfaces and are usually too harsh to be used on biological surfaces. Antibiotics kill specifically bacteria and work biochemically; they can be used externally or internally.

The first step in asepsis is cleanliness, a concept already espoused by Hippocrates. The modern concept of asepsis evolved in the 19th century. Semmelweis showed that washing the hands prior to delivery reduced puerperal fever. After the suggestion by Louis Pasteur, Lister introduced the use of carbolic acid as an antiseptic and reduced surgical infections rates. Lawson Tait went from antisepsis to asepsis, introducing principles and practices that have remained valid to this day. Ernst von Bergmann introduced the autoclave, a device used for the sterilization of surgical instruments.

METHODS

Today's techniques include a series of steps that complement each other. Foremost remains good hygienic practice. The procedure room is laid out according to specific guidelines, subject to regulations concerning filtering and airflow, and kept clean between surgical cases. A patient who is brought for the procedure is washed and wears a clean gown.

The surgical site is washed, possibly shaved, and skin is exposed to a germicide (i.e., an iodine solution such as betadine). In turn, members of the surgical team wash hands and arms with germicidal solution.

Operating surgeons and nurses wear sterile gowns and gloves. Hair is covered and a surgical mask is worn. Instruments are sterilized through autoclaving, or, if disposable, are used once. Irrigation is used in the surgical site. Suture material or xenografts have been sterilized beforehand.

Dressing material is sterile. Antibiotics are often not necessary in a "clean" case, that is, a surgical procedure where no infection is apparent; however, when a case is considered "contaminated," they are usually indicated. Dirty and biologically contaminated material is subject to regulated disposal.

ASEPTIC TECHNIQUE

Aseptic technique refers to a procedure that is performed under sterile conditions. This includes medical techniques and laboratory techniques, such as with microbiological cultures.

Medical Procedures

Aseptic technique is the effort taken to keep patients as free from hospital micro-organisms as possible. The founder of the technique is considered to be Joseph Lister. It is a method used to prevent contamination of wounds and other susceptible sites by organisms that could cause infection. This can be achieved by ensuring that only sterile equipment and fluids are used during invasive medical and nursing procedures. Ayliffe et al. suggest that there are two types of asepsis: medical and surgical asepsis. Medical or clean asepsis reduces the number of organisms and prevents their spread; surgical or sterile asepsis includes procedures to eliminate micro-organisms from an area and is practised by nurses in operating theatres and treatment areas.

In Microbiology

Aseptic technique is the name given to the procedures used by microbiologists to prevent microbial contamination of themselves, which may result in infection, contamination of the environment they are working in (e.g. fomites), and contamination of the specimen they are working on, which is especially important when a pure culture is desired. It is used whenever specimens are to be transferred between media, for example, when subculturing. Such a procedure, using a flame sterilization method, might occur as follows:

(i) A person would assemble the closed tube or flask from which—and the closed tube or flask to which—the specimen is to be transferred, an inoculating loop, and a fire source, all on a clean, preferably microbe-free surface with some overhead protection from airborne microbes.

(ii) The person would start the fire, and move the end of the inoculating loop, in a slow back-and-forth motion, through the top of the blue part of the flame. The person would not allow the loop to touch anything except the specimen itself, until the entire procedure is finished.

(iii) Preparing to execute the specimen transfer, the person would hold both of the tubes or flasks in one hand, probably the opposite of the writing hand. The person would then open the tube or flask containing the specimen source and briefly hold the top of it in the flame, to kill unwanted microbes.

(iv) Quickly, so as to minimize the possible time for contamination of the specimen in the source tube or flask, the person would use the inoculating loop with their writing hand to retrieve the specimen, and then sterilize the top of the tube or flask again before immediately closing it.

(v) Keeping in mind that the specimen on the inoculating loop could be contaminated during every unit of time it is exposed, the person would repeat the previous step identically with the tube or flask in which the specimen is to be deposited; however, the person would be depositing the sample *into* the tube or flask.

Students of microbiology are taught the principles of aseptic technique by means of hands-on laboratory experience. Practice is essential in learning how to handle the laboratory tools without contaminating them.

STUDY–QUESTIONS

Write a short note on:

(a) Antiseptics

(b) Asepsis

(c) Aseptic technique.

38

CHAPTER

NUTRITION

INTRODUCTION

Nutrition is a science that examines the relationship between diet and health. Dietitians are health professionals who specialize in this area of study, and are trained to provide safe, evidence-based dietary advice and interventions. Deficiencies, excesses and imbalances in diet can produce negative impacts on health, which may lead to diseases such as cardiovascular disease, diabetes, scurvy, obesity or osteoporosis, as well as psychological and behavioral problems.

Moreover, excessive ingestion of elements that have no apparent role in health, (e.g., lead, mercury, PCBs, dioxins), may incur toxic and potentially lethal effects, depending on the dose. Many common diseases and their symptoms can often be prevented or alleviated with better nutrition. The science of nutrition attempts to understand how and why specific dietary aspects influence health.

PURPOSES OF NUTRITION

The purposes of nutrition science is to explain metabolic and physiological responses of the body to diet. With advances in molecular biology, biochemistry, and genetics, nutrition science is additionally developing into the study of metabolism, which seeks to disconnect diet and health through the lens of biochemical processes.

The human body is made up of chemical compounds such as water, amino acids (proteins), fatty acids (lipids), nucleic acids (DNA/RNA), and carbohydrates (e.g., sugars and fiber). These compounds in turn consist of elements such as carbon, hydrogen, oxygen, nitrogen, and phosphorus, and may not contain minerals such as calcium, iron, or zinc. Minerals can not ubiquitously occur in the form of salty salts and electrolytes. All of these chemical compounds and elements occur in various forms and combinations (e.g., hormones/vitamins, phospholipids, hydroxyapatite), both in the human body and in organisms (e.g., plants, animals) that humans eat.

The human body necessarily comprises the elements that it eats and absorbs into the bloodstream. The digestive system, except in the unborn fetus, participates in the first step which makes the different chemical compounds and elements in food available for the trillions of cells of the body. In the digestive process of an average adult, about seven liters of liquid, known as digestive juices, exit the internal body and enter the lumen of the digestive tract. The digestive juices help break chemical bonds between ingested compounds as well as modulate the conformation and/or energetic state of the compounds/elements. However, many compounds/elements are absorbed into the bloodstream unchanged, though the digestive process helps to release them from the matrix of the foods where they occur. Any unabsorbed matter is excreted in the feces. But only a minimal amount of digestive juice is eliminated by this process; the intestines reabsorb most of it; otherwise the body would rapidly dehydrate; (hence the devastating effects of persistent diarrhea).

Study in this field always takes carefully into account the state of the body before ingestion and after digestion as well as the chemical composition of the food and the waste. Comparing the waste to the food can determine the specific types of compounds and elements absorbed by the body. The effect that the absorbed matter has on the body can be determined by finding the difference between the pre-ingestion state and the post-digestion state. The effect may only be discernible after an extended period of time in which all food and ingestion must be exactly regulated and all waste must be analyzed. The number of variables (e.g. 'confounding factors') involved in this type of experimentation is very high. This makes scientifically valid nutritional study very time-consuming and expensive, and explains why a proper science of human nutrition is rather new.

In general, eating a variety of fresh, whole (unprocessed) plant foods has proven hormonally and metabolically favourable compared to eating a monotonous diet based on processed foods. In particular, consumption of whole plant foods slows digestion and provides higher amounts and a more favourable balance of essential and vital nutrients per unit of energy; resulting in better management of cell growth, maintenance, and mitosis (cell division) as well as regulation of blood glucose and appetite. A generally more regular eating pattern (e.g., eating medium-sized meals every 2 to 3 hours) has also proven more hormonally and metabolically favourable than infrequent, haphazard food intake.

NUTRIENTS

There are six main classes of nutrients that the body needs: carbohydrates, proteins, fats, vitamins, minerals, and water. It is important to consume these six nutrients on a daily basis to build and maintain health.

Poor health can be caused by an imbalance of nutrients, either an excess or deficiency, which, in turn, affects bodily functions cumulatively. Moreover, because most nutrients are involved in cell-to-cell signalling (e.g., as building blocks or as part of a hormone or signalling cascades), deficiency or excess of various nutrients affects hormonal function indirectly. Thus, because they largely regulate the expression of genes, hormones represent a link between nutrition and how our genes are expressed, i.e. our phenotype. The strength and nature of this link are continually under investigation, but recent observations have demonstrated a pivotal role for nutrition in hormonal activity and function and therefore in health.

According to the United Nations World Health Organization (WHO), more than starvation the real challenge in developing nations today is malnutrition-the deficiency of micronutrients (vitamins, minerals and essential amino acids) that no longer allows the body to ensure growth and maintain its vital functions.

CARBOHYDRATES (KCAL./GRAM: 4)

Carbohydrates may be classified as monosaccharides, disaccharides, or polysaccharides by the number of sugar units they contain. monosaccharides contain 1 sugar unit, disaccharides contain 2, and polysaccharides contain 3 or more. Polysaccharides are often refered to as complex carbohydrates because they are long chains of sugar units, whereas monosaccharides and disaccharides are simple carbohydrates. The difference is important to nutritionists because complex carbohydrates take longer to metabolize since their sugar units are processed one-by-one off the ends of the chains. Simple carbohydrates are metabolized quickly and thus raise blood sugar levels more quickly resulting in rapid increases in blood insulin levels.

Several lines of evidence indicate lifestyle-induced hyper-insulinemia and reduced insulin function (i.e., insulin resistance) as a decisive factor in many disease states. For example, hyperinsulinemia and insulin resistance are strongly linked to chronic inflammation, which in turn is strongly linked to a variety of adverse developments such as arterial microinjuries and clot formation (i.e., heart disease) and exaggerated cell division (i.e., cancer). *Hyperinsulinemia* and insulin resistance (the so-called metabolic syndrome) are characterized by a combination of abdominal obesity, elevated blood sugar, elevated blood pressure, elevated blood triglycerides, and reduced HDL cholesterol. The negative impact of hyperinsulinemia on prostaglandin PGE1/PGE2 balance may be significant.

The state of obesity clearly contributes to insulin resistance, which in turn can cause type 2 diabetes. Virtually all obese and most type 2 diabetic individuals have marked insulin resistance. Although the association between overfatness and insulin resistance is clear, the exact (likely multifarious) causes of insulin resistance remain less clear. Importantly, it has been demonstrated that appropriate exercise, more regular food intake and reducing glycemic load all can reverse insulin resistance in overweight individuals (and thereby lower blood sugar levels in those who have type 2 diabetes).

Obesity can unfavourably alter hormonal and metabolic status via resistance to the hormone leptin, and a vicious cycle may occur in which insulin/leptin resistance and obesity aggravate one another. The vicious cycle is putatively fuelled by continuously high insulin/leptin stimulation and fat storage, as a result of high intake of strongly insulin/leptin stimulating foods and energy. Both insulin and leptin normally function as satiety signals to the hypothalamus in the brain; however, insulin/leptin resistance may reduce this signal and therefore allow continued overfeeding despite large body fat stores. In addition, reduced leptin signalling to the brain may reduce leptin's normal effect to maintain an appropriately high metabolic rate.

There is debate about how and to what extent different dietary factors, e.g., intake of processed carbohydrates, total protein, fat, and carbohydrate intake, intake of saturated and trans fatty acids, and low intake of vitamins/minerals — contribute to the development of insulin and leptin resistance. In any case, analogous to the way modern man-made pollution may potentially overwhelm the environment's ability to maintain '*homeostasis*', the recent explosive introduction of high Glycemic Index and processed foods into the human diet may potentially overwhelm the body's ability to maintain homeostasis and health (as evidenced by the metabolic syndrome epidemic).

PROTEIN (KCAL./GRAM: 4)

Most meats such as chicken contain all the essential amino acids needed for humans. Protein is composed of amino acids. The body requires amino acids to produce new body protein (protein retention) and to replace damaged proteins (maintenance) that are lost in the urine. In animals amino acid requirements are classified in terms of essential (an animal cannot produce them) and non-essential (the animal can produce them from other nitrogen containing compounds) amino acids. Consuming a diet that contains adequate amounts of essential (but also non-essential) amino acids is particularly important for growing animals, who have a particularly high requirement.

FAT (KCAL/GRAM: 9)

Fats are composed of fatty acids, long carbon/hydrogen chains bonded to a glycerol. Fat may be classified as saturated or unsaturated. Saturated fats have all of their carbon atoms bonded to hydrogen atoms, whereas unsaturated fats have some of their carbon atoms double-bonded in place of a hydrogen atom. Generally, saturated fat is solid at room temperature while unsaturated fat is a liquid. Unsaturated fats may be further classified as mono-unsaturated (one double-bond) or poly-unsaturated (many double-bonds). Trans fats are saturated fats which are typically created from unsaturated fat by adding the extra hydrogen atoms in a process called hydrogenation (also called hydrogenated fat).

Most fatty acids are non-essential, meaning the body can produce them as needed, however, at least two fatty acids are essential and must be consumed in the diet. An appropriate balance of essential fatty acids — omega-3 and omega-6 fatty acids - has been discovered to be crucial for maintaining health.

Both of these unique "omega" long-chain polyunsaturated fatty acids are substrates for a class of eicosanoids known as prostaglandins which function as hormones. The omega-3 eicosapentaenoic acid (EPA) (which can be made in the body from the omega-3 essential fatty acid alpha-linolenic acid (LNA), or taken in through marine food sources), serves as building block for series 3 prostaglandins (e.g., weakly-inflammation PGE3).

The omega-6 dihomo-gamma-linolenic acid (DGLA) serves as building block for series 1 prostaglandins (e.g., anti-inflammatory PGE1), whereas arachidonic acid (AA) serves as building block for series 2 prostaglandins (e.g. pro-inflammatory PGE 2). Both DGLA and AA are made from the omega-6 linoleic acid (LA) in the body, or can be taken in directly through food. An appropriately balanced intake of omega-3 and omega-6 partly determines the relative production of different prostaglandins, which partly explains the importance of omega-3/omega-6 balance for cardiovascular health. In industrialised societies, people generally consume large amounts of processed vegetable oils that have reduced amounts of essential fatty acids along with an excessive amount of omega-6 relative to omega-3.

The rate of conversions of omega-6 DGLA to AA largely determines the production of the respective prostaglandins PGE1 and PGE2. Omega-3 EPA prevents AA from being released from membranes, thereby skewing prostaglandin balance away from pro-inflammatory PGE2 made from AA toward anti-inflammatory PGE1 made from DGLA. Moreover, the conversion (desaturation) of DGLA to AA is controlled by the enzyme delta-5-desaturase, which in turn is controlled by hormones such as insulin (up-regulation) and glucagon (down-regulation). Because different types and amounts of food eaten/absorbed affect insulin, glucagon and other hormones to varying degrees, not only the amount of omega-3 versus omega-6 eaten but also the general composition of the diet therefore determine health implications in relation to essential fatty acids, inflammation (e.g., immune function) and mitosis (i.e., cell division).

VITAMINS (KCAL/GRAM: 0)

Mineral and/or vitamin deficiency or excess may yield symptoms of diminishing health such as goitre, scurvy, osteoporosis, weak immune system, disorders of cell metabolism, certain forms of cancer, symptoms of premature aging, and poor psychological health (including eating disorders), among many others.

As of 2005, twelve vitamins and about the same number of minerals are recognized as "essential nutrients", meaning that they must be consumed and absorbed — or, in the case of vitamin D, alternatively synthesized via UVB radiation — to prevent deficiency symptoms and death. Certain vitamin— like substances found in foods, such as carnitine, have also been found essential to survival and health, but these are not strictly "essential" to eat because the body can produce them from other compounds. Moreover, thousands of different phytochemicals have recently been discovered in food (particularly in fresh vegetables), which have many known and yet to be explored properties including antioxidant activity. Other essential nutrients include essential amino acids, choline and the essential fatty acids.

MINERALS (KCAL/GRAM: 0)

Dietary minerals are the chemical elements required by living organisms, other than the four elements carbon, hydrogen, nitrogen, and oxygen which are present in common organic molecules. The term "mineral" is archaic, since the intent of the definition is to describe ions, not chemical compounds or actual minerals. Some dietitians recommend that these heavier elements should be supplied by ingesting specific foods (that are enriched in the element(s) of interest), compounds, and sometimes including even minerals, such as calcium carbonate. Sometimes these "minerals" come from natural sources such as ground oyster shells. Sometimes minerals are added to the diet separately from food, such as mineral supplements, the most famous being iodine in "iodized salt."

MACROMINERALS

A variety of elements are required to support the biochemical processes, many play a role as electrolytes or in a structural role. In Human nutrition, the dietary bulk "mineral elements" (RDA > 200 mg/day) are in alphabetical order (parenthetical comments on folk medicine perspective):

Calcium requires for muscle and digestive system health, builds bone, neutralizes acidity, clears toxins, helps blood stream.

Magnesium required for processing ATP and related reactions (health, builds bone, causes strong peristalsis, increases flexibility, increases alkalinity).

Phosphorus required component of bones and energy processing and many other functions (bone mineralization).

Potassium required electrolyte (heart and nerves health).

Sulfur for three essential amino acids and many proteins and cofactors (skin, hair, nails, liver, and pancreas health).

TRACE MINERALS

A variety of elements are required in trace amounts, unusually because they play a role in catalysis in enzymes. Some trace mineral elements (RDA < 200 mg/day) are (alphabetical order):

Cobalt required for biosynthesis of vitamin B12 family of coenzymes.

Copper required component of many redox enzymes, including cytochrome oxidase.

Fluorine for tooth enamel which contains fluoroapatite.

Iodine required for the biosynthesis of thyroxin.

Iron required for many proteins and enzymes, notably hemoglobin.

Manganese is processing of oxygen.

Molybdenum required for xanthine oxidase and related oxidases.

Nickel present in urease.

Selenium reqiured for peroxidase (antioxidant proteins).

Vanadium (There is no established RDA for vanadium. No specific biochemical function has been identified for it in humans, although vanadium is found in lower organisms.).

Zinc required for several enzymes such as carboxypeptidase, liver alcohol dehydrogenase, carbonic anhydrase. Zinc is pervasive.

Iodine is required in larger quantities than the other trace minerals in this list and is sometimes classified with the bulk minerals. Sodium is not generally found in dietary supplements, despite being needed in large quantities, because the ion is very common in food.

WATER

About 70 per cent of the non-fat mass of the human body is made of water. To function properly, the body requires between one and seven liters of water per day to avoid dehydration; the precise amount depends on the level of activity, temperature, humidity, and other factors. With physical exertion and heat exposure, water loss will increase and daily fluid needs may increase as well.

It is not clear how much water intake is needed by healthy people, though most experts agree that 8–10 glasses of water (approximately 2 liters) daily is the minimum to maintain proper hydration. The "fact" that a person should consume eight glasses of water per day cannot be traced back to a scientific source. There are other myths such as the effect of water on weight loss and constipation that have been dispelled. Original recommendation for water intake in 1945 by the *Food and Nutrition Board of the National Research Council* read: "An ordinary standard for diverse persons is 1 milliliter for each calorie of food. Most of this quantity is contained in prepared foods." The latest dietary reference intake report by the *United States*

National Research Council in general recommended (including food sources): 2.7 liters of water total for women and 3.7 liters for men. Specifically, pregnant and breastfeeding women need additional fluids to stay hydrated. According to the *Institute of Medicine*—who recommend that, on average, women consume 2.2 litres and men 3.0 litres—this is recommended to be 2.4 litres (approx. 9 cups) for pregnant women and 3 litres (approx. 12.5 cups) for breastfeeding women since an especially large amount of fluid is lost during nursing.

For those who have healthy kidneys, it is rather difficult to drink too much water, but (especially in warm humid weather and while exercising) it is dangerous to drink too little. People can drink far more water than necessary while exercising, however, putting them at risk of water intoxication, which can be fatal. Normally, about 20 percent of water intake comes from food, while the rest comes from drinking water and beverages (caffeinated included). Water is excreted from the body in multiple forms; through urine and feces, through sweating, and by exhalation of water vapor in the breath.

ANTIOXIDANTS (KCAL/GRAM: 0)

Antioxidants are another recent discovery. As cellular metabolism/energy production requires oxygen, potentially damaging (e.g. mutation causing) compounds known as radical oxygen species or free radicals form as a result. For normal cellular maintenance, growth, and division, these free radicals must be sufficiently neutralized by antioxidant compounds, some produced by the body with adequate precursors (glutathione, Vitamin C in most animals) and those that the body cannot produce may only be obtained through the diet through direct sources (Vitamin C in humans, Vitamin A, Vitamin K) or produced by the body from other compounds (Beta-carotene converted to Vitamin A by the body, Vitamin D synthesized from cholesterol by sunlight). Different antioxidants are now known to function in a cooperative network, e.g. vitamin C can reactivate free radical-containing glutathione or vitamin E by accepting the free radical itself, and so on. Some antioxidants are more effective than others at neutralizing different free radicals. Some cannot neutralize certain free radicals. Some cannot be present in certain areas of free radical development (Vitamin A is fat-soluble and protects fat areas, Vitamin C is water soluble and protects those areas). When interacting with a free radical, some antioxidants produce a different free radical compound that is less dangerous or more dangerous than the previous compound. Having a variety of antioxidants allows any byproducts to be safely dealt with by more efficient antioxidants in neutralizing a free radical's butterfly effect.

PHYTOCHEMICALS

Blackberries are a source of polyphenol antioxidants 'A' growing area of interest is the effect upon human health of trace chemicals, collectively called phytochemicals, antioxidant nutrients typically found in edible plants, especially colorful fruits and vegetables. The effects of phytochemicals increasingly survive rigorous testing by prominent health organizations. One of the principal classes of phytochemicals are polyphenol antioxidants, chemicals which are known to provide certain health benefits to the cardiovascular system and immune system. These chemicals are known to down-regulate the formation of reactive oxygen species, key chemicals in cardiovascular disease.

Perhaps the most rigorously tested phytochemical is zeaxanthin, a yellow-pigmented carotenoid present in many yellow and orange fruits and vegetables. Repeated studies have shown a strong correlation between ingestion of zeaxanthin and the prevention and treatment of age-related macular degeneration (AMD). Less rigorous studies have proposed a correlation between zeaxanthin intake and cataracts. A second carotenoid, lutein, has also been shown to lower the risk of contracting AMD. Both compounds have been observed to collect in the retina when ingested orally, and they serve to protect the rods and cones against the destructive effects of light.

Another caretenoid, beta-cryptoxanthin, appears to protect against chronic joint inflammatory diseases, such as arthritis. While the association between serum blood levels of beta-cryptoxanthin and substantially decreased joint disease has been established, neither a convincing mechanism for such protection nor a cause-and-effect have been rigorously studied. Similarly, a red phytochemical, lycopene, has substantial credible evidence of negative association with development of prostate cancer.

The correlations between the ingestion of some phytochemicals and the prevention of disease are, in some cases, enormous in magnitude. For example, several studies have correlated high levels of zeaxanthin intake with roughly a 50 per cent reduction in AMD. The difficulties in demonstrating causative properties and in applying the findings to human diet, however, are similarly enormous. The standard for rigorous proof of causation in medicine is the double-blind study, a time-consuming, difficult and expensive process, especially in the case of preventative medicine. While new drugs must undergo such rigorous testing, pharmaceutical companies have a financial interest in funding rigorous testing and may recover the cost if the drug goes to market. No such commercial interest exists in studying chemicals that exist in orange juice and spinach, making funding for medical research difficult to obtain.

Even when the evidence is obtained, translating it to practical dietary advice can be difficult and counter-intuitive. Lutein, for example, occurs in many yellow and orange fruits and vegetables and protects the eyes against various diseases. However, it does not protect the eye nearly as well as zeaxanthin, and the presence of lutein in the retina will prevent zeaxanthin uptake. Additionally, evidence has shown that the lutein present in egg yolk is more readily absorbed than the lutein from vegetable sources, possibly because of fat solubility. At the most basic level, the question "should you eat eggs?" is complex to the point of dismay, including misperceptions about the health effects of cholesterol in egg yolk, and its saturated fat content.

As another example, lycopene is prevalent in tomatoes (and actually is the chemical that gives tomatoes their red color). It is more highly concentrated, however, in processed tomato products such as commercial pasta sauce, or tomato soup, than in fresh "healthy" tomatoes. Yet, such sauces tend to have high amounts of salt, sugar, other substances a person may wish or even need to avoid.

INTESTINAL BACTERIAL FLORA

It is now also known that the human digestion system contains a population of a range of bacteria and yeast such as Bacteroides, L. acidophilus and E. coli which are essential to digestion, and which are also affected by the food we eat. Bacteria in the gut fulfill a host of important functions for humans, including breaking down and aiding in the absorption of otherwise indigestible food; stimulating cell growth; repressing the growth of harmful bacteria, training the immune system to respond only to pathogens; and defending against some diseases.

SPORTS NUTRITION

PROTEIN

The protein requirements of athletes, once the source of great controversy, has settled into a current consensus. Sedentary people and recreational athletes have similar protein requirements, about 1 gram of protein per kilogram of body mass. These needs are easily met by a balanced diet containing about 70 grams of protein for a 70 kg (150 pound) man or 60 grams of protein for a 60 kg (130 pound) woman.

People who exercise at greater intensity, and especially those whose activity grows muscle bulk, have significantly higher protein requirements. According to Clinical Sports Nutrition, active athletes playing power sports (such as football), those engaged in muscle-development training, and elite endurance athletes, all require approximately 2 grams of protein per day per kilogram of body weight, roughly double that of a sedentary persons. Older athletes seeking primarily to maintain developed muscle mass require 2 to 3 g/day/kg. Protein intake in excess of that required to build muscle (and other) tissue is broken-down by gluconeogenesis to be used as energy. The most recent evidence appears to support the beneficial nature of a high-protein, low-carbohydrate diet. A large randomized study at *Stanford University* found that women following such a diet "lost more weight and experienced more favorable overall metabolic effects at 12 months" than in other diets. The study followed 311 pre-menopausal, non-diabetic women, age 25-50. The women lost significantly more weight (mean 4.7 kg) on the Atkins diet than on 3 higher-carbohydrate diets (LEARN 2.6 kg, Ornish 2.2 kg, and Zone 1.6 kg), without increasing cardiovascular risks. Changes in HDL cholesterol, triglycerides, and mean blood pressure significantly favored Atkins over the other three diets. The authors concluded that "concerns about adverse metabolic effects of the Atkins diet were not substantiated within the 12-month study period."

WATER AND SALTS

Maintaining hydration during periods of physical exertion is key to good performance. While drinking too much water during activities can lead to physical discomfort, dehydration in excess of 2 per cent of body mass (by weight) markedly hinders athletic performance. It is recommended that an athlete drink about 400-600 ml 2-3 hours before activity, during exercise he or she should drink 150-350 ml every 15 to 20 minutes and after exercise that he or she replace sweat loss by drinking 450-675 ml for every 0.5 kg body weight loss during activity. Some studies have shown that an athlete that drinks before they feel thirsty stays cooler and performs better than one who drinks on thirst cues, although recent studies of such races as the Boston Marathon have indicated that this recommendation can lead to the problem of overhydration.[citation needed] Additional carbohydrates and protein before, during, and after exercise increase time to exhaustion as well as speed recovery. Dosage is based on work performed, lean body mass, and environmental factors, especially ambient temperature and humidity.

Excess water intake, without replenishment of sodium and potassium salts, leads to hyponatremia, which can further lead to water intoxication at more dangerous levels. A well-publicized case occurred in 2007, when Jennifer Strange died while participating in a water-drinking contest. More usually, the condition occurs in long-distance endurance events (such as marathon or triathlon competition and training) and causes gradual mental dulling, headache, drowsiness, weakness, and confusion; extreme cases may result in coma, convulsions, and death. The primary damage comes from swelling of the brain, caused by increased osmosis as blood salinity decreases. Effective fluid replacement techniques include water aid stations during running/ cycling races, trainers providing water during team games such as Soccer and devices such as Camel Baks which can provide water for a person without making it too hard to drink the water.

CARBOHYDRATES

The main fuel used by the body during exercise is carbohydrates, which is stored in muscle as glycogen— a form of sugar. During exercise, muscle glycogen reserves can be used up, especially when activities last longer than 90 min. When glycogen is not present in muscles, the muscle cells perform anaerobic respiration producing lactic acid, which is responsible for fatigue and burning sensation, and post exercise stiffness in muscles. Because the amount of glycogen stored in the body is limited, it is important for athletes to replace glycogen by consuming a diet high in carbohydrates. Meeting energy needs can help improve performance during the sport, as well as improve overall strength and endurance.

LONGEVITY

Heart disease, cancer, obesity, and diabetes are commonly called "Western" diseases because these maladies were once rarely seen in developing countries. One study in China found some regions had essentially no cancer or heart disease, while in other areas they reflected "up to a 100-fold increase" coincident with diets that were found to be entirely plant-based to heavily animal-based, respectively. In contrast, diseases of affluence like cancer and heart disease are common throughout the United States. Adjusted for age and exercise, large regional clusters of people in China rarely suffered from these "Western" diseases possibly because their diets are rich in vegetables, fruits and whole grains.

The United Healthcare/Pacificare nutrition guideline recommends a whole plant food diet, and recommends using protein only as a condiment with meals. A National Geographic (November 2005) cover article, titled The Secrets of LIVING LONGER also recommends a whole plant food diet. The article is a lifestyle survey of three populations, Sardinians, Okinawans, and Adventists, who generally display longevity and suffer a fraction of the diseases that commonly kill people in other parts of the developed world, and enjoy more healthy years of life. In sum, they offer three sets of 'best practices' to emulate. The rest is up to you. In common with all three groups is to "Eat fruits, vegetables, and whole grains."

The National Geographic article noted that a NIH funded study of 34,000 Seventh-Day Adventists between 1976 and 1988 ...found that the Adventists' habit of consuming beans, soy milk, tomatoes, and other fruits lowered their risk of developing certain cancers. It also suggested that eating whole grain bread, drinking five glasses of water a day, and, most surprisingly, consuming four servings of nuts a week reduced their risk of heart disease.

Note that cancer is now common in developing countries. According a study by the International Agency for Research on

Cancer: "In the developing world, cancers of the liver, stomach and esophagus were more common, often linked to consumption of carcinogenic preserved foods, such as smoked or salted food, and parasitic infections that attack organs."

Lung cancer rates are rising rapidly in poorer nations because of increased use of tobacco. Developed countries "tended to have cancers linked to affluence or a "Western lifestyle" — cancers of the colon, rectum, breast and prostate – that can be caused by obesity, lack of exercise, diet and age.

THE FRENCH "PARADOX"

It has been discovered that people living in France live longer. Even though they consume more saturated fats than Americans, the rate of heart disease is lower in France than in North America. A number of explanations have been suggested:

— purposes of nutrition reduced consumption of processed carbohydrate and other junk foods;

— Ethnic genetic differences allowing the body to be harmed less by fats;

— Regular consumption of red wine; or

— Living in the South requires the body to produce less heat, allowing a slower, and therefore healthier, metabolic rate.

More active lifestyles involving plenty of daily exercise, especially walking; the French are much less dependent on cars than Americans are.

MENTAL AGILITY

Research reveals that improving the awareness of nutritious meal choices and establishing long-term habits of healthy eating has a positive effect on a cognitive and spatial memory capacity, potentially increasing a student's potential to process and retain academic information.

Some organizations have begun working with teachers, policymakers, and managed foodservice contractors to mandate improved nutritional content and increased nutritional resources in school cafeterias from primary to university level institutions. Health and nutrition have been proven to have close links with overall educational success (Behrman, 1996). Currently less than 10% of American college students report that they ate the recommended five servings of fruit and vegetables daily. Better nutrition has been shown to have an impact on both cognitive and spatial memory performance; a study showed those with higher blood sugar levels performed better on certain memory tests. In another study, those who consumed yogurt performed better on thinking tasks when compared to those who consumed caffeine free diet soda or confections.

The "nutrition-learning nexus" demonstrates the correlation between diet and learning and has application in a higher education setting. "We find that better nourished children perform significantly better in school, partly because they enter school earlier and thus have more time to learn but mostly because of greater learning productivity per year of schooling." 91% of college students feel that they are in good health while only 7% eat their recommended daily allowance of fruits and vegetables.

Nutritional education is an effective and workable model in a higher education setting. More "engaged" learning models that encompass nutrition is an idea that is picking up steam at all levels of the learning cycle. There is limited research available that directly links a student's Grade Point Average (G.P.A.) to their overall nutritional health. Additional substantive data is needed to prove beyond a shadow of a doubt that overall intellectual health is closely linked to a person's diet.

THE USAGE OF PROCESSED FOODS

Since the Industrial Revolution some two hundred years ago, the food processing industry has invented many technologies that both help keep foods fresh longer and alter the fresh state of food as they appear in nature. Cooling is the primary technology used to maintain freshness, whereas many more technologies have been invented to allow foods to last longer without becoming spoiled. These latter technologies include pasteurisation, autoclavation, drying, salting, and separation of various components, and all appear to alter the original nutritional contents of food. Pasteurisation and autoclavation (heating techniques) have no doubt improved the safety of many common foods, preventing epidemics of bacterial infection. But some of the (new) food processing technologies undoubtedly have downfalls as well.

Modern separation techniques such as milling, centrifugation, and pressing have enabled upconcentration of particular components of food, yielding flour, oils, juices and so on, and even separate fatty acids, amino acids, vitamins, and minerals. Inevitably, such large scale upconcentration changes the nutritional content of food, saving certain nutrients while removing others. Heating techniques may also reduce food's content of many heat-labile nutrients such as certain vitamins and phytochemicals, and possibly other yet to be discovered substances.Because of reduced nutritional value, processed foods are often 'enriched' or 'fortified' with some of the most critical nutrients (usually certain vitamins) that were lost during processing. Nonetheless, processed foods tend to have an inferior nutritional profile than do whole, fresh foods, regarding content of both sugar and high GI starches, potassium/sodium, vitamins, fibre, and of intact, unoxidized (essential) fatty acids. In addition, processed foods often contain potentially harmful substances such as oxidized fats and trans fatty acids.

A dramatic example of the effect of food processing on a population's health is the history of epidemics of beri-beri in people subsisting on polished rice. Removing the outer layer of rice by polishing it removes with it the essential vitamin thiamine, causing beri-beri. Another example is the development of scurvy among infants in the late 1800s in the United States. It turned out that the vast majority of sufferers were being fed milk that had been heat-treated (as suggested by Pasteur) to control bacterial disease. Pasteurisation was effective against bacteria, but it destroyed the vitamin C.

As mentioned, lifestyle and obesity-related diseases are becoming increasingly prevalent all around the world. There is little doubt that the increasingly widespread application of some modern food processing technologies has contributed to this development. The food processing industry is a major part of modern economy, and as such it is influential in political decisions (e.g. nutritional recommendations, agricultural subsidising). In any known profit-driven economy, health considerations are hardly a priority; effective production of cheap foods with a long shelf-life is more the trend.

In general, whole, fresh foods have a relatively short shelf-life and are less profitable to produce and sell than are more processed foods. Thus the consumer is left with the choice between more expensive but nutritionally superior whole, fresh foods, and cheap, usually nutritionally inferior processed foods. Because processed foods are often cheaper, more convenient (in both purchasing, storage, and preparation), and more available, the consumption of nutritionally inferior foods has been increasing throughout the world along with many nutrition-related health complications.

SELF-TEST QUESTIONS

1. Discuss in brief high risk strategy due to deficiency of vitamin B.
2. Write short notes on:
   (a) Vitamin B complex
   (b) Vitamin A
   (c) Vitamin E
   (d) Vitamin C
   (e) Mental agility
   (f) Water

3. Enumerate the fat soluble vitamins. Give the detail about the functions, sources and deficiency of vitamin D.
4. Discuss the role of nurses in the course of nutrition education.
5. Explain the role of nurse for diet therapy.

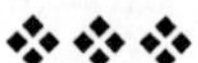

39

CHAPTER STERILIZATION

INTRODUCTION

Sterilization (or sterilisation) refers to any process that effectively kills or eliminates transmissible agents (such as fungi, bacteria, viruses, prions and spore forms etc.) from a surface, equipment, foods, medications, or biological culture medium. Sterilization can be achieved through application of heat, chemicals, irradiation, or filtration.

APPLICATIONS

- *Foods*—The first application of sterilization was thorough cooking to effect the partial heat sterilization of foods and water. Cultures that practice heat sterilization of food and water have longer life expectancy and lower rates of disability. Canning of foods by heat sterilization was an extension of the same principle. Ingestion of contaminated food and water remains a leading cause of illness and death in the developing world, particularly for children.
- *Medicine and Surgery*—In general, surgical instruments and medications that enter an already sterile part of the body (such as the blood, or beneath the skin) must have a high sterility assurance level. Examples of such instruments include scalpels, hypodermic needles and artificial pacemakers. This

is also essential in the manufacture of parenteral pharmaceuticals.

Heat sterilization of medical instruments is known to have been used in Ancient Rome, but it mostly disappeared throughout the Middle Ages resulting in significant increases in disability and death following surgical procedures.

Preparation of injectable medications and intravenous solutions for fluid replacement therapy requires not only a high sterility assurance level, but well-designed containers to prevent entry of adventitious agents after initial sterilization.

HEAT STERILIZATION

Steam Sterilization

A widely-used method for heat sterilization is the autoclave. Autoclaves commonly use steam heated to 121°C (250°F), at 103 kPa (15 psi) above atmospheric pressure. Solid surfaces are effectively sterilized when heated this temperature for at least 15 minutes or to 134°C for a minimum of 3 minutes. However, liquids and instruments packed in layers of cloth require a much longer time to reach a sterilizing temperature. After sterilization, autoclaved liquids must be cooled slowly to avoid boiling over when the pressure is released.

Proper autoclave treatment will inactivate all fungi, bacteria, viruses and also bacterial spores, which can be quite resistant. It will not necessarily eliminate all prions.

For prion elimination, various recommendations state 121–132°C (270°F) for 60 minutes or 134°C (273°F) for at least 18 minutes. The prion that causes the disease scrapie (strain 263 K) is inactivated relatively quickly by such sterilization procedures; however, other strains of scrapie, as well as strains of CJD and BSE are more resistant. Using mice as test animals, one experiment showed that heating BSE positive brain tissue at 134-138°C (273-280°F) for 18 minutes resulted in only a 2.5 log decrease in prion infectivity. (The initial BSE concentration in the tissue was relatively low). For a significant margin of safety, cleaning should reduce infectivity by 4 logs, and the sterilization method should reduce it a further 5 logs.

To ensure the autoclaving process was able to cause sterilization, most autoclaves have meters and charts that record or display pertinent information such as temperature and pressure as a function of time. Indicator tape is often placed on packages of products prior to autoclaving. A chemical in the tape will change color when the appropriate conditions have been met. Some types of packaging have built-in indicators on them.

Biological indicators ("bioindicators") can also be used to independently confirm autoclave performance. Simple bioindicator devices are commercially available based on microbial spores. Most contain spores of the heat resistant microbe *Bacillus stearothermophilus*, among the toughest organisms for an autoclave to destroy. Typically these devices have a self-contained liquid growth medium and a growth indicator. After autoclaving an internal glass ampule is shattered, releasing the spores into the growth medium. The vial is then incubated (typically at 56°C (132 °F)) for 48 hours. If the autoclave destroyed the spores, the medium will remain its original color. If autoclaving was unsuccessful the *B. sterothermophilus* will metabolize during incubation, causing a color change during the incubation.

For effective sterilization, steam needs to penetrate the autoclave load uniformly, so an autoclave must not be overcrowded, and the lids of bottles and containers must be left ajar. During the initial heating of the chamber, residual air must be allowed to escape as steam enters the autoclave chamber; otherwise the final temperature will be less than that of the entering steam. Indicators should be placed in the most difficult places for the steam to reach to ensure that steam actually penetrates there.

For autoclaving, as for all disinfection of sterilization methods, cleaning is critical. Extraneous biological matter or grime may shield organisms from the property intended to kill them, whether it physical or chemical. Cleaning can also remove a large number of organisms. Proper cleaning can be achieved by physical scrubbing. This should be done with detergent and warm water to get the best results. Cleaning instruments or utensils with organic matter, cool water must be used because warm or hot water may cause organic debris to coagulate. Treatment with ultrasound or pulsed air can also be used to remove debris.

Food

Although imperfect, cooking and canning are the most common applications of heat sterilization. Boiling water kills the vegetative stage of all common microbes. Roasting meat until it is well done typically completely sterilizes the surface. Since the surface is also the part of food most likely to be contaminated by microbes, roasting usually prevents food poisoning. Note that the common methods of cooking food do not sterilize food - they simply reduce the number of disease-causing micro-organisms to a level that is not dangerous for people with normal digestive and immune systems. Pressure cooking is analogous to autoclaving and when performed correctly renders food sterile. However, some foods are notoriously difficult to sterilize with home canning equipment, so expert recommendations should be followed for home processing to avoid food poisoning.

Food Utensils

Dishwashers often only use hot tap water or heat the water to between 49 and 60°C (120 and 140°F), and thus provide temperatures that could promote bacterial growth. That is to say, they do not effectively sterilize utensils. Some dishwashers do actually heat water up to 74°C (165°F) or higher; those often are specifically described as having sterilization modes of some sort, but this is not a substitute for autoclaving. Note that dishwashers remove food traces from the utensils by a combination of mechanical action (the action of water hitting the plates and cutlery) and the action of detergents and enzymes on fats and proteins. This removal of food particles thus removes one of the factors required for bacterial growth (food), and explains why items with cracks and crevices should either be washed by hand or disposed of: if the water cannot get to the area needing cleaning, the warm, moist, dark conditions in the dishwasher can actually promote bacterial growth.

Bathing

Bathing and washing are not hot enough to sterilize bacteria without scalding the skin. Most hot tap water is between 43 and 49°C (110 and 120°F), though some people set theirs as high as 55°C (130°F). Humans begin to find water painful at 41 to 42°C (106 to 108°F), which to many bacteria is just starting to get warm *enough* for them to grow quickly; they will grow faster, rather than be killed at temperatures up to 55°C (130°F) or more.

Other methods

Other heat methods include flaming, incineration, boiling, tindalization, and using dry heat.

Flaming is done to loops and straight-wires in microbiology labs. Leaving the loop in the flame of a Bunsen burner or alcohol lamp until it glows red ensures that any infectious agent gets inactivated. This is commonly used for small metal or glass objects, but not for large objects (see Incineration below). However, during the initial heating infectious material may be "sprayed" from the wire surface before it is killed, contaminating nearby surfaces and objects. Therefore, special heaters have been developed that surround the inoculating loop with a heated cage, ensuring that such sprayed material does not further contaminate the area.

Incineration will also burn any b organism to ash. It is used to sanitize medical and other biohazardous waste before it is discarded with non-hazardous waste.

Boiling in water for 15 minutes will kill most vegetative bacteria and viruses, but boiling is ineffective against prions and many bacterial and fungal spores; therefore boiling is unsuitable for sterilization. However, since boiling does kill most vegetative microbes and viruses, it is useful for reducing viable levels if no better method is available. Boiling is a simple process, and is an option available to most anyone most anywhere, requiring only water, enough heat, and a container that can withstand the heat; however, boiling can be hazardous and cumbersome.

Tindalization/Tyndallization named after John Tyndall is a lengthy process designed to reduce the level of activity of sporulating bacteria that are left by a simple boiling water method. The process involves boiling for a period (typically 20 minutes) at atmospheric pressure, cooling, incubating for a day, boiling, cooling, incubating for a day, boiling, cooling, incubating for a day, and finally boiling again. The three incubation periods are to allow heat-resistant spores surviving the previous boiling period to germinate to form the heat-sensitive vegetative (growing) stage, which can be killed by the next boiling step. This is effective because many spores are stimulated to grow by the heat shock. The procedure only works for media that can support bacterial growth - it will not sterilize plain water. Tindalization/tyndallization is ineffective against prions.

Dry heat can be used to sterilize items, but as the heat takes much longer to be transferred to the organism, both the time and the temperature must usually be increased, unless forced ventilation of the hot air is used. The standard setting for a hot air oven is at least two hours at 160°C (320°F). A rapid method heats air to 190°C (374°F) for 6 minutes for unwrapped objects and 12 minutes for wrapped objects. Dry heat has the advantage that it can be used on powders and other heat-stable items that are adversely affected by steam (for instance, it does not cause rusting of steel objects).

Prions can be inactivated by immersion in sodium hydroxide (NaOH 0.09N) for two hours plus one hour autoclaving (121°C/250°F). Several investigators have shown complete (>7.4 logs) inactivation with this combined treatment. However, sodium hydroxide may corrode surgical instruments, especially at the elevated temperatures of the autoclave.

CHEMICAL STERILIZATION

Chemicals are also used for sterilization. Although heating provides the most reliable way to rid objects of all transmissible agents, it is not always appropriate, because it will damage heat-sensitive materials such as biological materials, fiber optics, electronics, and many plastics.

Ethylene oxide (EO or EtO) gas is commonly used to sterilize objects sensitive to temperatures greater than 60°C such as plastics, optics and electrics. Ethylene oxide treatment is generally carried out between 30°C and 60°C with relative humidity above 30 per cent and a gas concentration between 200 and 800 mg/L for at least three hours. Ethylene oxide penetrates well, moving through paper, cloth, and some plastic films and is highly effective. Ethylene oxide sterilizers are used to process sensitive instruments which cannot be adequately sterilized by other methods. EtO can kill all known viruses, bacteria and fungi, including bacterial spores and is satisfactory for most medical materials, even with repeated use. However it is highly flammable, and requires a longer time to sterilize than any heat treatment. The process also requires a period of post-sterilization aeration to remove toxic residues. Ethylene oxide is the most common sterilization method, used for over 70 per cent of total sterilizations, and for 50 per cent of all disposable medical devices.

The two most important ethylene oxide sterilization methods are: (1) the gas chamber method and (2) the micro-dose method. To benefit from economies of scale, EtO has traditionally been delivered by flooding a large chamber with a combination of EtO and other gases used as dilutants (usually CFCs or carbon dioxide). This method has drawbacks inherent to the use of large amounts of sterilant being released into a large space, including air contamination produced by CFCs and/or large amounts of EtO residuals, flammability and storage issues calling for special handling and storage, operator exposure risk and training costs. Because of these problems a micro-dose sterilization method was developed in the late 1950s, using a specially designed bag to eliminate the need to flood a larger chamber with EtO. This method is also known as gas diffusion sterilization, or bag sterilization. This method minimize the use of gas.

Bacillus subtilis, a very resistant organism, is used as a rapid biological indicator for EO sterilizers. If sterilization fails, incubation at 37°C causes a fluorescent change within four hours, which is read by an auto-reader. After 96 hours, a visible color change occurs. Fluorescence is emitted if a particular (EO resistant) enzyme is present, which means that spores are still active. The color change indicates a pH shift due to bacterial metabolism. The rapid results mean that the objects treated can be quarantined until the test results are available.

Ozone is used in industrial settings to sterilize water and air, as well as a disinfectant for surfaces. It has the benefit of being able to oxidize most organic matter. On the other hand, it is a toxic and unstable gas that must be produced on-site, so it is not practical to use in many settings.

Chlorine bleach is another accepted liquid sterilizing agent. Household bleach consists of 5.25 per cent sodium hypochlorite. It is usually diluted to 1/10 immediately before use; however to kill *Mycobacterium tuberculosis* it should be diluted only 1/5. The dilution factor must take into account the volume of any liquid waste that it is being used to sterilize. Bleach will kill many organisms immediately, but for full sterilization it should be allowed to react for 20 minutes. Bleach will kill many, but not all spores. It is highly corrosive and may corrode even stainless steel surgical instruments.

Glutaraldehyde and formaldehyde solutions (also used as fixatives) are accepted liquid sterilizing agents, provided that the immersion time is sufficiently long. To kill all spores in a clear liquid can take up to 12 hours with glutaraldehyde and even longer with formaldehyde. The presence of solid particles may lengthen the required period or render the treatment ineffective. Sterilization of blocks of tissue can take much longer, due to the time required for the fixative to penetrate. Glutaraldehyde and formaldehyde are volatile, and toxic by both skin contact and inhalation. Glutaraldehyde has a short shelf life (<2 weeks), and is expensive. Formaldehyde is less expensive and has a much longer shelf life if some methanol is added to inhibit polymerization to paraformaldehyde, but is much more volatile. Formaldehyde is also used as a gaseous sterilizing agent; in this case, it is prepared on-site by depolymerization of solid paraformaldehyde. Many vaccines, such as the original Salk polio vaccine, are sterilized with formaldehyde.

Ortho-phthalaldehyde (OPA) is a chemical sterilizing agent that received Food and Drug Administration (FDA) clearance in late 1999. Typically used in a 0.55 per cent solution, OPA shows better myco-bactericidal activity than glutaraldehyde. It also is effective against glutaraldehyde-resistant spores. OPA has superior stability, is less volatile, and does not irritate skin or eyes, and it acts more quickly than glutaraldehyde. On the other hand, it is more expensive, and will stain proteins (including skin) gray in color.

Hydrogen peroxide is another chemical sterilizing agent. It is relatively non-toxic once diluted to low concentrations (although a dangerous oxidizer at high concentrations), and leaves no residue.

Sterrad sterilization chambers use hydrogen peroxide vapor to sterilize heat-sensitive equipment such as rigid endoscopes. A recent model can sterilize most hospital loads in as little as 20 minutes. The Sterrad has limitations with processing certain materials such as paper/linens and long thin lumens. Paper products cannot be sterilized in the Sterrad system because of a process called cellulostics, in which the hydrogen peroxide would be completely absorbed by the paper product.

Hydrogen peroxide and formic acid are mixed as needed in the Endoclens device for sterilization of endoscopes. This device has two independent asynchronous bays, and cleans (in warm detergent with pulsed air), sterilizes and dries endoscopes automatically in 30 minutes. Studies with synthetic soil with bacterial spores showed the effectiveness of this device.

Dry sterilization process (DSP) uses hydrogen peroxide at a concentration of 30-35 per cent under low pressure conditions. This process achieves bacterial reduction of 10-6...10-8. The complete process cycle time is just 6 seconds, and the surface temperature is increased only 10-15°C (18 to 27°F). Originally designed for the sterilization of plastic bottles in the beverage industry, because of the high germ reduction and the slight temperature increase the dry sterilization process is also useful for medical and pharmaceutical applications.

Peracetic acid (0.2 per cent) is used to sterilize instruments in the Steris system.

Prions are highly resistant to chemical sterilization. Treatment with aldehydes (e.g., formaldehyde) have actually been shown to increase prion resistance. Hydrogen peroxide (3 per cent) for one hour was shown to be ineffective, providing less than 3 logs (10-3) reduction in contamination. Iodine, formaldehyde, glutaraldehyde and peracetic acid also fail this test (one hour treatment). Only chlorine, a phenolic compound, guanidinium thiocyanate, and sodium hydroxide (NaOH) reduce prion levels by more than 4 logs. Chlorine and NaOH are the most consistent agents for prions. Chlorine is too corrosive to use on certain objects. Sodium hydroxide has had many studies showing its effectiveness.

RADIATION STERILIZATION

Methods exist to sterilize using radiation such as X-rays, gamma rays, or subatomic particles.

- Gamma rays are very penetrating and are commonly used for sterilization of disposable medical equipment, such as syringes, needles, cannulas and IV sets. Gamma radiation requires bulky shielding for the safety of the operators; they also require storage of a radioisotope (usually Cobalt-60), which continuously emits gamma rays (it cannot be turned off, and therefore always presents a hazard in the area of the facility).

- X-rays are less penetrating than gamma rays and tend to require longer exposure times, but require less shielding, and are generated by an X-ray machine that can be turned off for servicing and when not in use.
- Ultraviolet light irradiation (UV, from a germicidal lamp) is useful only for sterilization of surfaces and some transparent objects. Many objects that are transparent to visible light absorb UV. UV irradiation is routinely used to sterilize the interiors of biological safety cabinets between uses, but is ineffective in shaded areas, including areas under dirt (which may become polymerized after prolonged irradiation, so that it is very difficult to remove). It also damages many plastics, such as polystyrene foam.
- Subatomic particles may be more or less penetrating, and may be generated by a radioisotope or a device, depending upon the type of particle.

Irradiation with X-rays or gamma rays does not make materials radioactive. Irradiation with particles may make materials radioactive, depending upon the type of particles and their energy, and the type of target material: neutrons and very high-energy particles can make materials radioactive, but have good penetration, whereas lower energy particles (other than neutrons) cannot make materials radioactive, but have poorer penetration.

Irradiation is used by the United States Postal Service to sterilize mail in the Washington, DC area. Some foods (e.g. spices, ground meats) are irradiated for sterilization (see food irradiation).

STERILE FILTRATION

Clear liquids that would be damaged by heat, irradiation or chemical sterilization can be sterilized by mechanical filtration. This method is commonly used for sensitive pharmaceuticals and protein solutions in biological research. A filter with pore size 0.2 μm will effectively remove bacteria. If viruses must also be removed, a much smaller pore size around 20 nm is needed. Solutions filter slowly through membranes with smaller pore diameters. Prions are not removed by filtration. The filtration equipment and the filters themselves may be purchased as presterilized disposable units in sealed packaging, or must be sterilized by the user, generally by autoclaving at a temperature that does not damage the fragile filter membranes. To ensure sterility, the filtration system must be tested to ensure that the membranes have not been punctured prior to or during use.

To ensure the best results, pharmaceutical sterile filtration is performed in a room with highly filtered air (HEPA filtration) or in a laminar flow cabinet or "flowbox", a device which produces a laminar stream of HEPA filtered air.

STUDY–QUESTIONS

Write a short note on:

(a) Heat Sterilization

(b) Chemical sterilization

(c) Sterile filtration

(d) Radiation sterilization.

40

CHAPTER VIOLENT PATIENTS

INTRODUCTION

Emergency physicians encounter violent patients as predictably as they encounter airways. Fundamentally, the approach to violence in the ED is analogous to the approach to the airway. There are several routes to airways compromise, yet regardless of the cause, the physician must control the airway before subsequent treatment. Similarly, violent behavior is an endpoint for many different medical and psychiatric pathologies; the emergency physician must control the behavior, to prevent escalation and injury, before moving on to further evaluation.

At the same time, it is imperative that the physician suspect any decompensated behavior to be the result of a medical or surgical condition, until proven otherwise. Treatment of conditions that may cause agitation, such as hypoxia, may in fact resolve behavioral problems. But often, the behavior itself will need to be addressed before definitive care can take place.

The focus of this presentation is to review the emergent treatment of violent behavior, not to dwell on the pathologies that may have led to the behavior. Since the definitive medical or psychiatric diagnosis in these patients is often not possible in the emergency situation, it is imperative to have a clear management approach to behaviorally discontrolled patients.

DEFINITIONS AND EPIDEMIOLOGY

Violent behavior constitutes any set of actions that are forceful or directed enough to cause injury to the patient or others. In nature, violent behavior may be an appropriate response to a given set of environmental circumstances. Individual responses to environmental circumstance will be fashioned by many factors, such as personality characteristics, (or disorders), such as aggressiveness, poor impulse control, antisocial or manipulative traits. Emotions, especially fear, powerlessness, anger and rage play a key role in the propensity for violent response, and may be most amenable to verbal intervention. Agitation, or a state of psychomotor hyperactivity, and psychosis, a breakdown of rational perception, may be due to either medical or psychiatric causes.

However, any violent behavior in the ED usually constitutes maladaptive behavior and should be considered a pathologic state that could lead to morbidity or mortality. Appropriate prevention or intervention becomes warranted. A history of violence, regardless of diagnosis, is the most uniform predictor of violent behavior in the ED. Many ED's have a system for documenting and notifying ED staff about patients with prior violent visits to the ED.

As with the airway, recognition of the potential for deterioration, and preparation for decompensation are the best assurance for the safety patients and staff. Three progressive but integrated strategies are outlined: de-escalation, restraints and seclusion, and pharmacologic interventions. The "least restrictive alternative doctrine" dictates that the least invasive means be used to control the violent.

DE-ESCALATION

The apparent chaos of the ED may contribute to the behavioral deterioration of patients at risk, but there are environmental variables which can be addressed to help alleviate the potential for decompensation.Waiting times, frustrating for anyone, can be minimized. Placing at risk patients in a quiet or private exam room will decrease external stimuli. Patients may need to be separated from other loud or aggressive patients, friends or family. Alternatively, if cooperative, those same people can be enlisted for support. Show your concern for patient well-being by offering comfort in the form of warm clothing or blankets, a chair or stretcher, food or drink. Question patients early and directly about weapons or potential weapons, and remove them.

When talking to the patient, (verbal de-escalation), the overriding principle is that staff convey their professional concern for the well-being of the patient, that the staff is in control, and that no harm will come to the patient. When you are with the patient, be sure that you have a means of egress; you should be closer to the door than the patient, but aware that you don't convey a feeling of entrapment, and never locked in. Be aware of body language; crossed arms, hands behind the back, a forward leaning frontal posture, prolonged or intense eye contact can be perceived as threatening or challenging. Respect personal space.

When speaking to at risk patients it is important to maintain a calm, controlled tone. Never express anger or hostility, and never minimize or "write off" patient threats or feelings. Express your empathy and concern; statements such as, "I understand you are feeling frustrated, that you're having a hard time", and "you're here to get help, let's try to figure out what's going on", convey both. Emphasize that they are safe, that the staff is there for them. However, you also need to clearly define limits for patient behavior, and consequences of their actions. Provide reasonable alternatives to aggressive behavior. It is crucial that your staff be consistent in their approach; manipulative patients may attempt to split staff who do not have a unified strategy.

Always be alert for changes in patient mood, loud or aggressive speech or actions, increasing psychomotor activity, which may signal impending loss of control. The ultimate gauge for impending danger is the care giver's visceral perceptions; if one feels unsafe or threatened in the face of a potentially hostile patient, it is best to abort the interaction until interventions are instituted to restore confidence. Security personnel or local police can be a show of force that may dissuade inappropriate behaviors. They can also be instrumental in the ultimate implementation of physical restraints/containment.

Sometimes, in spite of your best efforts at de-escalation, patient behavior will deteriorate. If less restrictive efforts are unsuccessful, restraints, seclusion and/or medication may used in response to emergent or imminently dangerous behavior. 24

Once the decision has been made to proceed with restraints or seclusion there must be sufficient trained personnel so that the procedure can be carried out safely and effectively if physical force becomes warranted. At all times the staff must convey confidence, calmness, and proceed with implementation as if it were a routine procedure. Overtly violent encounters are stressful for both patients and staff and can contribute to deterioration of morale, depression, and anxiety. It is appropriate to have some type of debriefing that offers the opportunity for staff to discuss the event and the associated feelings.

SECLUSION/RESTRAINTS

Seclusion can be useful for agitated patients by decreasing the external stimuli and permitting the patient "time-out" to regain behavioral control. A seclusion room must be safe, above all, and free of objects that could be used to injure self or others. Medical conditions which are unstable and require close physical interactions or monitoring preclude the use of seclusion.

Prior to seclusion, it is imperative that potentially dangerous items be removed. At first the door can remain open, but if agitation continues the door is locked for safety. The patient must always be aware of the consequences of his behavior; and be given periodic opportunities to comply with defined behavioral parameters in order to be released from seclusion. Medications can be offered to avoid further restrictive measures. The patient in seclusion should be checked no less than every 15 minutes or, if available, monitored by closed-circuit television. Staff must clearly document the need for seclusion, intervening steps, and medications given.

Restraints—The implementation of restraints is a disheartening procedure, but it is often the best option, generally reserved for those situations where there is the potential for imminent harm to patient or staff through patient behavior. Again, once the decision is made, the overriding principles are that it be done swiftly and humanely, and that the patient be reassured that it is felt to be in their best interest.

The implementation of physical restraints is a dangerous procedure, both for staff and patient. It should never be attempted unless there is sufficient manpower to ensure that it can be done with a minimum of struggle. A minimum of 5 staff members is recommended, one for each limb and an extra or team leader. The presence of staff may also assist in the calming the patient, thus aborting the need for restraints. But once the decision is made to proceed, implementation must be completed and negotiations temporarily suspended. The team leader, just as in team resuscitation, will oversee the others and ensure completeness. It is usually best that the physician avoid physical participation in subduing a combative patient as this may corrupt the therapeutic relationship. If possible, provide the patient or family with an ongoing explanation of the reasons for the procedure, and what to expect. Secure all four limbs firmly to the bedframe, snug without impairing circulation (allow one finger space between the skin and the restraint). Elevate the patients' head slightly to minimize the risk of aspiration.

Hospital policies should address the frequency and parameters of patient monitoring while in restraints, i.e., skin integrity, vital signs, pulses, etc. Once the patient is controlled, conduct a thorough physical exam, if not yet completed. Evaluate the patient periodically to asses the need for continued restraints. The chart should reflect the reasons for restraints, why less restrictive methods were not utilized, medications given, course of treatment and response. After the patient is in control, the staff can decide to remove the restraints one limb at a time, while monitoring the patient for behavioral control.

MEDICATIONS

Pharmacologic management of the violent or agitated patient may serve as primary therapy, or as an adjunct to the other efforts. Whenever possible, the patient is given choices, which can allow them to regain some measure of control. Oral administration will presumably address control issues and best retain dignity for all, but if parenteral routes are agreeable, the effects will be more rapid. There are times that pharmacologic therapies are necessary in addition to physical restraint. This would include continued high risk behavior, such as spitting, biting, disruptive verbal threats, and struggling against the restraints and medical care, i.e., blood drawing and other testing. This is especially true where there is a primary medical condition that can be complicated by continued struggle or agitation.

Clearly, medical conditions that may contribute to agitation, such as pain or hypoxia, need to be addressed concomitantly. Physicians are often hesitant to give sedating medications for fear of complications or obscuring the physical exam. That said, the risk of over sedation is outweighed by the risk of continued struggle, for instance, in the intoxicated patient with a c-spine injury.

Antipsychotic medications, alternately referred to as neuroleptics or psychotropics, were developed in the 1940's. Maintenance therapy with these medications revolutionized our management of the mentally ill. These same medications, given rapidly, in large doses, were found effective in acute control of behavior; by the 1970's, rapid tranquilization was well defined in the psychiatric literature, and more recently in the emergency literature. The goal of rapid tranquilization is simply to control behavior, without over sedation, without loss of airway or cardiovascular stability, such that definitive evaluation and care can be completed. It is not diagnosis specific; it is effective for violent behavior due to psychiatric, emotional, or medical causes.

ANTI-PSYCHOTICS

The psychotropic medications are broadly classified as high potency, such as haloperidol, and low potency, such as chlorpromazine. All of the antipsychotics are effective in controlling psychotic features of any etiology, and they all have in common a therapeutic index that makes them safe. The predominant side effects of the low potency medications are anticholinergic and sedating, while the high potency medications cause more extrapyramidal side effects.

The primary action of neuroleptics results from dopamine receptor blockade in the CNS. It is presumed that dopamine antagonism in the cortex and limbic system is clinically expressed as reduced interest in the environment, decreased response to both internal and external stimuli, and inhibition of self-motivated and exploratory behavior. Extrapyramidal effects, namely dystonia, akathisia and tardive dyskinesia, are ascribed to the interference with dopamine in the basal ganglia. The anticholinergic activity and alpha blocking effects of these drugs may result in postural hypotension, tachycardia, urinary retention, dry mouth, and constipation, which can usually be managed conservatively in the acute setting. Tardive dyskinesia is due to long term therapy, and not an issue in the acute setting. (NMS) is a rare side effect.

Haloperidol—Haloperidol has become the standard for rapid tranquilization due to its strength and desirable side effect profile; it is a powerful antipsychotic with minimal sedating and cardiovascular effects. It may be given orally (PO) or intramuscular (IM), and though not FDA approved for intravenous (IV) use, it is commonly given by that route with no reported complications. Peak serum levels are achieved 20 to 40 minutes after IM administration, at 3 to 6 hours when given orally, and the half-life is 10 to 19 hours. When used for rapid tranquilization, halperidol is dosed at 5 to 10 mgs PO, IM, or IV, every 10 to 30 minutes, and titrated to desired effect.Dosing starts with 2 mg in the elderly or those with comorbidity. It has repeatedly been shown safe and effective for control of behavior in the acute setting, both in the psychiatric and emergency literature.

The predominant side effect is acute dystonia, usually manifested as torticollis, opisthotonos or oculogyric crisis. Rarely, airway protection becomes an issue. Dystonia is most commonly seen in the first 24 hours, in young healthy individuals, and not dose related. Akathisia, or the subjective feeling of restlessness, or "crawling out of one's skin", is less common, but probably underdetected because it is subjective, or misdiagnosed as breakthrough agitation. This can occur in the first weeks of therapy, most commonly in elderly women. Fortunately, both of these effects are relieved quickly with diphenhydramine, 25-50 mg IM or IV, or benztropine, 2 mg PO or IM. Relief usually occurs in minutes and is complete. Repeat doses can be given, and for those few that do not respond, benzodiazepines may be used. The symptoms can recur after initial relief, and this needs to be anticipated when patients are transferred or discharged.

Antipsychotic medications in general can lower the seizure threshold in animal studies and alter EEG patterns. However, there are no reports of induced seizures clearly due to haloperidol despite its documented use in high risk populations, such as alcoholics and post-ictal patients.26 Since antipsychotics have anticholinergic properties and a quinidine like effect, their use in overdoses of medications having similar properties is cautioned.

Droperidol—Droperidol is a butyrophenone distinct from haloperidol by a single substitution on the piperidine ring. It has been used for years in Europe as an antipsychotic, and as an adjunct for anesthesia in the U.S. for its sedating and antiemetic properties. Only recently has it been used in U.S. psychiatric and emergency practice. It is given either IM or IV, at a dose of 2.5 to 10 mg, titrated to effect, with onset of clinical effect in just minutes after IM administration, and a half-life of 2 to 4 hours. The safety and efficacy of droperidol in acute behavior control has been documented in both the psychiatric and emergency literature with dosing up to 50 mg. In comparison to haloperidol, droperidol was found more effective at equal doses given IM, though the advantage appeared to fade with the IV route.

BENZODIAZEPINE AND COMBINATION PHARMACOTHERAPY

Benzodiazepines (BNZ) have been used for years in psychiatric practice as an adjunctive therapy for behavior control in mania, psychosis and agitation. They are the drug of choice in agitation due to withdrawal states and catecholamine toxidromes such as cocaine or amphetamine ingestions. Currently, the most commonly studied BNZ is lorazepam which has the advantage of safety, rapid IM absorption, and reliability.

Rapid tranquilization combining a benzodiazepine and antipsychotic offers the advantage of minimizing the amount of any single drug given and combining the sedation of the benzodiazepine with the behavioral modification of the antipsychotic. Historically, the available sedatives were chlorpromazine and barbiturates; by adding a barbiturate, the dosage of chlorpromazine could be decreased, minimizing it's propensity to cause hypotension. The introduction of BNZs provided a safer adjunct, and allowed for a lower antipsychotic dose and less extrapyramidal side effects, possibly due to their own muscle relaxant properties. Studies have shown that a 5 mg. Haloperidol in combined with 2-4 mg lorazapam is more effective than either drug alone in controlling behavior in the emergency setting.

Rapid tranquilization has been shown to be safe and effective. Titratability is a key concept. Rare reports of complications do not support the trepidation that many physicians feel. Side effects are uncommon and, if anticipated, will rarely cause excessive anxiety for the physician or life-threat for the patient. There is arguably a trend, supported by the literature, towards using droperidol or combination therapy, when compared to haloperidol used alone. Droperidol is superior to haloperidol when given IM due to its rapid absorption and shorter half-life, and may have a lower incidence of extrapyramidal side effects. This is significant in the emergency setting due to the difficulties in obtaining IV access in the agitated patient. It is unclear that there is any superiority when given IV. Combination therapy allows the reduction of dosing of both of the component medications, mitigating side effect potential, and offers efficacy at least equal to the single drugs. Ultimately, however, the choice of medication for behavior control is far less important, and less complicated, than the decision to use medication.

STUDY–QUESTIONS

Write a short note on:

(a) Violent Patients

(b) Antipsychotics

(c) Restraints

(d) Medications.

41 CHAPTER

SIGNS OF DEATH

If we know what these distant signs of death are.... we shall be warned to make preparations that will benefit our future life. The signs of death are of two kinds: distant and close. The distant signs can be experienced even when we are not suffering from any particular illness. They are experienced between six and three months before we die, and are of three kinds: bodily signs, mental signs, and dream signs. They do not necessarily indicate that we shall soon die, but if they persist this means that death is probably imminent. If we know what these distant signs of death are, we shall know when we are experiencing them, and so we shall be warned to make preparations that will benefit our future life. We shall know that it is time to make sure that we are engaging in pure Dharma practice and to apply any methods we have learnt for extending our life span, such as the practices of Amitayus and White Tara. If these are not successful we should definitely apply the practice of powa.

DISTANT SIGNS OF DEATH

Some of the distant bodily signs of death are the following: while we are passing urine or excrement we continuously hiccup; we can no longer hear the buzzing sound of our inner ear when we block our ears; when we apply pressure against our fingernails and then release it the blood does not quickly return; during sexual intercourse, if we are a woman we release white drops instead of red and if we are a man we release red drops instead of white; for no reason we cannot taste things; for no reason we cannot smell things; our exhaled breath is cold – when we blow on our hand it feels cold instead of warm; our tongue shrinks and feels rolled or swollen, and when we poke it out we can no longer see its tip; in the dark when we press the top of our eyeball with our finger so that the eyeball protrudes a little we can no longer see colourful shapes and patterns; we hallucinate a sun at night; when we sit in the sun in the morning we can no longer see in our shadow streams of energy flowing from the crown of our head; saliva no longer forms in our mouth; the end of our nose becomes pinched; black marks appear on our teeth; our eyeballs sink further into the hollows of our eyes.

Distant mental signs of death include: a change in our usual temperament, for example, we become aggressive when we are usually kind and gentle, or we become gentle when we are usually aggressive and ill-tempered; for no reason we begin to dislike the place where we live, our friends, or other objects of attachment; we feel sad for no reason; our wisdom and intelligence become less clear and less powerful.

Distant dream signs include repeated dreams that we are falling from a high mountain, that we are naked, or that we are travelling south on our own across a desert.

SIGNS OF APPROACHING DEATH

When confronted with approaching death, many of us wonder when exactly will death occur. Many of us ask the question, "How much time is left?". This can often be a difficult question to answer. The dying do not always cooperate with the predictions of the doctors, nurses or others who tell family members or patients how much time is left.

Hospice staff have frequently observed that even the predictions by physicians about the length of time from the original diagnosis till death is often inaccurate. Many families report that "the doctor told us he [the patient] only had so much time left, and he's lived much longer than that." ... or a similar story. Statistical averages do not tell us exactly how long a particular patient has to live; they can only serve as a general guideline or point of reference.

Although statistical averages do not help much in an individual case, there are specific signs of approaching death which may be observed, and which do indicate that death is approaching nearer. Each individual patient is different. Not all individuals will show all of these signs, nor are all of the signs of approaching death always present in every case.

Depending on the type of terminal illness and the metabolic condition of the patient, different signs and symptoms arise. An experienced physician or hospice nurse can often explain these signs and symptoms to you. If you have questions about changes in your loved one's condition, ask your hospice nurse for an explanation, that is one of the reasons she is serving you.

There are two phases which arise prior to the actual time of death: the "pre-active phase of dying," and the "active phase of dying." On average, the pre-active phase of dying may last approximately two weeks, while on average, the active phase of dying lasts about three days.

We say "on average" because there are often exceptions to the rule. Some patients have exhibited signs of the preactive phase of dying for a month or longer, while some patients exhibit signs of the active phase of dying for two weeks. Many hospice staff have been fooled into thinking that death was about to occur, when the patient had unusually low blood pressure or longer periods of pausing in the breathing rhythym. However, some patients with these symptoms can suddenly recover and live a week, a month or even longer. Low blood pressure alone or long periods of pausing in the breathing (apnea) are not reliable indicators of imminent death in all cases. God alone knows for sure when death will occur.

SIGNS OF THE PREACTIVE PHASE OF DYING

- Increased restlessness, confusion, agitation, inability to stay content in one position and insisting on changing positions frequently (exhausting family and caregivers)
- Withdrawal from active participation in social activities
- Increased periods of sleep, lethargy
- Decreased intake of food and liquids
- Beginning to show periods of pausing in the breathing (apnea) whether awake or sleeping
- Patient reports seeing persons who had already died
- Patient states that he or she is dying
- Patient requests family visit to settle "unfinished business" and tie up "loose ends"
- Inability to heal or recover from wounds or infections
- Increased swelling (edema) of either the extremities or the entire body

SIGNS OF THE ACTIVE PHASE OF DYING

- Inability to arouse patient at all (coma) or, ability to only arouse patient with great effort but patient quickly returns to severely unresponsive state (semi-coma)
- Severe agitation in patient, hallucinations, acting "crazy" and not in patient's normal manner or personality
- Much longer periods of pausing in the breathing (apnea)
- Dramatic changes in the breathing pattern including apnea, but also including very rapid breathing or cyclic changes in the patterns of breathing (such as slow progressing to very fast and then slow again, or shallow progressing to very deep breathing while also changing rate of breathing to very fast and then slow)
- Other very abnormal breathing patterns
- Severely increased respiratory congestion or fluid buildup in lungs
- Inability to swallow any fluids at all (not taking any food by mouth voluntarily as well).

- patient states that he or she is going to die
- patient breathing through wide open mouth continuously and no longer can speak even if awake
- urinary or bowel incontinence in a patient who was not incontinent before
- marked decrease in urine output and darkening color of urine or very abnormal colors (such as red or brown)
- blood pressure dropping dramatically from patient's normal blood pressure range (more than a 20 or 30 point drop)
- systolic blood pressure below 70, diastolic blood pressure below 50
- patient's extremities (such as hands, arms, feet and legs) feel very cold to touch
- patient complains that his or her legs/feet are numb and cannot be felt at all
- cyanosis, or a bluish or purple coloring to the patients arms and legs, especially the feet and hands)
- patient's body is held in rigid unchanging position.

Although all patients do not show all of these signs, many of these signs will be seen in some patients. The reason for the tradition of "keeping a vigil" when someone is dying is that we really don't know exactly when death will occur until it is obviously happening. If you wish to "be there" with your loved one when death occurs, keeping a vigil at the bedside is part of the process.

Always remember that your loved one can often hear you even up till the very end, even though he or she cannot respond by speaking. Your loving presence at the bedside can be a great expression of your love for your loved one and help him to feel calmer and more at peace at the time of death.

STUDY-QUESTION

Write a short note on sign of death.

***

42

CHAPTER

SEXUAL ASSAULT

INTRODUCTION

Sexual assault is any physical contact of a sexual nature without voluntary consent. When sexual assault associated with rape, it is much broader and the specifics may vary according to social, political or legal definition. According to the U.S. Department of Health and Human Services, sexual assault includes inappropriate touching, vaginal, anal, and oral penetration, sexual intercourse, rape, attempted rape, and child molestation plus torturing the victim with many sexual ways.

Perpetrators may include, but are not limited to, strangers, acquaintances, superiors, legal entities (as in the case of torture), or family members. Both male and female sex predators can commit sexual assault against same-sex or opposite-sex victims or both. Generally, victims are more likely to be assaulted by an acquaintance (such as a friend or co-worker) or a family member than by a complete stranger. The act is sometimes accomplished by force sufficient to cause physical injury. More often, the act is accomplished by psychological coercion alone, with no overt physical injuries to the victim. However, even when no lasting physical injury is sustained, the psychological damage done by this form of intimate violation may be substantial. Psychological damage is often particularly severe when sexual assault is committed by parents against children due to the incestuous nature of the assault.

WHO IS VULNERABLE

Anyone is a potential victim of sexual assault, although females are at a higher risk of victimization than men. A person who is the victim of sexual assault may require assistance from medical and law enforcement resources. Medical and law enforcement professionals strongly recommend that a victim call for help and report what has happened.

Medical professionals are concerned for the well-being of the victim, who may need immediate medical attention, not only for injuries, but against sexually transmitted disease, and possibly to avoid unwanted conception. In many locations, EMTs, emergency room nurses and doctors are trained to help rape victims. Some emergency rooms have rape kits which are used to collect evidence.

"A victim of sexual assault should be offered prophylaxis for pregnancy and for sexually transmitted diseases, subject to informed consent and consistent with current treatment guidelines. Physicians and allied health practitioners who find this practice morally objectionable or who practice at hospitals that prohibit prophylaxis or contraception should offer to refer victims of sexual assault to another provider who can provide these services in a timely fashion." Police are charged with the enforcement of the laws forbidding sexual assault and to gather evidence to identify and prosecute the offender. Further, police provide safety advice and prevention tips, to prevent people from becoming victims of sexual assault.

REDUCING THE RISK OF SEXUAL ASSAULT

Police agencies routinely offer safety tips and advice for reducing the risk of sexual assault. Many argue that there are risk factors for sexual assault that lie with the victim; that is, certain behaviors by the victim exist may increase the chance of sexual assault.

While it is widely accepted that the victim is not to blame, for would-be victims of sexual assault, there are a variety of precautions that may be taken to minimize the chance of falling victim to sexual predators. The advice given is extensive, and vary in specifics, they all tend to include certain precautions:

- Avoid being alone in public, particularly at night, or in dark and/or isolated places.
- Maintain situational awareness. Be aware of other persons.
- Keep personal information (such as name, address and telephone numbers) on your person, and not on key-chains.
- Keep your vehicle and home locked.
- Avoid isolated places such as deserted parking lots or stairwells in office buildings as much as possible.
- If a motorist asks for assistance, stand a distance from the vehicle.
- Be alert. Never sleep in public—including buses, cabs and benches. Have car and house keys ready before you reach the door.
- Walk facing traffic.
- Trust your instincts—if you feel you are being followed, if you have suspicions about a minor auto accident, or being stopped by a police official, keep driving to a well-lit, populated area before stopping. In the case of a police officer, in the United States and many other countries, a driver who does so for their own safety cannot be further penalized for evading arrest or failing to stop (provided they do so eventually).
- Don't allow yourself to be alone with someone whom you do not know or trust. This may prevent stranger sexual assault (2 per cent of all assaults), although will not prevent the more common types of assault such as acquaintance sexual assault.
- If you are in trouble or feel you are in danger, don't be afraid to attract help any way you can. Scream, yell or run away to safety.

- If you choose to carry any type of weapon for self-protection, give careful consideration to your ability and willingness to use it. Remember there is always the chance that it could be taken away and used against you.

STUDY–QUESTIONS

Write a short note on sexual assult.

INDEX

A

Absorbtion 113
Accident 209
Accidental poisoning 353
Adolescence and adulthood 165
Agonal respiration 406
Air safety 217
Ambulance 321
Antibiotics 509
Antioxidants 545
Antiseptic 527
Appendicitis 485
Asepsis 531
Aseptic technique 532
Asphyxia 407
Asthma 140
Audible warnings 330
Autonomic Nervous System 132

B

Back pain 570
Bandages 269
Bites and stings 243
Bowel obstruction 492
Bowman's capsule 146
Breathing 136
Bronchi 135
Burn 169
Burns Dressings 179

C

Car accident 213
Cardiac arrhythmia 421
Cardiogenic shock 433
Central nervous system 127
Cerebrum 129
Chemical sterilization 563
Chilblains 284
Child abuse 350
Children with burns 355
Chronic bronchitis 141
Chronic kidney disease (CKD) 448
Community emergencies 340
Concealed pregnancy 403
Contusion and concussion injury 373
Convulsion or seizure 455
Corneal abrasion 372
Coronary circulation 118

D

Deep burns 172
Dental problems 394

Depth of unconsciousness 230
Diabetic coma 466
Dialysis 450
Diaphragm 135
Different types of ambulances 322
Digestive system 105
Disaster management 340
Diseases of the Ear 386
Dislocations 252
Distant signs of death 579
Drowning 236
Drug overdose 490

E

Ear 384
Earthquakes 341
Eclampsia 438
Electrocardiogram 123
Emergency 305
Emergency action principles (EAP) 309
Emergency department 311
Emergency management 310
Emergency services 342
Emphysema 141
ENT 384
Excretion 144
External genitals 155

F

Facial and dental emergencies 391
Faeces and defecation 113
Febrile convulsion 354
Female reproductive system 154
Figure of eight bandage 275
Fire 226
Fire explosions 340
First aid 2
Floods 341
Forebrain 129
Foreign bodies in the ear 385
Fracture 248
Fracture healing 251
Fractures and children 250
Frostbite 287

G

Gastrointestinal tract 106
Golden rules of first aid 12

H

Haemorrhage or bleeding 187
Head Injury 202
headache 496
Heat exhaustion 278
Heat sterilization 558
Heat stroke 278
Hepatitis 477
Hernia 518
Hoarseness and stridor in children 391
Hormones and female cycles 155
human circulatory system 116
Human crutch 293
Hypothalamus 129
Hypothermia 289
Hypovolemia 435

I

Inflammation of the eye 375
Injuries 182
International agencies 344
Intestinal bacterial flora 548

K

Kidney 144

L

Loading stretcher 299
Lost tampons 403

M

Malnutrition 483
Man-made hazards 337
Meningitis 458
Metabolic acidosis 471
Metabolic emergencies 461
Micturition 148
Midbrain 130
Migraine 499
Minor burns and scalds 174
Modern vehicles 324

N

Natural disasters 336
Nervous system 126
Neurogenic shock 437
Non-penetrating eye injury 370
Nose 387
Nose bleeds 388
Nutrients 537

P

Pancreas 112
Penetrating eye injury 373
Personal emergencies 311
Physiological changes in elderly people 359
Pneumonia 140
Poisoning 237
Psychology of ageing 361
Pulse 120

R

Radiation casualties 345
Radiation injury 373
Radiation sterilization 556
Recurrent bandage 275
Reducing the risk of sexual assault 585
Respiratory system 133
Road traffic accidents 210
road-traffic crash 213
Road-traffic safety 213
Roller bandages 274

S

Seclusion/restraints 572
Slings 270
Smart wheelchair 300
Spinal cord 130
Sports nutrition 548
sprains 186
Sterile filtration 567
Sterilization 557
Stomach 109
Stress amongest women 397
Sudden infant death dyndrome (SIDS) 356
sunburn 281
Superficial burns 173
Systemic circulation 116

T

Throat 389
toothache 507
Trauma during pregnancy 399
Travel sikcness 515
Triangular bandage 269
Types of disaster 336

U

Ultra filteration 147
Unconsciousness 229
Urinary tract in infections 150
Urine 149
urine concentration 148

V

Venous system 124

W

Wound closure 194
Wounds 183

NOTES

NOTES

NOTES

NOTES